PLURAL+PLUS

COMPANION WEBSITE

Purchase of *Clinical Management of Swallowing Disorders, Fourth Edition* comes with complimentary access to supplementary materials on a PluralPlus companion website.

The companion website is located at:

http://www.pluralpublishing.com/publication/cmsd4e

STUDENTS:

To access the **student** materials, you must register on the companion website and log in using the access code below.*

Access Code: CMSD4E-C7WLP6M

INSTRUCTORS:

To access the **instructor** materials, you must contact Plural Publishing, Inc. to be verified as an instructor and receive your access code.

> Email: information@pluralpublishing.com
> Tel: 866-758-7251 (toll free) or 858-492-1555

Note for students: If you have purchased this textbook used or have rented it, your access code will not work if it was already redeemed by the original buyer of the book. Plural Publishing does not offer replacement access codes for used or rented textbooks.

Look for this icon throughout the text, directing you to supplementary videos available on the companion website.

Clinical Management of Swallowing Disorders

FOURTH EDITION

Clinical Management of Swallowing Disorders

FOURTH EDITION

Thomas Murry, PhD, CCC-SLP
Ricardo L. Carrau, MD, FACS
Karen M.K. Chan, PhD

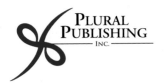

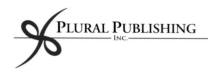

5521 Ruffin Road
San Diego, CA 92123

e-mail: info@pluralpublishing.com
Website: http://www.pluralpublishing.com

Typeset in 10.5/13 Garamond by Flanagan's Publishing Services, Inc.
Printed in Korea by Four Colour Print Group
20 19 18   2 3 4 5

Library of Congress Cataloging-in-Publication Data

Names: Murry, Thomas, 1943- author. | Carrau, Ricardo L., author. | Chan,
    Karen M. K., author.
Title: Clinical management of swallowing disorders / Thomas Murry, Ricardo L.
    Carrau, Karen M.K. Chan.
Description: Fourth edition. | San Diego, CA : Plural Publishing, [2018] |
    Includes bibliographical references and index.
Identifiers: LCCN 2016033816| ISBN 9781597569347 (alk. paper) | ISBN
    1597569348 (alk. paper)
Subjects: | MESH: Deglutition Disorders—diagnosis | Deglutition
    Disorders—therapy
Classification: LCC RC815.2 | NLM WI 250 | DDC 616.3/1—dc23
LC record available at https://lccn.loc.gov/2016033816

Contents

Preface

Clinical Management of Swallowing Disorders, Fourth Edition, has been a core swallowing textbook for the past 15 years. The *Fourth Edition* is now updated with full color images, video examples of normal swallowing and actual patients, and improved tables. This text addresses the needs of students who will treat swallowing disorders as well as those clinicians who currently treat swallowing disorders in hospitals, rehabilitation centers, nursing homes, and private outpatient clinics. *Clinical Management of Swallowing Disorders, Fourth Edition,* examines the diagnosis and treatment of swallowing disorders in children and adults. The text emphasizes team management, swallowing safety, nutrition, behavioral treatments, and surgical options. A significant number of changes have been added to bring the reader up to date in all aspects of the management of swallowing disorders. Dr. Karen Chan from the University of Hong Kong, who currently teaches swallowing disorders, has joined Drs. Murry and Carrau as an author for this *Fourth Edition.* She brings an international flavor and a broad range of knowledge to the text.

The essential aspects of dysphagia management are presented in a format that both beginners and clinicians needing a practical update on dysphagia will find useful. Because of our daily clinical involvement treating swallowing disorders in major teaching institutions and teaching this information to students, we saw a need to revise and update the text that continues to be well accepted by clinicians, students, and teachers. This book addresses clinical issues at the current level of clinical understanding. The material contained in the *Clinical Management of Swallowing Disorders, Fourth Edition,* derives from a vast storehouse of recent knowledge and academic pursuits, along with our daily experiences from our multispecialty swallowing disorder clinics and research activities. Since the third edition was published, new evidence has demonstrated the importance of early intervention and aggressive treatment of dysphagia. Outcome data are now available to show the importance of proper assessments and treatments to deter and prevent aspiration and improve patients' quality of life. The *Fourth Edition* addresses clinical issues through clinical evidence and case studies. We have distilled the complexity of the pathophysiology of dysphagia to a practical level that can be absorbed by students and clinicians. Practical treatment options for a wide variety of swallowing problems with medical, surgical, and behavioral treatment models are concisely presented.

Throughout the book, certain terms are highlighted. These terms, which are germinal to the understanding of swallowing, are briefly explained in the text and some of the terms are further expanded in the Glossary. However, the reader may want to pursue these in greater depth, thus, the reason for highlighting them. We have tried to maintain the focus on treatment of swallowing disorders and have purposely avoided long discussions on the causes and complications of many neuromuscular diseases and neurological conditions that result in dysphagia. Rather, we have focused on the essentials of assessments and treatment of swallowing in those patients.

We now work in 3 separate universities, but we continue to share a philosophy that focuses on a multispecialty treatment approach based on sound research where available, consistent clinical methods, and the review of the outcomes of treatment to enhance our future clinical care. In most chapters, video examinations of case examples are provided.

Chapter One presents the clinical scope of dysphagia—who has dysphagia, the indications for intervention, the importance of treating dysphagia, and the relationship of dysphagia to associated medical conditions. A review of the extent of swallowing disorders in hospitals, nursing homes, and otherwise healthy individuals is provided. Video examples of normal swallowing are part of this chapter. There are almost no medical conditions or diseases in which swallowing disorders do not occur. While many swallowing disorders may be temporary, the need to intervene early and address them must be considered in light of the primary disease or disorder.

Chapter Two reviews the essential anatomy and function of the swallowing mechanism. We have chosen to present a summary of normal swallowing anatomy along with a concise review of the contributions of the cranial nerves rather than an extensive anatomic and neuroanatomic description of swallowing in keeping with the clinical focus of this text. The contributions of the cranial nerves are presented in tables that the clinician can easily access for later use. In the *Fourth Edition*, the current understanding of the interaction of the phases of swallowing is discussed. In this addition, we have added a review of the sensory information that, in the past, has been given little or no attention in much of the swallowing literature.

Chapter Three has been extensively revised to provide current reviews and descriptions of swallowing disorders that arise from various neurological and head and neck disorders and diseases. Definitions of aspiration and aspiration pneumonia are given. An updated list of diseases with their major associated swallowing problems along with video examples is found in this chapter. An array of tables accompanies this chapter, which provides quick access to diseases and disorders and the swallowing problems associated with these disorders. In addition, the effects of medication on swallowing are discussed.

In **Chapter Four**, we present an updated overview of swallowing disorders arising from surgical interventions. With the increasing number of in-office and operating room surgical procedures, there is a greater need to understand those procedures and how they will affect swallowing in the short and long terms. The effects of surgery to the head, neck, and upper airway always produce a swallowing disorder. While many of these problems are temporary, the swallowing team must acutely manage them. The authors relate their daily experiences in the team management of these disorders. Long-term swallowing disorders arising from oral cancer or skull base surgical procedures are treated from the swallowing clinician's reference. Indications for aggressive and conservative surgical treatments and follow-up management are presented in this chapter.

Chapter Five has been extensively revised to focus on the clinical swallow evaluation (CSE), the starting point for swallowing management. We begin this chapter with an extensive review of commonly used clinician-based screening protocols and patient self-assessment tools. This then becomes the basis for subsequent testing and management. The different components of a full clinical swallow evaluation (CSE) are then described in the sequence of how they may appear in a typical evaluation session. While the CSE is rarely the only evaluation of swallowing, it is an essential first step in the management process. Moreover, our experience with the CSE has led us to identify appropriate instrumental tests to be done subsequently to identify additional tests and consultations early in the treatment process.

Chapter Six is a completely new chapter in the *Fourth Edition* that focuses on the instrumental evaluation of swallowing. Importance is placed upon the indications for instrumental tests and criteria for test selection. We have updated the procedures and recommendations for different instrumental tests based on recent evidence. Video examples of modified barium swallow (MBS) examinations and flexible endoscopic evaluations of swallowing (FEES) are included to illustrate the use of these instruments.

Chapter Seven presents the nonsurgical treatment approaches to swallowing. This chapter starts with an introduction to evidence-based practice and a multidisciplinary approach to swallowing therapy. This chapter has been revised extensively based on the plethora of current information that has been developed since the third edition was published. Techniques are divided in compensatory swallowing therapy and rehabilitative swallowing therapy. *Note*: these terms are specifically defined in the *Fourth Edition*. Since the majority of treatments for swallowing disorders are nonsurgical, this important chapter outlines exercises for improving oral motor strength, bolus propulsion, and swallowing safety. Extensive references to evidence for various procedures are provided. Recent developments in the use of electrical stimulation and cortical neuromodulating methods are reviewed and discussed in light of new evidence for their use.

Chapter Eight addresses nutrition and the collaboration with nutrition specialists. The importance of working with a registered dietitian is now becoming more important in light of the various food options and food consistencies for patients. A unique aspect of this chapter is the explanation of the properties of liquids and foods that clinicians can understand. The introduction to rheology as a characteristic of foods and liquids is presented. Although the terms are new to speech-language pathologist, they are part of the everyday activities in a swallowing clinic. The latest framework for foods and drinks developed by the International Dysphagia Diet Standardization Initiative (IDDSI) is fully described with current evidence. Nonoral feeding methods are also presented with current evidence. Malnutrition and dehydration, 2 factors that affect recovery from dysphagia, are discussed in

relation to specific populations. A completely new section on ethical considerations has been added to this chapter.

Chapter Nine has been revised and expanded to include the assessment of pediatric swallowing disorders. In Chapter Nine, the focus is on a thorough assessment of the infant and the swallowing disorders that occur at birth and in childhood. The case history takes on a special importance since it includes the parents and others who may be involved with the birth, growth, and development of the child. The anatomy and physiology of the child is discussed with attention to developmental milestones of feeding and eating. The importance of the child's ever-changing behavior as it relates to eating is outlined. A survey of the most common disorders that have an effect on eating and swallowing are discussed.

Chapter Ten is a new chapter for the *Fourth Edition*. In this chapter, we explore the feeding and swallowing treatment options for infants and children. Although swallowing safely is the underlying concern for all children, there are specific issues regarding feeding that must be taken into account depending on the underlying diagnosis. Children with birth disorders, genetic disorders, and developmental disorders require special attention in order to facilitate proper growth and nutrition needs. Various neonate and child syndromes and disorders will be presented with the focus on specific needs related to swallowing and feeding.

Chapter Eleven provides a description of the most common surgical procedures for treating swallowing disorders that are not amenable to direct or indirect nonsurgical treatment. As with previous chapters, modifications to the surgical literature required revision of this chapter to identify new surgical techniques that focus on preventing aspiration and improving vocal fold closure. This chapter offers the clinician an understanding of the surgical procedures used to manage aspiration from conservative vocal fold medialization techniques to extensive procedures such as laryngotracheal separation. Although the surgical procedures are briefly described, the importance of decision making by the dysphagia team in planning surgery is emphasized. This chapter combines the surgical procedures with the prosthetic management of swallowing disorders.

Following removal of essential swallowing organs, the need for a multispecialty team to manage structural rehabilitation has become increasingly important. Dysphagia clinicians are now routinely recruited to work with an oral prosthodontist to ensure maximum swallowing and communication functions are restored. This includes the understanding of oral prosthodontics as well as other biomechanical and adaptive devices to aid the patient to swallow safely.

Chapter Twelve presents our philosophical approach to the organization of a multidisciplinary swallowing center with examples of how the multidiscipline team works in the swallowing center. The center combines clinicians trained to manage swallowing and voice disorders in one center since the diagnosis and treatment may involve treating both issues concurrently. Cases are presented to show the value of a comprehensive swallowing that includes voice specialists as well. The contributions of the speech-language pathologist and otolaryngologist in the diagnosis and treatment phases are described.

The concept of a unified center implies efficiency, comprehensiveness, and timeliness in the clinical management process of patients who will benefit from a combined management approach.

A **glossary** is included to help the beginning swallowing therapist quickly find important terms. The glossary in the *Fourth Edition* has been completely revised and includes explanations of the terms as they relate to swallowing and other disease conditions.

This text evolved from our clinical and research interests to improve the treatment of swallowing disorders and from our daily involvement in treating those disorders emanating from a variety of medical conditions, diseases, and disorders. We have translated our clinical experiences into a series of chapters that contain information that we draw upon daily. The *Clinical Management of Swallowing Disorders, Fourth Edition,* offers the student and the practicing clinician a textbook of the current procedures for the management of pediatric and adult swallowing disorders.

Acknowledgments

The authors acknowledge the contributions by colleagues in the various disciplines who diagnose and treat swallowing disorders. We have maintained a multidiscipline approach to the treatment of dysphagia over our careers and, through the references in this edition, we acknowledge all of those individuals who manage swallowing disorders in a multidisciplinary format.

The authors are deeply indebted to Marie-Pierre Murry for her work in reviewing the final version of the text, for preparing the glossary which includes extended details as they relate to both swallowing and the underlying disease process and for her unending encouragement while completing the fourth edition.

The authors acknowledge the dedication of Kalie Koscielak and Linda Shapiro, Plural Publishing Inc., who patiently attended to the details of the figures, video legends, and table headings. They worked early and late to bring this version together.

Heartfelt thanks to the Chan's and Ko's family for their professional support and encouragement throughout the preparation of the *Fourth Edition*. Special thanks to Tina Cheung from the Swallowing Research Laboratory, Division of Speech and Hearing Sciences, the University of Hong Kong for her editorial work and table revisions.

We also acknowledge Ivy Cheng, Dai Pu and Kelly Ho, graduate students at the Swallowing Research Laboratory, Division of Speech and Hearing Sciences, the University of Hong Kong, and to Dr. Brianna Crawley and Dr. Rebecca Howell for specific video selections.

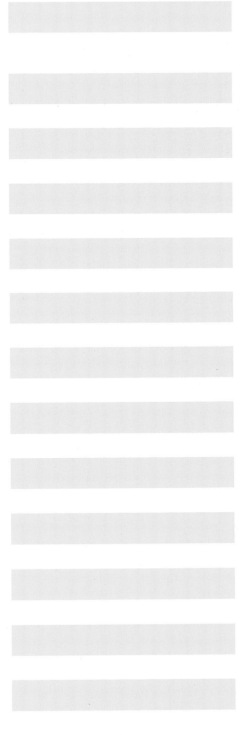

Video List

Chapter 1

Video 1–1. Normal flexible endoscopic evaluation of swallowing (FEES).

Video 1–2. Normal modified barium swallow examination (MBS also known as videofluoroscopic examination of swallowing [VFSS]).

Video 1–3. FEES examination of a patient with a history of dysphagia.

Video 1–4. MBS showing a trace of the barium flowing down into the airway after the majority of the bolus is swallowed.

Chapter 2

Video 2–1. Patient with difficulty initiating the proper sequence and thus resulting in significant pooling of the bolus.

Video 2–2. VFSS exam of a patient following CVA.

Chapter 3

Video 3–1. Penetration obtained during transnasal flexible endoscopy.

Video 3–2. Aspiration and cough.

Video 3–3. FEES with aspiration and no cough and the bolus at the level of the larynx.

Video 3–4. VFSS with silent aspiration.

Video 3–5. CVA, right vocal fold paralysis, poor cough, and poor laryngeal elevation.

Video 3–6. Patient with mid-stage Parkinson's disease working to achieve a swallow.

Video 3–7. Effects of inflammation and mucositis several years after XRT.

Chapter 4

Video 4–1. Videofluoroscopic study with the residue of food in the mouth after each swallow.

Video 4–2. Patient with partial glossectomy attempting to swallow with the bolus in the front of his mouth.

Chapter 6

Video 6–1. FESST exam. In this exam the endoscope is seen delivering a pulse of air to the aryepiglottic fold prior to delivering food to the patient.

Video 6–2. FEES video of an individual who had penetration on both liquid and solid materials but produced a cough to clear the penetrated boluses.

Video 6–3. Sample of MBS taken at the lateral position of an individual who had delayed swallow reflex.

Video 6–4. MBS of a 74-year-old man who was 6 years post stroke and had pharyngeal residue after swallow.

Video 6–5. MBS of a 66-year-old man who was 2 years post stroke and had reduced laryngeal elevation and trace aspiration of thin liquid.

Video 6–6. MBS of a 68-year-old man who was 4 years post stroke and had silent aspiration.

Chapter 7

Video 7–1. Patient swallows a liquid bolus and also a cracker.

Video 7–2. Shaker exercise.

Chapter 9

Video 9–1. Child who presented with a behavioral problem related to feeding. Note the movement in the larynx.

Chapter 12

Video 12–1. Patient with Parkinson's disease reporting the feeling of food remaining in his throat.

Video 12–2. Patient with Parkinson's disease who is being treated with breathing exercises using a breath trainer.

Video 12–3. Exam with the lesion on the right vocal fold.

Video 12–4. Patient following radiation therapy for an oral pharyngeal cancer.

Video 12–5. Young child with autism spectrum disorder with excessive residue.

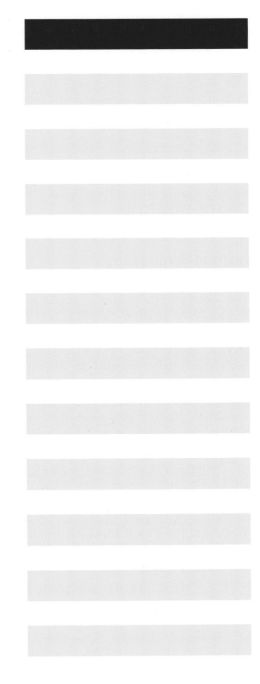

Introduction to and Epidemiology of Swallowing Disorders

A Look at the Chapter

In this chapter, normal and disordered swallowing are defined with video examples. Terminology is reviewed as it relates to normal and abnormal swallowing. The impact of a swallowing disorder on quality of life is presented with examples with a look toward tools for assessing quality of life. Those tools are more specifically reviewed in Chapter 5. We also introduce self-assessment as a tool for studying dysphagia. This is followed by the epidemiology of swallowing disorders. Epidemiology refers to both prevalence and cause of a disorder. In this chapter, we focus on prevalence. Causes will be taken up in later chapters.

INTRODUCTION

Normal Swallowing

The normal swallow is a rapid and overlapping sequence of neurologically controlled movements involving the muscles of the oral cavity, pharynx, larynx, esophagus, and stomach. Although most individuals take normal swallowing for granted, everyone experiences an abnormal swallow at some time in life, most likely resulting in an episode of a sudden choking sensation. However, in a normal, healthy person, this is usually resolved quickly by a cough or throat clearing.

When the muscles of the swallowing organs or the nerves that govern these organs are disordered, disrupted, damaged, or destroyed, swallowing can no longer be normal. However, because of the neuroplasticity of the swallowing organs and their ability to develop compensatory strategies, individuals with neurological or muscular damage to the swallowing organs can still swallow certain types of foods and liquids safely. Video 1–1 is an example of a normal flexible endoscopic evaluation of swallowing (FEES). Video 1–2 is an example of a normal **modified barium swallow** examination (MBS also known as videofluoroscopic swallow study [VFSS]).

Note the fluid movement and the speed of the bolus as it travels to the esophagus.

Abnormal Swallowing

Abnormal swallowing includes difficulty with swallowing or the total inability to swallow, referred to as dysphagia and aphagia, respectively.

*The global definition of **dysphagia** is simply "difficulty in swallowing."*

When someone cannot swallow at all, the term **aphagia**, or "inability to swallow anything," is used. The terms dysphagia and aphagia refer to swallowing saliva, liquids, foods, and medications of all consistencies. Dysphagia may also include such problems as foods or liquids "sticking" in the throat or regurgitation of swallowed liquids or foods. Swallowing difficulties may arise from mechanical problems of the swallowing mechanism, neurological disorders, gastrointestinal disorders, or loss of organs due to surgery or traumatic injury. Dysphagia and aphagia may also involve the disruption of the timing of the events needed to swallow normally.

Video 1–3 is a FEES examination of a patient with a history of dysphagia. Note that the food colored green remains in the area above the vocal folds and is not swallowed. It may ultimately be aspirated if the patient does not cough it out. Video 1–4 is an example of an MBS showing a trace of the barium flowing down into the airway after the majority of the bolus is swallowed. In a patient with a weak cough or pulmonary disease, this can lead to aspiration pneumonia.

Impact of Swallowing Disorders on Quality of Life

It is estimated that in the United States alone, 300,000 to 600,000 people with clinically significant dysphagia are diagnosed annually.[1,2] Nearly 70% of these patients are older than 60 years of age.[2] The true incidence of dysphagia may not be known, as it is often a condition following a primary diagnosis.

Since dysphagia is a *symptom*, it is often not listed as the principal diagnosis if the physician has only documented the underlying cause. However, according to the *International Classification of Diseases, Tenth Revision* (ICD-10), the appropriate code for dysphagia can be listed as a secondary diagnosis following stroke, esophagitis, and other diseases of the neurological system or gastroesophageal pathway.[3]

Swallowing disorders, even when subtle, eventually take a toll on quality of life. Because eating is a natural part of social interaction, daily nutrition, and general health, the importance of normal swallowing cannot be overstated. Swallowing affects quality of life in a number of ways, regardless of the severity of the problem. Table 1–1 summarizes common effects that dysphagia has on the quality of life.

Aspiration

Aspiration is a condition in which foods, liquids, pills, or oropharyngeal secretions pass into the airway below the level of the true vocal folds. This happens occasionally to most people; but in the absence of injuries to the muscles or nerves of swallowing, most people have the ability to sense the food or liquid in the airway and cough it out. When there is an injury or damage to the swallowing mechanism and aspiration is frequent or extensive, there is a higher risk of lung infections, dehydration, and malnutrition, and the enjoyment of eating diminishes; thus, quality of life also diminishes.[4,5]

Dehydration

Dehydration is the state when there is not enough water in the body to maintain a healthy level of fluids in the body's tissues. Even in an otherwise healthy person, lack of adequate water intake can lead to dehydration. Water is an essential element for all individuals as it replaces fluid losses from bowel movements, urination, and also from general physical exercise. A general rule of thumb is to

TABLE 1–1. Effects of Dysphagia on Quality of Life

A. Functional Limitations

1. Limitations on the types of food that a patient can swallow safely
2. Patients may be limited to a specific diet of foods that they do not like
3. Time required to swallow and finish a meal may be longer
4. Oral structures may limit the types of food to swallow
5. Some foods may cause the patient to choke
6. Awareness due either to visual or conscious limitations restrict eating
7. Gastric structures or functions may limit amount or type of foods

B. Activities and Participation

1. Patients on a nonoral diet may be reluctant to attend events where food is served
2. Foods related to cultural or religion may not be available to patient
3. Ability to hold and use straw or utensils may limit eating/drinking
4. Ability to eat in a group setting may limit activities
5. Ability to prepare meals may reduce food intake

C. Environmental Factors

1. Changes in room lighting or sound may limit eating
2. Proper eating arrangements may be limited due to room spaces
3. Eating in public may present unwanted attention
4. Use of personal care providers may be needed during mealtimes
5. Ability to prepare food may be limited

replace body fluids with 3 quarts of water per day. For patients with neurological impairments who may be at risk for aspiration when swallowing liquids, fluid intake may require constant monitoring. Other factors such as medications that have dehydrating side effects, as discussed in Chapter 3, may impact one's ability to swallow. For example, when there is not enough natural saliva in the mouth, chewing becomes more difficult, food does not easily form a bolus, and particles may break apart and require multiple swallows. Payne et al reported that dysphagia patients are at high risk for dehydration, which represents a common cause of morbidity and rehospitalization in this group.[6] Patients with dysphagia should be evaluated frequently for signs of dehydration and, if present, further evaluation of other nutritional deficiencies may be warranted.

Malnutrition

Malnutrition is the condition that occurs when your body does not get enough nutrients due to the inability to ingest food safely, the reluctance to eat or fear of eating/drinking due to past swallowing problems, or the inability to digest or absorb ingested nutrients. Once a person is unable to ingest food safely, his or her ability to maintain health decreases. This is especially important for patients who are recovering from extensive surgeries, strokes, or other debilitating diseases and will require extensive rehabilitation. Once malnutrition develops, its treatment may be as important as any other part of the rehabilitation process. Recovery from malnutrition has been shown to help in the rehabilitation process, including in the treatment of dysphagia, leading to improvement in the patient's quality of life. The specifics of nutrition are reviewed in Chapter 8.

Weight Loss

There is a great preoccupation with weight loss in our society. Extensive weight loss either induced or without reason, requires attention from the dysphagia team. Significant weight loss is associated with the loss of muscle mass, which may produce weakness severe enough to change the daily activities of an individual. Moreover, weight loss may

affect coordination of muscles especially in repeated activities such as swallowing. Weight loss associated with starvation, whether intentional or not, may lead to damage of other vital organs, namely the heart. When unplanned weight loss develops, a swallowing disorder should be suspected. Weight loss should not be so extensive that it affects quality of life nor should it continue beyond normal weight ranges.

> *The impact of weight loss on various medical conditions or postsurgical recovery has been shown to slow or delay recovery.*

A recent survey of studies related to weight loss suggests the importance of monitoring food and liquid intake.[7] The factors most consistently associated with weight loss were depression, poor oral intake, swallowing issues, and eating/chewing dependency. Staffing factors were associated with weight loss in most studies.

> *The factors most consistently associated with a low body mass index (BMI) included immobility, poor oral intake, chewing problems, dysphagia, female gender, and older age. The factors most consistently associated with poor nutrition included impaired function, dementia, swallowing/chewing difficulties, poor oral intake, and older age.*

Temporary nonoral feeding arrangements are now more commonly used to stabilize weight during recovery from severe diseases and disorders and to speed up such recovery.[8,10]

Types of Pneumonia

Not all pneumonia is the result of dysphagia or aphagia. Infections, poor health, and lack of proper posthospital care may lead to other types of pneumonia. Clinicians who treat swallowing disorders must be aware of these, as aspiration may play a part in their cause.

Aspiration Pneumonia. When pulmonary infection results from acute or chronic aspiration of fluids, foods, or oral secretions from the mouth or from fluids arising in the stomach and flowing into the airway, **aspiration pneumonia** develops. This is a potentially life-threatening condition and requires significant medical attention. However, not all aspiration leads to pneumonia. Studies report that 28% to 36% of asymptomatic healthy older adults demonstrate trace aspiration on a FEES and up to 45% of normal adults demonstrate aspiration of oropharyngeal secretions during sleep.[4] Nonetheless, aspiration pneumonia creates significant morbidity and may account for up to 70% of community-acquired pneumonia in elderly patients.[11]

Nosocomial Pneumonia. **Nosocomial pneumonia**, also called hospital-acquired pneumonia, is usually the result of bacterial infections acquired during the first 48 to 72 hours following admission to a hospital. Nosocomial pneumonia is often the cause of death following admission to an intensive care unit. Factors such as old age, aspiration of saliva, fever, and gastric contents rising and falling into the airway (gastric reflux) are common causes of nosocomial pneumonia.

Community-Acquired Pneumonia. **Community-acquired pneumonia (CAP)** is an infection of the lungs in people who have not been hospitalized. It is a disease that can affect people of all ages and is often the leading cause of death in countries where vaccination against diseases has not been established.

In CAP, the patient may appear to be swallowing normally but, due to fever or breathing difficulty, the lungs slowly absorb fluids, resulting in infection.

CAP is treated with antibiotics and may require rehospitalization. In undeveloped countries, CAP can occur in patients who have recently been hospitalized and discharged without proper follow-up.[11]

Other Impacts of Swallowing Disorders on Quality of Life

General Health

The inability to swallow correctly may lead to a decline in general health. This may be slow or rapid and is usually, but not always, associated with other diseases. For individuals with systemic diseases such as **Parkinson's disease**, diabetes mellitus, or high blood pressure, dysphagia may decline slowly. For disorders such as gastroesophageal reflux and autoimmune disorders, dysphagia may initially be sporadic and will increase as the severity of the primary problem increases.[12] With the onset of dysphagia, the body is not able to cope as well with the primary disease. Moreover, the primary disease may be exacerbated by the dysphagia.

Psychological Well-Being

Eating is a social function as well as a nutritional necessity. When an illness or disease is further compounded by dysphagia, the natural social functions in which food plays a role are limited.[13] The person with a swallowing disorder can no longer participate seamlessly in the social interactions that surround meals. He or she is no longer able to eat in his or her normal location (home, for example) or with the same individuals that he or she has dined in the past. The meal is now in a clinical setting or in a setting with a caregiver following a prescribed diet that may include foods that are new to the individual and not part of his or her lifelong diet. In controlled settings such as a hospital or nursing home, the diet to adhere to is one that will allow the patient to regain health rather than a diet whose primary purpose is enjoyment.

Financial Well-Being

The financial impact caused by dysphagia can be significant if there is a need for special foods, supplemental feeding, primary **enteral** or **parenteral nutrition**, dysphagia therapy, special gadgets and appliances to aid in the preparation of meals, or the need for others to assist with feeding. Some or all of these expenses may be paid for by insurance; however, the costs of all dysphagia-related management issues may be substantial and may continue for extended periods of time, straining the financial condition of the patient, his or her family, and the economic welfare of the patient. Limitations brought by insurance capitation or personal financial abilities often compromise ideal rehabilitation strategies.

The true financial impact of dysphagia remains unknown, as research has not yet determined the total cost of major events such as aspiration pneumonia and hospital readmissions or the cost-benefit ratio for the early identification and management of swallowing disorders. Conventional wisdom suggests that early intervention may prevent extensive comorbidities that result from the interaction of swallowing disorders with other diseases or disorders; clinical research ultimately will lead to the confirmation of methods of dysphagia rehabilitation.

NEED FOR EARLY INTERVENTION

"Not everything that counts can be counted."

Dennis Burket, as quoted in Kitchen Table Wisdom *by R. N. Remen*[14]

Quality of Life

There is only limited, albeit strong and intuitively correct, evidence that the diagnosis and treatment of dysphagia are efficacious from the standpoint of significantly reducing aspiration pneumonia. Most of the evidence that exists is based on studies of stroke patients, although, as pointed out in later in Chapters 5, 7, and 8, there also is evidence derived from research on patients undergoing treatment for cancers of the head and neck. The limited evidence suggests that, in the acute care setting, dysphagia management is accompanied by reduced pneumonia rates. Furthermore, the use of a complete **clinical swallow evaluation (CSE)** appears to be cost effective.[1] Others have found dysphagia management to be useful in the rehabilitation of swallowing disorders in other populations. Wasserman et al[15] have shown that, regardless of the underlying diagnosis, accurate reporting of the clinical swallow evaluation information and an early aggressive treatment program are efficacious in reducing the length of hospital stays in patients undergoing major surgery for head and neck cancer. Additionally, development of valid screening procedures, such as the scale created by Foster and colleagues[16] may offer further basis for early treatment of patients with dysphagia. They administered a screening instrument for dysphagia to 299 inpatients and found that the scale provided a means for targeting patients for early swallowing assessment and intervention.

McHorney and colleagues[17,18] presented early versions of 2 quality-of-life assessments to determine the need and value of treating swallowing disorders. The SWAL-QOL is a validated, 44-item tool and described in detail in Chapter 5. The SWAL-CARE is a 15-item tool that assesses quality of care and patient satisfaction and is also described in Chapter 5. The SWAL-QOL and SWAL-CARE may help clinicians to focus on the patient's treatment and determine treatment effectiveness. The work of McHorney[18] found that the SWAL-QOL and SWAL-CARE were related primarily to oral transit duration and total swallow duration.

In general, the lack of control groups, the undefined effects of diseases, and the lack of long-term follow-up data limit the statements that can be made about the true effects of early dysphagia intervention. Nonetheless, the clinical evidence gathered by those treating patients with dysphagia on a day-to-day basis suggests that intervention improves quality of life. The lack of prospective, controlled, randomized research should not suggest that swallowing programs using the CSE or other programs such as the MBS (see Chapter 6) or the FEES (see Chapter 6) should not be continued. On the contrary, studies such as that by Odderson et al[19] and Mahler et al[20] provide strong arguments for continued early intervention in dysphagia. Early on, Odderson et al looked at pneumonia rates before and after initiating a CSE program in a hospital setting.

Aspiration pneumonia rates in stroke patients were substantially reduced after an early intervention swallowing program was initiated compared to pneumonia rates before the program was started.

Mahler and colleagues[20] studied Parkinson's disease and found that a program focusing on strengthening laryngeal closure and cough showed prolonged positive effects on speech and swallowing. Additional research is needed to provide further evidence for programs that focus on dysphagia intervention to include a data acquisition format that offers an opportunity to assess their contribution to reduction of aspiration pneumonia, length of hospital stays, and readmissions to hospitals due to swallowing-related problems.

EPIDEMIOLOGY

Dysphagia can be caused by many different disorders, including natural aging, neurological diseases, head injury, degenerative diseases, systemic diseases, autoimmune disorders, neoplasms, and infections. Treatment modalities such as surgery, radiation therapy, and medications can also lead to dysphagia. Chronic reflux laryngitis, often overlooked, may also interfere with normal swallowing. Patients with head or neck cancer have a variable presentation. They often have significant dysphagia at the time of initial presentation, and their swallowing function also often suffers as a result of treatment, although some deficits improve with time. Patients with Parkinson's disease suffer from dysphagia that becomes more severe as the disease progresses. Because of these varied and often compounded etiologies, it may not be possible to ascertain the true incidence of any particular category of disorder. In addition to these factors, there is no single test that is 100% accurate for diagnosing dysphagia or its primary cause.

Swallowing disorders may arise as comorbidities of other disorders or as precursors to more significant diseases and disorders. Moreover, the incidence of swallowing disorders may vary depending on the type of diagnostic evaluation. Table 1–2 shows the incidence of oropharyngeal dysphagia in patients who exhibited aspiration during videofluoroscopic and flexible endoscopic examinations.[3,21,22]

The incidence of swallowing disorders following a stroke remains high; however, with the advent of improved assessment techniques, the treatment process following evidence of aspiration is now better understood. If all of the tests for examination of swallowing are considered, the true incidence of swallowing disorders may be substantially higher. When the swallowing disorder accompanies other medical conditions, the primary condition may be affected by the swallowing disorder. Conversely, a swallowing disorder may be the symptom of another neurological disease or condition requiring

TABLE 1–2. Incidence of Oropharyngeal Dysphagia in Patients Who Exhibited Aspiration During Videofluoroscopic Examination and Flexible Endoscopic Evaluation of Swallowing[a]

Cause of Dysphagia	Number (%) of Patients
Head and neck oncologic surgery	59 (36)
Cerebrovascular accident	47 (29)
Cardiac-related event[b]	294 (22)
Closed head injury	12 (7)
Spinal cord injury	10 (6)
Degenerative neurologic disease[c]	9 (6)
Adductor vocal fold paralysis	7 (4)
Zenker diverticulum	4 (2)
Generalized weakness	5 (3)
Cerebral palsy	3 (2)
Central nervous system involvement from AIDS	Unknown
Craniotomy (for aneurysm repair)	2 (1)
Undetermined	4 (2)

[a]Adapted and modified from Rasley et al.[21]

[b]Data derived from Aviv et al.[22]

[c]Includes Parkinson disease, motor neuron disease, and multiple sclerosis.

treatment. Thus, the exact incidence of swallowing disorders remains unknown.

Cerebrovascular Accidents (CVAs) and Neurological Diseases

Stroke is the third leading cause of death in the United States. Approximately 500,000 new cases are reported yearly and 150,000 individuals die of CVAs every year. Prospective studies have demonstrated an incidence of dysphagia as high as 41.7% in the first month after a CVA. The overall rate of aspiration resulting from a CVA is approximately 33.3%. One-half of these patients will aspirate silently (with no obvious clinical symptoms or signs). As many as 20% die of aspiration pneumonia in the first year after a CVA, and 10% to 15% will die of aspiration pneumonia after the first year following the stroke. In general, the larger the area of ischemia, the more significant is the swallowing disorder. Although the site of lesion does not always correlate with the type and severity of the swallowing disorder, brainstem strokes produce dysphagia more frequently than cortical strokes. Table 1–3 shows the epidemiological data compiled from the Agency for Healthcare Policy and Research and Quality (AHRQ) for neurological diseases including stroke.[1]

Specific information concerning stroke suggests that a left cerebral infarction increases the risk of aspiration pneumonia compared to a right-side CVA.[23] A recent study by Flowers et al looked at the co-occurrence of dysphagia, dysarthria, and aphasia. They found estimates of the incidence of dysphagia, dysarthria, and aphasia were 44%, 42%, and 30%, respectively.[24] The highest co-occurrence of any two impairments was 28% for the presence of both dysphagia and dysarthria. Ten percent of all the 221 patients studied had all 3 impairments. The highest predictors were nonalert level of consciousness for dysphagia, symptoms of weakness for dysarthria, and right-sided symptoms for aphasia.

Dementia

Dementia refers to the inability to carry out tasks due to the loss of brain function. The loss of func-

tions depends on the part of the brain that is damaged. Dysphagia is common in elderly patients with **dementia**. According to videofluoroscopic reports, normal swallowing function is found in only 7% of patients with dementia. This group of patients is the most difficult to assess with any type of functional study, due to their dementia. The effectiveness of therapeutic maneuvers that require patient cooperation is also low. Nonoral nutrition alternatives must be considered in patients with dementia and dysphagia. Recurrences of aspiration pneumonia, continued weight loss, and/or refusal to eat are the key indications for implementing nonoral nutrition alternatives.

Elderly Population

Seventy to 90% of elderly patients, even those without known neurological disease, have some degree of swallowing dysfunction, if not true dysphagia. Objective functional tests are necessary to rule out specific diseases and to assess the risk of aspiration. As many as 50% of elderly patients have difficulty eating, leading to nutritional deficiencies with associated weight loss, increased risk of falling, poor healing, and increased susceptibility to other illnesses. Weight loss, increased length of meals, depression, and general complaints of fatigue are often observed in this group prior to the diagnosis of a swallowing disorder.

Head and Neck Oncology

The presence of a tumor in the upper aerodigestive tract may affect swallowing by

1. Mechanical obstruction due to bulk or extraluminal compression
2. Decreased pliability of the soft tissue due to neoplastic infiltration
3. Direct invasion leading to paralysis of important pharyngeal or laryngeal muscles
4. Loss of sensation (taste, feel) caused by nerve injury
5. Pain

TABLE 1–3. Epidemiological Data From the Published Literature: Neurological Diseases and the Rate of Dysphagia Within Each

Disease	Prevalence (per 100 000)	Incidence (per 100 000)	Study	Reason	Diagnosed Occurrence of Dysphagia (%)	Study	Reason
Stroke	NA	145	Brown et al. (25)	Mayo Clinic	VFSS: 74.6	Daniels et al. (35)	Median of VFSS studies
		289	Modan and Wagener (26)	Mayo Clinic seemed low: this provides an upper estimate	CSE: 41.7	DePippo et al. (36)	Median of CSE studies[a]
Parkinson disease	106.9	13	Mayeux et al. (27)	Only number on general population that included elderly	VFSS: 69.1	Bushmann et al. (37); Fuh et al. (38)	Mean of 2 studies in which L-dopa was withheld
Alzheimer disease	259.8	NR	Beard et al. (28)	Only published number	VFSS: 84	Horner et al. (39)	Only published number
Multiple sclerosis	170.8	NR	Wynn et al. (29)	Only number; Mayo Clinic	NR	NA	NA
Motor neuron disease	170.8	6.2	Lilienfeld et al. (30)	Only published number	51.2 (method not reported)	Leighton et al. (40)	Exam, not survey
Amyotrophic lateral sclerosis	NR	1.8	McGuire et al. (31)	Exam, not survey	29 (method not reported)	Litvan et al. (41)	Only published number
Progressive supranuclear palsy	1.39	1.1	Golbe et al. (32); Bower et al. (33)	Only published number	VFSS: 55.6	Kagel, Leopold (42)	Only published number
Huntington disease	1.9	0.2	Kokmen et al. (34)	Only published number	VFSS: 100		

Abbreviations: CSE, bedside swallowing evaluation; NA, not applicable; NR, not reported; VFSS, videofluoroscopic swallowing study (also known as the modified barium swallow [MBS]).
[a]Now referred to in this text as the clinical swallow evaluation (CSE).

6. Factors related to desire for eating (appetite and craving)

Treatments for squamous cell carcinoma, namely, surgery, radiation, or chemotherapy, produce dis-abilities that are usually proportional to the volume of the resection and/or the radiation field. Surgery produces division and fibrosis of muscles and anesthetic areas due to the transection or extirpation of afferent neural fibers and/or receptors.

*Radiation therapy leads to **xerostomia** (dryness of the mouth), which, in many cases, is permanent and a main source of swallowing complaints made by patients.*

Irradiation also produces fibrosis of the oropharyngeal and laryngeal musculature. Chemotherapy may lead to weakness, nausea, or reduced sensory processes and may add to immediate radiation side effects such as mucositis, the thickening of mucus in the mouth, pharynx, and esophagus. Although newer types of radiation treatment known as **intensity modulated radiation therapy** (IMRT) have been used recently and are described more fully in Chapter 3, the results still impact swallowing both in the short term and long term.

Swallowing function after radiation treatment appears to be related to both site and stage of disease. In general, patients with so-called anterior tumors, such as on the floor of the mouth or anterior oral tongue, have better posttreatment outcomes regarding swallowing than do patients with posterior tumors, such as on the oropharynx or hypopharynx. Reconstructive methods also influence the swallowing outcome. Patients who are reconstructed with primary closure have fewer problems swallowing than patients who are reconstructed with bulky insensate flaps.

Hospitalized Patients

The incidence of swallowing disorders in patients admitted to critical care units is increased by the need for endotracheal and nasogastric intubation and tracheotomy, the use of sedatives, impaired consciousness, and the debilitated status of many of the patients requiring critical care.

Acute care patients should be assessed for swallowing disorders within the first 24 hours of hospitalization. In many hospitals, a standing order exists for a CSE of the acute patient within 24 hours of admission. Patients requiring mechanical ventilation are at higher risk for aspiration pneumonia. The mortality of nosocomial pneumonia is estimated to be 20% to 50% for hospitalized patients. Hospital costs due to nosocomial infection may exceed $22,000 per occurrence.

Nursing Home Residents

Studies carried out in nursing homes have demonstrated that 40% to 60% of the residents have clinical evidence of dysphagia. This number appears to be increasing in recent years. Smith et al[43] suggest that the high number of nursing home residents with dysphagia is due, at least in part, to discharging patients with swallowing disorders from acute care settings into institutional care.

The prevalence of all types of pneumonia has been estimated to be 2%, although it is unknown how many of these patients developed pneumonia as a result of aspiration. The death rate for patients diagnosed with pneumonia in a nursing home and admitted to acute care centers may exceed 40% of all readmissions.

Cardiac-Related Conditions

The number of patients seen in major medical centers for cardiac-related conditions is always increasing, due to the life-sustaining procedures available in emergency settings and the types of surgical treatment available to patients following cardiac events. In 2004, a large cohort of patients (1340) with swallowing disorders was examined by Aviv and colleagues[44] in an effort to identify safety and comfort factors related to assessment of swallowing disorders using the flexible endoscopic examination of swallowing with sensory testing (FEESST) procedure in inpatients and outpatients. The largest patient subgroup, as might be expected, included poststroke patients; however, surprisingly, the second-largest group included patients with cardiac-related events (22.2%). The majority of cardiac-related cases in the acute, inpatient setting had undergone open heart surgery (almost 60% of cases), followed by patients who had had heart attacks and those with congestive heart failure and newly diagnosed arrhythmias. The authors found that a large percentage of these patients had significant vagal nerve sensory dysfunctions when tested with FEESST and thus were at risk for **silent aspiration**—that is, aspiration without sensing the need to cough.

Gastroesophageal Reflux and Laryngopharyngeal Reflux

Over the past 15 to 20 years, reflux disease has been shown to be a common cause of swallowing disorders. Belafsky reported that the most common cause of dysphagia complaints was related to reflux disease.[45] Gastroesophageal and laryngopharyngeal reflux are discussed in detail in Chapter 3. In short, acid from the stomach rises into the esophagus and often to the level of the larynx creating a burning in the chest or a feeling of a lump in the throat leading to a delayed or disrupted normal swallow.

Other Conditions

Patients may present to an outpatient facility with numerous problems that include difficulty with swallowing or the inability to swallow. Other swallowing disorders may also be identified when a patient is hospitalized for the care of other conditions. Table 1–4 outlines the most common conditions that may indicate a swallowing disorder is also present. The true incidence of swallowing disorders in patients presenting with these problems is unknown.

In infants and young children, swallowing problems are often overlooked until a nutritional or failure to thrive condition exists. Infant and childhood dysphagia have evolved into a separate area of study thanks to increased neonatal care, better instrumentation to study the problem, and findings of the importance of nutrition to improve other coexisting problems in young children. The main causes of sucking, swallowing, and feeding disorders are lesions of the brainstem such as malformations of the posterior fossa, neonatal brainstem tumors, agenesis of cranial nerves, lesions of the posterior brain, craniovertebral anomalies and syndromes that involve rhombencephalic development such as Pierre Robin sequence, CHARGE syndrome, and so on.

TABLE 1–4. Conditions That May Lead to or Are Directly Related to Swallowing Disorders

Type of Condition	Common Examples
Congenital	Dysphagia lusoria
	Tracheoesophageal fistula
	Laryngeal clefts
	Other foregut abnormalities
Inflammatory	Gastroesophageal reflux disease (GERD)
	Laryngopharyngeal reflux (LPR)
Infections	Lyme disease
	Neuropathies/encephalitis
	Chagas disease
	HIV
Trauma	Central nervous system trauma
	Upper aerodigestive tract
	Blunt traumatic injuries to the oral, laryngeal, and/or esophageal organs
	Burns
Endocrine	Goiter
	Hypothyroid
	Diabetic neuropathy
Neoplasia	Oral cavity and contents
	Upper aerodigestive tract
	Thyroid
	Central nervous system
Systemic	Autoimmune disorders
	Dermatomyositis
	Scleroderma
	Sjögren disease
	Amyloidosis
	Sarcoidosis
Iatrogenic	Surgery
	Chemotherapy
	Other medications
	Radiation

Suprabulbar lesions, neuromuscular disorders, peripheral esophageal, digestive, and laryngeal anomalies and dysfunctions can also be involved.[46]

The main principles of the management of congenital sucking, swallowing, and feeding disorders are discussed in Chapters 9 and 10.

Burns

The true incidence of swallowing disorders caused by burns is not well documented. Although burns may occur in the oral cavity, pharynx, or esophagus, unless the burns are extreme in the oral cavity and pharynx, they usually resolve with no significant swallowing disorder. However, burns in the esophagus may lead to esophageal strictures.[47] Examination of the esophagus with endoscopy and ultrasound has improved the morbidity associated with esophageal burn disorders; nonetheless, patients often need recurring dilation and possibly esophageal stents to maintain nutrition. Late reconstructive surgery, mainly using colon transposition, offers the best results in referral centers, either in children or adults, but such a difficult surgical procedure is often unavailable in developing countries.[48] Continuous long-term monitoring is important as strictures may re-form and esophageal cancer may develop, which is rare but possible.

SUMMARY

Swallowing disorders have a significant effect on a patient's quality of life, including the patient's physical, financial, and psychological well-being. These effects are highlighted in this chapter and discussed in depth by Treats within the framework of the World Health Organization's International Classification of Functioning, Disability, and Health.[49] Dysphagia leads to a number of complicating factors, whether the patient is generally healthy or is recovering from a neurological event, cancer, or other surgery. The inability to swallow leads to weight loss, weakness, and, in severe cases, complicating medical problems.

Although research is somewhat limited, there appears to be a general clinical consensus that early intervention in dysphagia through proper diagnosis and treatment may reduce the comorbidities and thus shorten the length and cost of the hospital stay.

Treatment of swallowing disorders varies according to the underlying pathophysiology and status of the patient. Outpatients with minor problems are generally cooperative and willing to make adjustments in lifestyle and diet to improve their swallowing disorder. Hospitalized patients may be severely deconditioned or their cognitive status may limit their cooperation in the rehabilitation process. The patient with dysphagia presents a unique opportunity for team diagnosis and treatment. The remainder of this text explores the methods and approaches to treating swallowing disorders.

DISCUSSION QUESTIONS

1. With which groups of patients might the SWAL-QOL and SWAL-CARE be most useful? In what groups might its use be limited?
2. What are some of the significant negative effects of a swallowing disorder on an otherwise healthy person?
3. There is a rising awareness of reflux disease reported among otolaryngologists and speech-language pathologists (SLPs). What evidence exists to suggest the need for SLP involvement?
4. What are the complications that might exist with a patient with dementia when conducting a CSE prior to treatment?
5. Dementia presents unique problems to the clinician treating dysphagia. Why?

STUDY QUESTIONS

1. Aspiration refers to
   A. Liquid or food caught in the throat
   B. Liquid or food passing into the airway below the vocal folds
   C. Coughing after swallowing liquids or foods
   D. Inability to cough when choking on liquids or foods

2. Malnutrition develops when
   A. A person has not drunk enough water
   B. A person fails to eat a balanced diet
   C. A person does not take in the proper amount of protein calories
   D. A person goes on a crash diet not approved by a physician

3. In today's society, weight loss
   A. Is desirable when people are hospitalized
   B. May have negative effects on hospitalized patients
   C. Is usually recommended for overweight people when they are hospitalized
   D. Improves swallowing ability

4. The clinical swallowing evaluation
   A. Provides the basis for deciding what type of foods to give a patient with a swallowing disorder
   B. Provides the clinician with the patient's underlying swallowing problem
   C. Reduces the need for an instrumental swallowing examination
   D. May be used as a screening tool for identifying patients at risk for a swallowing disorder

5. Silent aspiration
   A. Occurs rarely in patients following strokes
   B. May be reduced using thickened consistencies of food
   C. Cannot be adequately identified during a clinical swallow evaluation
   D. Does not affect patients after their acute recovery period from a CVA

REFERENCES

1. US Department of Health and Human Services. Archived EPC Evidence Reports. 1999. Agency for Healthcare Research and Quality. Diagnosis and treatment of swallowing disorders (dysphagia) in acute-care stroke patients. Evidence report/technology assessment (Summary) pp. Assessment: No. 8. Rockville, MD: Agency for Health Care Policy and Research; 1999: AHCPR Publication 99-EO24.1–6.

2. Sura L, Madhavan A, Carnaby G, et al. Dysphagia in the elderly: management and nutritional considerations. *Clin Interv Aging.* 2012;7:287–298.

3. Center for Medicare and Medicaid Services 2015. https://www.cms.gov/medicare/coding.

4. Leder SB, Suiter DM. An epidemiologic study on aging and dysphagia in the acute care hospitalized population: 2000–2007. *Gerontology.* 2009;55:714–718.

5. Todd JT, Stuart A, Lintzenich CR, Wallin J, Grace-Martin K, Butler SG. Stability of aspiration status in healthy adults. *Ann Otol Rhinol Laryngol.* 2013;122(5):289–293.

6. Payne C, Wiffen PJ, Martin S. Interventions for fatigue and weight loss in adults with advanced progressive illness. *Cochrane Database Sys Rev.* 2012. doi:10.1002/14651858.CD008427.pub2.

7. Tamura BK, Bell CL, Masaki KH, Amella EJ. Factors associated with weight loss, low BMI, and malnutrition among nursing home patients: a systematic review of the literature. *J Am Med Dir Assoc.* 2013;14(9):649–655. doi:10.1016/j.jamda.2013.02.022. Epub 2013 Apr 30.

8. Feng X, Todd T, Hu Y, et al. Age-related changes of hyoid bone position in healthy older adults with aspiration. *Laryngoscope.* 2014;124:E231–E236.

9. Huxley EJ, Viroslav J, Gray WR, Pierce AK. Pharyngeal aspiration in normal adults and patients with depressed consciousness. *Am J Med.* 1978;64:564–568.

10. Mercuri A, Lim Joon D, Wada H, Rolfo A, Khoo V. The effect of an intensive nutritional program on daily set-up variations and radiotherapy planning margins of head and neck cancer patients. *J Med Imaging Rad.* 2009;53(5):500–505.

11. Dimopoulos G, Matthaiou DK, Karageorgopoulos DE, Grammatikos AP, Athanassa Z, Falagas ME. Short- versus long-course antibacterial therapy for community-acquired pneumonia: a meta-analysis. *Drugs.* 2008;68(13):1841–1854.

12. Marcason W. What are the primary nutritional issues for a patient with Parkinson's disease? *J Am Diet Assoc.* 2009;109(7):1316–1319.

13. Leslie P, Carding PC, Wilson JA. Investigation and management of chronic dysphagia. *Br Med J.* 2003;326:433–436.

14. Remen RN. *Kitchen Table Wisdom.* New York, NY: Penguin; 1996.

15. Wasserman T, Murry T, Johnson JT, Myers EN. Management of swallowing in supraglottic and extended supraglottic laryngectomy patients. *Head Neck.* 2001;23(12):1043–1048.

16. Foster CB, Gorga D, Padial C, et al. The development and validation of a screening instrument to identify hospitalized medical patients in need of early functional rehabilitation assessment. *Qual Life Res.* 2004;13(6):1099–1108.

17. McHorney CA, Robbins J, Lomax K, et al. The SWAL-QOL and SWAL-CARE outcomes tool for oropharyngeal dysphagia in adults: III. Documentation of reliability and validity. *Dysphagia.* 2002;17(2):97–114.

18. McHorney CA, Martin-Harris B, Robbins J, Rosenbek J. Clinical validity of the SWAL-QOL and SWAL-CARE outcome tools with respect to bolus flow measures. *Dysphagia*. 2006;21(3):141–148.

19. Odderson IR, Keaton JC, McKenna BS. Swallow management in patients on an acute stroke pathway: quality is cost effective. *Arch Phys Med Rehabil*. 1995;76(12):1130–1133.

20. Mahler LA, Ramig, LO, Fox C. Evidence-based treatment of voice and speech disorders in Parkinson's disease. *Curr Opin Otolaryngol Head Neck Surg*. 2015;23(3):209–215.

21. Rasley A, Logemann JA, Kahrilas P, Rademaker AW, Pauloski BR, Dodds WJ. Prevention of barium aspiration during videofluoroscopic swallowing studies: value of postural change. *Am J Roentgenol*. 1993;160:1005–1009.

22. Aviv JE, Di Tullio MR, Homma S, et al. Hypopharyngeal perforation near-miss during transesophageal echocardiography. *Laryngoscope*. 2004;114(5):821–826.

23. Yamamoto K, Koh H, Shimada H, Takeuchi J, Yamakawa M, Miki T. Cerebral infarction in the left hemisphere compared with the right hemisphere increases the risk of aspiration pneumonia. *Osaka City Med J*. 2014;60(2):81–86.

24. Flowers HL, Silver FL, Fang J, Rochon E, Martino R. The incidence, co-occurrence and predictors of dysphagia, dysarthria and aphasia after first-ever acute ischemic stroke. *J Commun Disord*. 2013;46(3):238–248.

25. Brown RD, Whisnant JP, Sicks JD, O'Fallon WM, Wiebers DO. Stroke incidence, prevalence, and survival: secular trends in Rochester, Minnesota, through 1989. *Stroke*. 1996;27(3):373–380.

26. Modan B, Wagener DK. Some epidemiological aspects of stroke: mortality/morbidity trends, age, sex, race, socioeconomic status. *Stroke*. 1992;23(9):1230–1236.

27. Mayeux R, Marder K, Cote, LJ, et al. The frequency of idiopathic Parkinson's's disease by age, ethnic group, and sex in northern Manhattan, 1988–1993. *Am J Epidemiol*. 1995;142(8):820–827.

28. Beard CM, Kokmen E, Offord K, Kurland LT. Is the prevalence of dementia changing? *Neurology*. 1991;41(12):1911–1914.

29. Wynn DR, Rodriguez M, O'Fallon WM, Kurland LT. A reappraisal of the epidemiology of multiple sclerosis in Olmsted County, Minnesota. *Neurology*. 1990;40(5):780–786.

30. Lilienfeld DE, Sprafka JM, Pham DL, Baxter J. Parkinson's's and motoneuron disease morbidity in the Twin Cities metropolitan area: 1979–1984. *Neuroepidemiology*. 1991;10(3):112–116.

31. McGuire V, Longstreth WT Jr, Koepsell TD, van Belle G. Incidence of amyotrophic lateral sclerosis in three counties in western Washington state. *Neurology*. 1996;47(2):571–573.

32. Golbe LI, Davis PH, Schoenberg BS, Duvoisin RC. Prevalence and natural history of progressive supranuclear palsy. *Neurology*. 1988;38(7):1031–1034.

33. Bower JH, Maraganore DM, McDonnell SK, Rocca WA. Incidence of progressive supranuclear palsy and multiple systems atrophy in Olmsted County, Minnesota, 1976 to 1990. *Neurology*. 1997;49(5):1284–1288.

34. Kokmen E, Ozekmekci FS, Beard CM, O'Brien PC, Kurland LT. Incidence and prevalence of Huntington's disease in Olmsted County, Minnesota (1950 through 1989). *Arch Neurol*. 1994;51(7):696–698.

35. Daniels SK, McAdam CP, Brailey K, Foundas AL. Clinical assessment of swallowing and prediction of dysphagia. *Am J Speech-Lang Pathol*. 1997;6:17–24.

36. DePippo KL, Holas MA, Reding MJ. Respiration and relative risk of medical complications following stroke. *Arch Neurol*. 1994;51(10):1051–1053.

37. Bushmann M, Dobmeyer SM, Leeker L, Perlmutter JS. Swallowing abnormalities and their response to treatment in Parkinson's's disease. *Neurology*. 1989;39(10):1309–1314.

38. Fuh JL, Lee RC, Wang SJ, et al. Swallowing difficulty in Parkinson's's disease. *Clin Neurol Neurosurg*. 1997;99(2):106–112.

39. Horner J, Alberts MJ, Dawson DV, Cook GM. Swallowing in Alzheimer's disease. *Alzheimer Dis Assoc Disord*. 1994;8(3):177–189.

40. Leighton SE, Burton MJ, Lund WS, Cochrane GM. Swallowing in motor neuron disease. *J Roy Soc Med*. 1994;87(12):801–805.

41. Litvan I, Sastry N, Sonies BC. Characterizing swallowing abnormalities in progressive supranuclear palsy. *Neurology*. 1997;48(6):1654–1662.

42. Kagel MC, Leopold NA. Dysphagia in Huntington's disease: a 16-year retrospective. *Dysphagia*. 1992;7(2):106–114.

43. Smith TL, Sun MM, Pippin J. Research and professional briefs: characterizing process control of fluid viscosities in nursing homes. *J Am Diet Assoc*. 2005:104(6):969–971.

44. Aviv JE, Murry T, Zschommler A, Cohen M, Gartner C. Flexible endoscopic evaluation of swallowing with sensory testing: patient characteristics and analysis of safety in 1340 consecutive examinations. *Ann Otol Rhinol Laryngol*. 2005;114(3):173–176.

45. Belafsky PC. Laryngopharyngeal reflux: the ENT perspective. *Gastroenterol Hepatol*. 2009;5(7):485–506.

46. Abadie V, Couly G. Congenital feeding and swallowing disorders. *Handb Clin Neurol*. 2013;113:1539–1549.

47. Cabral C, Chirica M, de Chaisemartin C, et al. Caustic injuries of the upper digestive tract: a population observational study. *Surg Endosc*. 2012;26(1):214–221.

48. Contini S, Scarpignato C. Caustic injury of the upper gastrointestinal tract: a comprehensive review. *World J Gastroenterol*. 2013;19(25):3918–3930.

49. Treats, T. Use of the ICF in dysphagia management. *Semin Speech Lang*. 2007;28:323–333.

Anatomy and Function of the Swallowing Mechanism

A Look at the Chapter

A thorough understanding of how dysphagia occurs and how it is treated requires an understanding of the anatomy of the swallowing organs. This chapter focuses on the aspects of the anatomy and physiology of the swallowing systems, but it is not intended to be a comprehensive study of head, neck, digestive, and respiratory anatomy and physiology. That is beyond the scope of a textbook for swallowing disorders. In this chapter, knowledge of anatomy and physiology with specific orientation to the swallowing organs is presented. This chapter also includes an understanding of the neurological correlates to normal and disordered swallowing. Video examples are included.

INTRODUCTION

Assessment and treatment of swallowing disorders require an understanding of the anatomy of the swallowing mechanisms and their function during the swallow. Although treatment of swallowing disorders includes many other aspects of care, such as quality of life and nutrition, knowing the mechanisms that allow one to swallow normally and why they may be swallowing abnormally is the basis for treating the disorders. This chapter provides a functional review of the structures involved in swallowing and their relationships during the act of swallowing.

Within each phase of swallowing, specific nerves carry out motor and sensory control. The result is a highly coordinated and interrelated series of events that pass the food or liquid to the stomach for digestion. In addition to this chapter, Ludlow provides an extensive review of the sensory and motor control mechanisms for voice, speech, and swallowing.[1] Table 2–1 outlines these components of the normal swallowing mechanism.[2] The key afferent and efferent neural responsibilities for each of the swallowing mechanisms are shown in Table 2–2.

TABLE 2–1. Functional Components of the Normal Swallowing Mechanism[a]

A. Oral Cavity—Responsible for bolus containment and preparation
1. Containment
a. Lips: closure after bolus intake
b. Cheeks: adequate tension to assist in lip closure
2. Bolus Preparation
a. Teeth: mastication
b. Tongue: driving force to initially propel the bolus
c. Gingival and buccal gutters: channel the bolus
d. Soft palate: contact with tongue
B. Oropharynx
1. Oropharyngeal Propulsion Pump
a. Soft palate
b. Lateral pharyngeal walls
c. Base of tongue
2. Velopharyngeal Function
a. Soft palate: elevates as tongue propels
b. Tongue elevation: necessary for propulsion
C. Hypopharynx
1. Muscular Propulsion
a. Pharyngeal constrictors
b. Piriform sinuses
c. Cricopharyngeal function
2. Larynx
a. Closure: glottis, ventricular folds, epiglottis
b. Pharyngeal squeeze
c. Hyoid elevation
D. Esophagus
1. Upper Esophageal Sphincter Opening
2. Primary Peristaltic Wave
3. Secondary Peristaltic Wave

[a]Adapted from Murry and Carrau.[2(p20)]

ANATOMY OF THE SWALLOWING MECHANISM

The anatomy of the swallowing mechanism can generally be divided into 4 major divisions: (1) oral, (2) pharyngeal, (3) laryngeal, and (4) esophageal.

TABLE 2–2. Contributions of Cranial Nerves to the Oral and Pharyngeal Phases of Deglutition[a]

Structure	Afferent	Efferent
Lips	V2 (maxillary), V3 (lingual)	VII
Tongue	V3 (lingual)	XII
Mandible	V3 (mandibular)	V (muscles of mastication), VII
Palate	V, IX, X	IX, X
Buccal region/cheeks		V (muscles of mastication), VII
Tongue base	IX	XII
Epiglottis (lingual surface)	IX	X
Epiglottis (laryngeal surface)	X (internal branch of superior laryngeal nerve)	X
Larynx (to level of true vocal folds)	X (internal branch of superior laryngeal nerve)	X
Larynx (below true vocal folds)	X (recurrent laryngeal nerve)	X
Pharynx (naso- and oro-)	IX	X (except for stylopharyngeus, which is innervated by IX)
Pharynx (hypo-)	X (internal branch of superior laryngeal nerve)	X

[a]Adapted with permission from Aviv.[3]

Within each of those divisions, specific actions take place to hold the food in the mouth, chew the food, and then pass it through the oropharynx to the esophagus where it enters the stomach. It would be a mistake to ignore any of these areas individually before describing how they interact because each may directly or indirectly lead to swallowing problems and aspiration of foods or liquids.

Oral Cavity

The oral cavity is responsible for gathering foods and liquids and preparing them for transit. The important aspects include chewing the food, mixing it with saliva, and then advancing the bolus to the posterior oral cavity. As food enters the oral cavity, the buccinators and orbicularis oris muscles help to seal the lips and keep the food on the tongue. Posteriorly, the soft palate lowers and creates a seal to prevent early leaking or spillage into the oro-

pharynx, an important part of maintaining airway protection.[4]

The tongue takes over quickly once food is in the oral cavity. The tongue is made up of intrinsic muscles and extrinsic muscles that do this work. Specific motions are activated to coordinate tongue motion. Loss or injury to one or more of the muscles will cause swallowing to be disrupted.[5] For example, if there is damage to the hypoglossal nerve on one side, the tongue is likely to direct the bolus from the strong side to the weak side. Food can pocket in the cheek. Hypoglossal damage can be seen with tongue deviation during protrusion.

Both gender and age likely influence the speed and accuracy of swallowing. Inamoto et al found that gender, height, and age each had effects on swallowing.[6] They found that the volumes of the larynx and hypopharynx were significantly greater in men than women. Especially with age, they found that the volumes of these cavities decreased. They also found smaller space in the piriform sinuses in the aging adult for both genders as both men and women aged. The volumes in these cavities should be considered when adjusting for bolus size and texture during swallowing assessments and treatments. The oral portion of the tongue is innervated by the hypoglossal nerve (CN XII). This portion of the tongue remains under voluntary control of the central nervous system. The base of the tongue sometimes thought of as the back of the tongue is controlled by the vagus nerve (CN X) primarily through the glossopharyngeal muscle.

The sensory nervous system of the tongue plays a role in swallowing. Taste receptors are found on the oral portion of the tongue and at the base of the tongue. Five basic taste sensations exist: sweet, sour, salty, bitter, and identified more recently, "zest."[7]

The tongue directs the bolus and provides the driving force for swallowing. This driving force can be measured by a number of strategies, such as the Iowa Oral Performance Instrument (IOPI). The tongue is highly mobile and rests on a sling of muscles attached to the mandible, maxilla, and tongue base.[8] Because of its mobility, it can control and move food rapidly when there are no injuries to the muscles or nerves of the tongue.

The tongue requires moisture to aid in the grinding and chewing processes. Natural saliva provides that moisture. Six paired major exocrine glands, parotid, submandibular, and sublingual, secrete saliva and open via ducts into the oral cavity. As many as 300 minor salivary glands also provide discharge of saliva fluids into the oral cavity. Normal salivary flow requires good hydration (water) to maintain ideal function of the tongue.

Pharynx

The pharynx begins at the posterior portion of the oral and nasal cavities and extends to the esophagus. As shown in Figure 2–1, it lies behind the larynx and trachea and provides direct passage to the stomach. The normal pharynx consists of a series of constrictor muscles that sequentially drive the food inferiorly to the stomach. Of significance is the cricopharyngeus muscle located at the base of the pharyngeal constrictors. This muscle maintains contraction during respiration but relaxes during swallowing to allow the larynx to elevate and the food to pass into the esophagus. Scarring, fibrosis, or nerve injury can lead to cricopharyngeal dysfunction that may result in aspiration despite normal oral and laryngeal function.

Larynx

The larynx is often thought to be the main organ of swallowing. However, while it is an important organ, it works in conjunction with the oral and pharyngeal phases of swallowing. Indeed, the larynx functions as an organ of respiration, phonation, and deglutition. Adjunctively, it aids in lifting and defecation by closing tightly and building pressure to help in those 2 activities.

The larynx shares the swallowing passageway for both airway and deglutitive functions; thus, it requires specific anatomic and physiologic adaptation for each function. In the normal individual, the larynx helps to regulate the passage of either air to or from the lungs or food and liquid into the esophagus. For swallowing, the larynx elevates and moves anteriorly. This movement can be impaired as a result of radiation, surgery, or central nervous system damage as in a cerebrovascular accident (CVA). Placing one finger over the thyroid prominence allows one to grossly feel this elevation during a dry swallow. Without this movement, foods and especially liquids are likely to enter the trachea leading to aspiration. Without a strong cough to clear the foods, continued entry of liquids or foods into the airway may lead to aspiration pneumonia.

Esophagus

The esophagus is a tube that connects the pharynx to the stomach. It begins at the base of the cricopharyngeus muscle and enters the stomach through the diaphragm muscle. The esophagus serves as a conduit to pass food through the thoracic cavity into the abdominal cavity for digestion and absorption. In describing the function of the esophagus, Pope

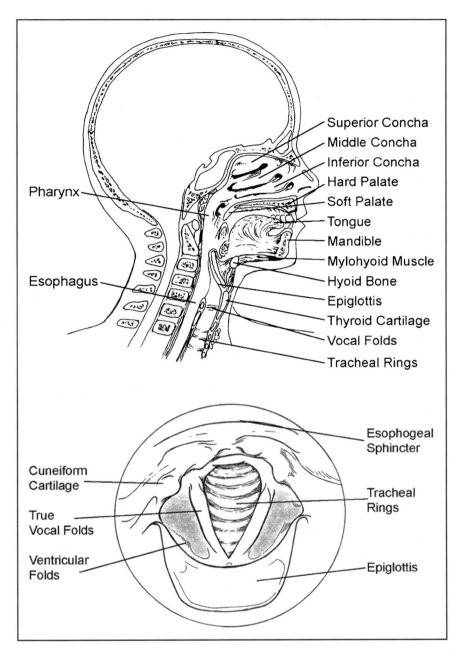

FIGURE 2–1. An overview of the nasopharynx, oropharynx, and laryngopharynx and the region of the vocal folds. Reproduced with permission from Sapienza and Hoffman Ruddy.[9]

reported on the description and function of the esophagus describing a series of peristaltic waves following the relaxation of the cricopharyngeus muscle.[10] A wide variety of disease processes may affect the muscles of the esophagus, with scleroderma representing the most common.

THE NORMAL SWALLOW

Traditionally, the normal swallow has been described as a series of 4 phases that relate to the passage of the **bolus** through specific anatomic structures. These phases are the oral preparatory, oral, pharyngeal, and esophageal. See Videos 1–1 and 1–2 for examples of normal swallowing.

> *The phases of swallowing were generally thought to occur sequentially; however, studies have shown that the oral and pharyngeal phases are interdependent.*[11]

Martin-Harris and colleagues originally presented evidence obtained from measuring the onset of the swallow and specific respiratory timing patterns associated with swallowing.[12] Using confirmatory factor analysis, they concluded that there is an overlap between the start of the oral and pharyngeal phases of swallowing. They identified 4 distinct patterns of breathing and swallowing that relate to age. They also identified 4 functional units of swallowing that overlap. They found that the onset of laryngeal closure and onset of hyoid excursion were strongly related and formed the first functional unit in the swallow. Also noted was that these events always occurred prior to the opening of the pharyngoesophageal segment. For most of their subjects, however, the hyoid returned to its rest position after breathing resumed. Thus, the interrelationships between breathing and swallowing demonstrated an overlap at the onset and offset of the swallow task.[13] The video examples from Chapter 1 (Videos 1–1 and 1–2) show the interrelated actions of swallowing in normal subjects.

In order to understand bolus preparation and bolus transit, the phases of swallowing will be described sequentially. Nonetheless, the reader should remember that theses phases overlap and normal swallowing involves the integration of phases. Moreover, it is also important to understand the interaction between the organs of swallowing and respiration function prior to, during, and after swallowing. These temporal relationships may affect bolus transit, retention and/or penetration, and aspiration.

Oral Phase

The oral phase of swallowing involves mastication and bolus transfer. These 2 functions usually operate sequentially; as mastication is completed, the bolus is then transferred. For the swallow to be normal, the anatomical structures of the upper aerodigestive system must be intact, and their function in sequence with each other must be appropriately timed. This requires the integrity of both the motor and sensory nervous systems. The 2 parts of the oral phase, mastication and bolus transfer, are reviewed separately in order to better understand both.

Mastication

The oral preparatory function involves mastication and bolus formation. The lips are essential for retaining the food in the oral cavity and for directing the food back to the tongue and teeth for bolus mastication and transfer. The movements of the tongue, mandible, dentition, soft palate, and muscles of the buccal cavity are temporally integrated to grind and position the food.

During the mastication and bolus preparation segment, the tongue arranges the bolus in a way that allows it to be moved to a location and position where it can be chewed. In the normal swallow, this usually results in the food being placed in the region of the molar teeth. At this point, the food is reduced through mastication, mixed with saliva, and forms the bolus that eventually will be swallowed.

At this time, factors such as taste, temperature, and the viscosity and size of bolus are sensed, and appropriate lip, tongue, buccal, and dental manipulations are carried out to finally prepare the bolus.

The trigeminal nerve (cranial nerve [CN] V), through its second and third divisions, provides sensory and motor innervations, respectively, to the muscles of mastication. Sensory information related to taste is mediated by CN VII (anterior two-thirds of the tongue) and CN IX (posterior one-third of the tongue).

Bolus Transfer

The food bolus is transported via the action of the tongue and its interaction with the palate, tongue, teeth, and cheeks. The oral segment is primarily a delivery system. Contact of the back of the tongue with the soft palate retains the bolus in the oral cavity, preventing early spillage into the pharynx. Once the bolus is prepared, it is positioned posteriorly on the tongue. The velum then elevates as the lips and buccal muscles contract to build pressure and reduce the volume of the oral cavity. The posterior tongue is depressed, and the anterior and middle portions of the tongue differentially elevate and begin the propulsion of the bolus to the oropharynx.

It should be emphasized that the tongue is the primary manipulator of food during the oral phase. Any injury or surgical treatment to the tongue will affect the oral phase of swallowing. Injury to the lips may complicate the problems in the oral phase. If lip closure and the maintenance of lip pressure are inadequate, the oral phase of swallowing will be affected due to lack of bolus containment. If normal bolus transit does not occur due to either a lack of lip closure or a lack of pressure buildup, there is a high probability that materials will be found in the cricopharyngeus area after the swallow is completed. When the food is properly masticated and formed into a bolus, the entire bolus is propelled into the oropharynx by the action of the tongue and the pressure buildup supported by adequate lip seal. This leads to the next stage of swallowing.

It is clear that with damage to the cranial nerves involved in swallowing, the oral phase of swallowing becomes abnormal, which may lead to further abnormalities as the bolus reaches or fails to reach the next phase in a coordinated manner. In the oral phase of swallowing, results from functional magnetic resonance imaging (fMRI) studies have revealed that the primary motor and sensory areas of the brain, as well as the anterior cingulate cortex and insular cortex, are active in healthy adults.[10]

Pharyngeal Phase

The pharyngeal phase of swallowing begins when the bolus reaches the level of the anterior tonsillar pillars. Normal function of the pharyngeal phase is dependent on the consistency of the bolus, the size of the bolus, and whether swallowing is a single or continuous event. A small well-organized bolus may pass the anterior faucial arches rapidly, whereas a poorly organized bolus will extend from the oral cavity into the oropharynx, requiring continuous interaction of the pharyngeal mechanisms.

The pharyngeal phase of swallowing is independent of both the oral and esophageal phases of swallowing. It can be stimulated to function externally in humans and certain animals.

The pharyngeal phase of swallowing involves the complex interaction of the tongue, velopharynx, and larynx. As the tongue elevates, velopharyngeal closure begins. This activity triggers the forward motion of the laryngeal structures to increase the opening of the upper esophageal sphincter. The larynx also elevates, all of which leads to relaxation of the cricopharyngeus musculature. When these actions occur with appropriate temporal integration, the bolus moves through the pharyngeal segment without penetration/aspiration into the airway. This activity is considered to be involuntary. An endoscopic view of the hypopharynx with residual bolus remaining is shown in Figure 2–2. The material in the cricopharyngeus indicates that a portion of the bolus did not pass into the esophagus.

Table 2–3, adapted from Simonian and Goldberg[14] summarizes the signs and possible causes of dysphagia and its treatment according to the phases of swallowing. More detailed descriptions of the treatment options are offered in Chapters 7 and 10.

Esophageal Phase

The **esophageal body** is a muscular tube extending 20 to 25 cm in length from its origin just caudal to the cricopharyngeus muscle to its termination at the gastric cardia. The esophagus shortens by about 10% through longitudinal muscle contractions during swallowing. Although the primary function of the esophageal body is passage of injected materials

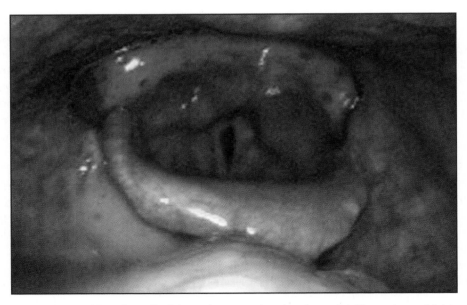

FIGURE 2–2. View from flexible endoscope showing the epiglottis and vocal folds shortly after the bolus has passed into the upper esophagus. *Note.* There is no food in the airway although some remains in the valleculae.

from the pharynx to the stomach, recent studies indicate that the esophagus is not merely a hollow, passive conduit for food transport. Rather, it has several active functions for acid control and mucosal protection.

Peristalsis, or sequential contraction of the esophagus and relaxation of the lower esophageal sphincter, characterizes the esophageal phase of swallowing. The bolus is propelled through the esophagus by contraction above and relaxation below the bolus. This relaxation is referred to as **descending inhibition**.

Primary peristalsis occurs when a swallow induces peristaltic activity, whereas **secondary peristalsis** refers to the initiation of a propagated contraction wave in the absence of a swallow. Initiation of secondary peristaltic contractions is involuntary and normally is not sensed. Ultimately, in a normal swallow, the bolus passes from the proximal to the distal esophagus and into the stomach.

Phase Relationships

It is clear from previous research[11,12] that the phases of swallowing involve a type of parallel processing from the cortex to the peripheral nervous system.

Problems during any one phase of swallowing may lead to problems during other phases. As will be pointed out in the remainder of this chapter, central nervous system structures control the motor sequencing of the transfer of the bolus from the lips to the stomach. However, these central processes require the coordination of the peripheral nervous system to carry out the functional passage of the bolus to the stomach. The phase relationships in swallowing are somewhat variable, affected by the type, size, and consistency of the bolus. Video 2–1 presents a patient with difficulty initiating the proper sequence and thus results in significant pooling of the bolus. Similarly this is shown in a VFSS exam of a patient following CVA in Video 2–2.

Even in the normal individual, the order of events and especially the timing of those events may not be entirely consistent. Moreover, the timing of events may vary for an individual depending on the conditions under which he or she is swallowing (distraction, multiple swallows, rapid swallows, etc). Nonetheless, Martin-Harris and colleagues have suggested an approximate order for the events of the normal swallow to be initiated.[15,16] The course of these events and the variation in timing are variable, but they follow the pattern recently described by Rosenbek and Jones[17] and outlined in Table 2–4.

TABLE 2–3. Diagnosis of Dysphagia Showing Signs of Cranial Nerve Deficits and Treatment Options

Type	Signs	Possible Causes	Treatment Options
Oral Preparatory	Lip flaccidity Labial leakage	CN V	Place food
Oral	Buccal pocketing	Facial weakness Surgical revision	Oral motor exercises, present food to stronger side
	Labored mastication	Lack of dentition Poor cognition	Modify food texture
	Premature spill	Lingual weakness	Chin-tuck position Modify food texture
Pharyngeal	Delayed swallow initiation	Poor oral phase Vagus nerve dysfunction Prolonged intubation	Thermal stimulation Posterior tongue strengthening
	Decreased laryngeal elevation	Tracheotomy Nasogastric tube Suprahyoid muscle	Tracheotomy cuff deflation, d/c NGT Edema
	Multiple swallow pattern	Decreased pharyngeal peristalsis/contraction	Alternate liquid and solid swallows
	Cough/throat clear immediately after the swallow	Aspiration secondary to decreased epiglottic deflection Poor oral phase Tracheoesophageal fistula (rare)	Supraglottic swallow Modify food texture
	Delayed cough, throat clear	Aspiration after the swallow secondary to pooling in the pharynx	Utilize dry swallow, alternating liquid and more solid swallows
	Change in vocal quality	Penetration to the level of the vocal cords Vocal cord weakness	NPL Modify food texture
Esophageal	Significantly delayed aspiration	Reflux, stricture	Medication Modify foods GI referral

[a]Adapted and revised with permission from Simonian and Goldberg.[14(p367)]

CRANIAL NERVES INVOLVED IN SWALLOWING

Vagus Nerve (CN X)

The vagus nerve provides motor and sensory innervation to the palate, pharynx, esophagus, stomach, and respiratory tract and is intimately involved in the regulation of blood pressure. Central contributions include motor innervation from the nucleus ambiguus and sensory innervation from the nucleus solitarius.

Recurrent Laryngeal Nerve (RLN)

This nerve innervates all of the muscles of the larynx, except the cricothyroid. It is responsible for glottic closure during swallowing.

TABLE 2–4. Events in a Normal Swallow Are Initiated in Approximately This Order[a]

Apnea onset
Oral bolus transport
Hyoid excursion
Laryngeal closure
Maximum laryngeal closure
PES opening
Maximum hyoid excursion
Laryngeal opening
Swallowing inspiration
Apnea onset
Last PES opening
Hyoid return

Abbreviation: PES, pharyngoesophageal segment.

[a]Reprinted with permission from Rosenbek and Jones.[17]

Superior Laryngeal Nerve (SLN)

The SLN bifurcates into 2 major divisions: an internal and an external division. The external division innervates the cricothyroid muscle, which retracts the posterior cricoid facet from the thyroid lamina, tensing the vocal fold and thus lengthening the anterior-to-posterior dimension of the glottis and changing the vocal pitch.

The internal branch of the SLN provides mucosal touch and proprioceptive sensory input from the supraglottic larynx, cricoarytenoid joints, posterior aspect of the larynx, and the pharyngeal mucosa in the piriform sinuses. Loss of sensation due to damage to the SLN results in anesthesia of the supraglottis and piriform sinuses, which leads to aspiration.

Despite secretions into the trachea, patients do not cough when the SLN is not functional. Jafari et al[18] found evidence that damage to the SLN alone without additional lesions in the brain or airway obstructions or diseases can result in aspiration. They suggested that following various conservative laryngeal surgeries, SLN injury was a main factor in dysphagia and aspiration.

Trigeminal Nerve (CN V)

The third division of the trigeminal nerve supplies sensory innervation to the tongue (lingual nerve) and to the inferior alveolus, buccal mucosa, and the lower lip (inferior alveolar nerve). Although sensation of the base of the tongue is supplied through CN IX (glossopharyngeal nerve), innervation of the oral tongue is conferred via the lingual nerve. The trigeminal nerve also supplies motor innervation to the mastication muscles, including those with mandibular and maxillary insertions.

Glossopharyngeal Nerve (CN IX)

This nerve provides sensory innervation to the oropharynx and the base of the tongue and supports taste fibers at the base of tongue. Its motor innervation is to the stylopharyngeus muscle.

Hypoglossal nerve (CN XII) controls critical movements of the tongue. Since the tongue is the primary mover of the bolus while in the mouth, these movements contribute significantly to the overall swallowing process. Problems with the hypoglossal nerve lead to the inability to move the bolus in place for chewing and for transmitting the bolus to the oropharynx. If there is damage to CN XII, the tongue may be weak or paralyzed. Speech becomes disrupted. If paralysis is present, the tongue deviates to the paralyzed side. Eventually, the tongue will begin to atrophy or shrink if the hypoglossal nerve is paralyzed, causing further problems with the bolus while in the oral cavity and making speech almost unintelligible. When CN XII is damaged because of strokes, infections, or tumors, it can become weak or paralyzed which can in turn lead to problems with communication, chewing, or swallowing.

SPHINCTERS

Swallowing can be visualized as the passage of the bolus through a series of dynamic chambers. These chambers are separated by sphincters (gates) that help to prevent spillage of the material before it enters the next chamber.

Sphincters maintain a watertight closure that aids in building up the pressure in the particular chamber to facilitate the propulsion of the bolus into the next chamber. Damage to any of the sphincters may affect disruption of the normal swallow.

The specific sphincter actions of the upper aerodigestive tract involved in swallowing are discussed below. Sphincter relaxation in a normal swallow generally precedes the onset of pharyngeal transit (bolus entry into the pharynx) and the initiation of swallow. Manometric studies have proven useful in interpreting the actions of the upper esophageal sphincter in the act of swallowing.[19,20] During a swallow of more than 5 cc of fluid, failure to coordinate the onset of pharyngeal transit (entry of the bolus into the pharynx) with the onset of swallow gestures can result in nasal reflux, aspiration, or regurgitation. In other swallows, however, particularly those associated with mastication, the linguopalatal sphincter may open repeatedly to allow small amounts of the bolus into the oropharynx and valleculae long before swallow sequence is initiated. Opening of the linguopalatal sphincter usually coincides with the onset of pharyngeal transit (bolus entry into the pharynx) and the initiation of the swallow.

Velopharyngeal Sphincter

Failure to close the velopharyngeal sphincter results in leakage of the bolus or air into the nasopharynx and a diminished ability to generate appropriate oropharyngeal pressures to propel the bolus through the oropharynx. Data by Pauloski and colleagues[20] in a study of manometry and fluoroscopy showed that increased tongue base activity resulted in increased pressure on the bolus, resulting in a more efficient swallow that was characterized by shorter transit times and better bolus clearance.

Laryngeal Sphincter

Laryngeal closure occurs in a sequential fashion, with approximation of the true vocal folds (CN X) preceding false vocal folds approximation, and finally approximation of the arytenoids to the peti-

ole of the epiglottis. Failure to close the supraglottic and glottic sphincters during the swallow results in penetration and aspiration and in decreased ability to generate adequate hypopharyngeal pressures to propel the bolus through the pharyngoesophageal segment and into the esophagus.

Upper Esophageal Sphincter

The upper esophageal sphincter (UES) is a tonically contracted group of skeletal muscles separating the pharynx from the esophagus. The major component of the sphincter is the cricopharyngeus muscle. At rest, the sphincter is in a state of **tonic contraction** that minimizes the entrance of air into the gastrointestinal tract during respiration. Equally important is its function to prevent the entry of refluxed material from the esophagus into the pharynx.

The tonically contracted UES relaxes during the pharyngeal peristaltic sequence. The relaxation begins after the onset of swallowing and lasts 0.5 to 1 second. The onset of the pharyngeal peristaltic wave is marked by apposition of the soft palate to the pharyngeal wall, generating a contraction that lasts over 0.1 second and generates a pressure greater than 180 mm Hg. Pharyngeal peristalsis transverses the oropharynx and hypopharynx at about 15 cm/sec and reaches the UES in about 0.7 second. After the relaxation phase, the sphincter contracts with an increase in force, in which the pressure may exceed twice the pressure of the resting tone for approximately a second prior to returning to baseline.

Poor coordination of the pharyngoesophageal segment may occur due to neurological deficits such as recurrent laryngeal nerve paralysis or brainstem stroke. Inadequate elevation of the hyoid-laryngeal complex and/or weakness of the pharyngeal constrictors also affect the function of the pharyngoesophageal segment as a sphincter.

Lower Esophagus

The lower esophagus is a specialized segment of smooth tubular muscle extending 20 to 25 cm in length from its origin just caudal to the cricopharyngeus muscle to its termination at the gastric cardia. It relaxes to permit the bolus to enter the gastric cavity and contracts to prevent gastroesophageal reflux in its resting state. Gross and histological examinations of the lower esophageal sphincter have failed to identify a specific sphincteric structure. Compared to adjacent structures, the lower esophageal muscle also possesses an increased sensitivity to many excitatory agents, suggesting a greater influence on sphincter tone by nerves and hormones.

CENTRAL NEURAL CONTROL OF SWALLOWING

Normal deglutition, the act of swallowing, is initiated voluntarily. Central neural control of swallowing can be divided into cortical and subcortical components. **Neural control** is composed of a very complex interaction of afferent sensory neurons, motor neurons, and interneurons that control voluntary and involuntary/reflexive actions of swallowing.

Cortical regulation includes centers in both hemispheres of the brain with representation for the pharynx and the esophagus. These cortical areas have interhemispheric connections and projections to the motor nuclei of the brainstem. Bilateral hemispheric stimulation produces a greater response than unilateral impulses, and this response is intensity and frequency dependent. Both motor and premotor cortical areas are involved in the initiation of swallowing or at least have the potential to modulate the contraction of the pharyngeal and esophageal musculature. Input from these cortical areas to the pharynx, however, seems greater than input to the esophagus. Similarly, afferent impulses from the pharynx, largely from the superior laryngeal nerve and glossopharyngeal nerve, have greater effects on cortical areas than those from the upper esophagus via the recurrent laryngeal nerve.

The "swallowing center," identified as an area within the reticular system of the brainstem that comprises the nucleus ambiguus (cranial nerves IX, X, and XI) and the nucleus of the tractus solitarius (cranial nerves VII, IX, and X) interact with other nuclei of the cranial nerves (V, IX, X, and XII).

The collection of brainstem nuclei coordinates the swallow sequence, acting as **the central pattern generator**" (sequential or rhythmic activities that are initiated by neural elements without external feedback).

Cranial nerve deficits cause changes in function that range from minor to life threatening. Table 2–5 summarizes the findings of deficits to the cranial nerves.

TABLE 2–5. Clinical Results after Cranial Nerve Injury

Cranial Nerve	Clinical Result of Injury
V—Trigeminal nerve (motor)	Slight weakness in mastication
VII—Facial nerve	Slight weakness in bolus control, weak lip closure
IX—Glossopharyngeal nerve (sensory)	Failure to trigger the pharyngeal stage of the swallow, premature spill of material from the mouth into the airway
IX—Glossopharyngeal nerve (motor)	Deficit from loss of function not great secondary to intact function of other elevators of the larynx
X—Superior laryngeal nerve (sensory)	Loss of protective glottic closure and cough reflex protecting airway from material on the supraglottic larynx
X—Vagus nerve (motor)	Inadequate velopharyngeal closure, nasal regurgitation, Incomplete clearing of residue in the hypopharynx, pooling of material above the level of the vocal folds, aspiration once the vocal folds open Inadequate glottic closure during pharyngeal transit
XII—Hypoglossal nerve	Bolus control problems; crippled swallow if bilateral

Source: Adapted and modified with permission from Perlman A, Schulze-Delrieu K. *Deglution and Its Disorders.* San Diego, CA: Singular Publishing;1997:354.

Impulses from afferent fibers arising from pharyngeal receptors respond to touch, pressure, chemical stimuli, and water and provide the means to elicit the pharyngeal swallow. Miller has described this as "the most complex all-or-none reflex in the mammalian central nervous system."[21] Thus, sensory impulses from the pharynx serve to adjust the frequency and intensity of the contraction of the pharyngeal musculature and direct the protective reflexes of the laryngeal sphincter.

Similarly, at the cortical level, impulses from sensory receptors from the oral cavity provide the central nervous system with information regarding touch, pressure, texture, shape, temperature, chemicals, and taste. Automatic adjustments and voluntary movements are combined to prepare the bolus before swallowing.

RESPIRATION AND DEGLUTITION

The respiratory system and its neurological control exert a strong influence on swallowing. The vocal folds are expected to completely adduct during a normal swallow. At that time, respiration stops. This is known as swallowing **apnea**. The prevention of aspiration relies on the apneic event occurring at the proper time. The ability of the vocal folds to close and of the respiratory system to clear the airway with a strong cough when food or liquids fall below the vocal folds aids in prevention of aspiration.

The study of apnea events and respirometric activity during the act of swallowing offers additional clues to the understanding of aspiration. Normal deglutition causes an abrupt decrease in airflow, leading to a variable interval of apnea, the time of which is dependent on the size of the bolus and whether the swallow is spontaneous or cued. Normal swallowing is most often followed by a period of expiration,[13] but other patterns of respiration have been found. The course of normal swallowing generally follows a pattern as that described in Table 2-4.

Martin-Harris and colleagues have identified 4 basic apnea patterns in normal swallowing. They are described in Table 2–6. The EX/EX pattern was found to be the most common pattern in the healthy group studied during the 5-mL-cup drinking task.[13]

TABLE 2–6. Four Patterns of Respiration Coordination in Swallowing

1. EX/EX	Expiration, apnea event, expiration
2. IN/EX	Inspiration, apnea event, expiration
3. EX/IN	Expiration, apnea event, inspiration
4. IN/IN	Inspiration, apnea event, inspiration

Abbreviations: EX, exhalation; IN, inhalation.

It should be pointed out that when the 3 non-EX/EX patterns were combined, a significant age difference was found between the EX/EX and the non-EX/EX patterns. In addition, the authors noted that the duration of the apnea event varied with the age of the individuals. It appears that there is an apnea event for the normal swallow, but the event may vary depending on the state of the patient, the bolus, and the age of the patient. One would suspect that paramedian posturing of the vocal folds is a common characteristic of normal swallowing to aid in the apneic event. This has been shown to be true in the work of Tabaee et al who showed confirmed clear paramedian vocal fold closure during swallow using flexible nasendoscopy.[22]

Although earlier in this chapter the act of swallowing was described in phases in order to facilitate understanding of the anatomical structures that are involved in swallowing, there is sufficient evidence to suggest that the involuntary and voluntary phases of swallowing actually occur simultaneously rather than serially. Abnormal respiratory coordination of the laryngeal closure and apnea lead to disruption in swallowing, and this lack of coordination may play a significant role in swallow-induced aspiration. After each swallow, there is a respiratory cycle "reset"; that is, the swallow causes the normal respiratory pattern to restart with exhalation after each swallow.

The onset of the apneic event has also been studied by Perlman and colleagues.[23] Using respirometric data combined with videofluoroscopy, they demonstrated that respiratory events of swallowing were occurring simultaneously in the oral cavity, base of tongue, valleculae, piriform sinuses, upper esophageal sphincter, and esophagus using respirometric data combined with videofluoroscopy. Thus, respiratory flow begins to subside from the onset of activity ongoing in the oral cavity.

Kelly and colleagues[24] examined normal healthy subjects during sleep and wakefulness and found that although expiration is usually associated with volitional (awake) swallows, reflexive swallows (those during sleep) are more variable and occurred during the expiratory-inspiratory cusp more often than did volitional swallows. Onset of vocal fold adduction also preceded the initiation of peristalsis in the nasopharynx and its propagation to the oropharynx. Thus, it is apparent that abnormal coordination of the laryngeal motion with bolus transport will lead to disruption in swallowing, and this lack of coordination may play a significant role in swallow-induced aspiration.

Once the vocal folds are completely adducted, respiration stops. Thus, the study of respirometric activity during the act of swallowing offers additional clues to the understanding of aspiration. Normal deglutition causes an abrupt decrease in air. It appears that there is an apnea event for normal swallow but that event may vary on the state of the patient, the bolus type and size, and the age of the patient.[25]

Earlier, Shaker and colleagues[26] demonstrated that vocal fold adduction occurs prior to the onset of hyoid bone movement, base of tongue movement, and submental surface myoelectric activity. Onset of vocal fold adduction also preceded the initiation of peristalsis in the nasopharynx and its propagation to the oropharynx. They concluded that it is apparent respiratory adjustments are an ongoing activity of each swallowing event.

SUMMARY

Both the cortical and subcortical pathways are important to the initiation and completion of swallowing. Oral musculature is represented symmetrically between the 2 hemispheres; laryngeal and esophageal muscles are asymmetrically represented. Most individuals, however, have a dominant swallow hemisphere.

A thorough knowledge of the anatomical structures and physiological functions of the structures involved in swallowing is necessary to understand the complexity of swallowing. The physiology of swallowing includes the interaction of sensory and motor functions and the interaction of the voluntary and involuntary aspects of swallowing. Traditionally, it was thought that swallowing occurred in sequential phases, beginning with chewing. Involuntary phases of swallowing are the responsibility of the brainstem. The studies by Miller,[21] Martin-Harris,[13] and Perlman[23] provide evidence of the interaction between the involuntary and voluntary aspects of swallowing. Nonetheless, the interaction between these aspects is not yet fully understood. In addition, recent evidence suggests that the oral and oropharyngeal phases are interdependent. Moreover, evidence from sensory testing obtained from studies of the superior laryngeal nerve suggests that the role of sensation obtained from studies of the superior laryngeal nerve may be more important than originally considered. In future chapters, the role of sensory testing as an integral part of the swallowing evaluation will be presented.

DISCUSSION QUESTIONS

1. What additional information of the oropharyngeal swallow does fMRI provide?
2. What is the importance of parallel processing of swallowing compared to the traditional phases of swallowing?

STUDY QUESTIONS

1. The primary afferent control of the tongue, lips, and mandible is via cranial nerve
   A. VII
   B. X
   C. V
   D. XI

2. The oral phase of swallowing liquid varies with
   Age   **T F**
   Type of bolus   **T F**
   Quality of dentition   **T F**
   Discuss why each answer is true or false.

3. Sensory and motor integration of the phases of swallowing suggest that
   A. Each phase of the swallow must be completed before the next one begins
   B. It is impossible to determine when one phase of swallow ends and the next begins
   C. Voluntary and involuntary aspects of swallowing may occur in parallel
   D. Unless the voluntary oral phase of swallowing is completed, the involuntary phases cannot begin

4. The involuntary phases of swallowing are regulated
   A. By unilateral cortical representation
   B. By unilateral brainstem representation
   C. By bilateral brainstem representation
   D. By sensory and motor branches of cranial nerve X

REFERENCES

1. Ludlow CL. Recent advances in laryngeal sensorimotor control for voice, speech and swallowing. *Curr Opin Otolaryngol Head Neck Surg.* 2004;12:160–165.
2. Murry T, Carrau RL. *Clinical Management of Swallowing Disorders.* San Diego, CA: Plural Publishing; 2006.
3. Aviv J. The normal swallow. In: Carrau RL, Murry T, eds., *Comprehensive Management of Swallowing Disorders.* San Diego, CA: Plural Publishing; 2006; Tables 3–1 and 3–2.
4. Dodds, W. The physiology of swallowing. *Dysphagia,* 1989;3(4):171–178.
5. Furuta M, Komiya-Nonaka M, Akifusa S, et al. Interrelationship of oral health status, swallowing function, nutritional status, and cognitive ability with activities of daily living in Japanese elderly people receiving home care services due to physical disabilities. *Community Dent Oral Epidemiol.* 2013;41(2):173–181.
6. Inamoto Y, Saitoh E, Okada S, et al. Anatomy of the larynx and pharynx: effects of age, gender and height revealed by multidetector computed tomography. *J Oral Rehab.* 2015: 1–8 doi:10:1111/joor.12298.
7. Eibling D. Anatomy and physiology of swallowing. In: Carrau R, Murry T, Howell R, eds. *Comprehensive Management of Swallowing.* 2nd ed. San Diego, CA: Plural Publishing; 2015; 2:11–27.
8. Adams VI, Mathisen B, Baines S, Lazarus C, Callister R. A systematic review and meta-analysis of measurements of tongue and hand strength and endurance using the Iowa Oral Performance Instrument (IOPI). *Dysphagia.* 2013 Sep;28(3):350–369.
9. Sapienza C, Hoffman Ruddy B. *Voice Disorders.* 2nd ed. San Diego, CA: Plural Publishing; 2013.p.32
10. Pope CE. The esophagus for the non esophagologist. *Am J Med.* 1997;103:19s–22s.
11. Martin-Harris B, Michel Y, Castell DO. *Physiologic model of oropharyngeal swallowing revisited.* Paper presented at: AAO-HNS Annual Meeting; September 20, 2004; New York, NY.
12. Martin-Harris B, Brodsky MB, Michel Y, et al. MBS Measurement Tool for Swallow Impairment—MBSImp: establishing a standard. *Dysphagia.* 2008;23:392–405.
13. Martin-Harris B, Brodsky MB, Michel Y, Ford CL, Walters B, Heffner J. Breathing and swallowing dynamics across the adult lifespan. *Arch Otolaryngol Head Neck Surg.* 2005;131(9):762–770.
14. Simonian MA, Goldberg AN. Swallowing disorders in the critical care patient. In: Carrau RL, Murry T, eds. *Comprehensive Management of Swallowing Disorders.* San Diego, CA: Singular Publishing; 1999:367–368.
15. Martin-Harris B. Temporal coordination of pharyngeal and laryngeal dynamics with breathing during swallowing: single liquid swallows. *J Appl Physiol.* 2003;94:1735–1743.
16. Martin-Harris B, Michel Y, Castell DO. Physiologic model of oropharyngeal swallowing revisited. *Otolaryngol Head Neck Surg.* 2005;133:234–240.
17. Rosenbek JC, Jones H. *Dysphagia in Movement Disorders.* San Diego, CA: Plural Publishing; 2009:12.
18. Jafari S, Prince RA, Kim Dy. Paydarfar D. Sensory regulation of swallowing and airway protection: a role for the internal superior laryngeal nerve in humans. *J Physiol.* 2003;550:287–304.
19. Hila A, Castell JA, Castell DO. Pharyngeal and upper esophageal sphincter manometry in the evaluation of dysphagia. *J Clin Gastroenterol.* 2001;33:355–361.
20. Pauloski BR, Rademaker AW, Lazarus C, Boeckxstaens G, Kahrilas PJ, Logemann JA. Relationship between manometric and videofluoroscopic measures of swallow function in healthy adults and patients treated for head and neck cancer with various modalities. *Dysphagia.* 2009 Jun;24(2):196–203.
21. Miller AJ. *The Neuroscientific Principles of Swallowing and Dysphagia.* San Diego, CA: Singular Publishing; 1998.
22. Tabaee A, Johnson PE, Gartner CJ, Kalwerisky K, Desloge RB, Stewart MG. Patient-controlled comparison of flexible endoscopic evaluation of swallowing with sensory testing (FEESST) and videofluoroscopy. *Laryngoscope.* 2006 May;116(5):821–825.
23. Perlman AL, Ettema SL, Barkmeier J. Respiratory and acoustic signals associated with bolus passage during swallowing. *Dysphagia.* 2000;15(2):89–94.
24. Kelly BN, Huckabee ML, Cooke N. The coordination of respiration and swallowing for volitional and reflexive swallows: a pilot study. *J Med Speech-Lang Path.* 2006;14(2):67–77.

25. Diaz Gross R, Atwood CW, Ross SB, Olszewski JW, Eichhorn KA. The coordination of breathing and swallowing in chronic obstructive pulmonary disease. *Am J Respir Care*. 2009;179:559–565.

26. Shaker R, Dodds WJ, Dantas RO, et al. Coordination of deglutitive closure with oropharyngeal swallowing. *Gastroenterology*. 1990;98:1478–1484.

Chapter 3

Swallowing Disorders Arising From Neurological Disorders and Other Diseases

"Let food be thy medicine and medicine be thy food."

—Hippocrates

CHAPTER OUTLINE

A Look at the Chapter

Dysphagia can occur for many reasons. It may be the result of a sickness such as pneumonia or due to injury from burns, intubation, or other surgery such as anterior cervical spine surgery. Dysphagia may also be the result of damage to the neurological system such as a stroke or to the neuromuscular system such as Parkinson's disease or one of the many types of muscle dystrophy. In this chapter, the causes leading to dysphagia are described. Students should keep in mind that diseases and injuries to the swallowing organs and nerves may be mild and resolve over time, or they may be severe and increase in severity over time. The speech-language pathologist may be the primary provider of services to the patient and must be aware of the changes that take place as a result of changes that occur due to the underlying disease or simply due to factors that occur with aging.

INTRODUCTION

The act of swallowing is a complex activity that requires the interaction of sensory and motor mechanisms. A swallowing problem occurs when there is a weakness or loss of neural control or traumatic damage to the structures involved in any part of the swallowing process. Beginning with weakness in the tongue or cheek muscles through any part of the anatomy down to and including the stomach, disruption along this aerodigestive channel will cause swallowing to be abnormal. Conditions or diseases such as a stroke or Parkinson's disease or other nervous system disorders reduce the safety of swallowing and may lead to mortality. Diseases such as cancer resulting in the surgical removal of organs or nerves or requiring radiation or chemotherapy to treat the disease may also cause dysphagia. Although the true incidence of all swallowing problems is unknown since they often occur in the context of other diseases, it has been estimated that at least 35% of patients over the age of 75 have an associated swallowing problem related to injury or damage to one or more of the organs of swallowing, muscle atrophy, cognitive decline, or other disorders and diseases. This includes all patients treated for head or neck cancer. They will be expected to have a temporary or permanent swallowing disorder. The true incidence may be substantially higher in the elderly since many feel that changes in what or how they swallow is simply age related.[1,2] Virtually all patients in advanced stages of Parkinson's disease experience swallowing problems and aspiration pneumonia. Wang reported that swallowing disorders are the primary cause of death in patients with Parkinson's disease.[3]

In the previous chapter, the normal swallow was described as three interactive events, **bolus preparation**, **airway protection**, and **bolus propulsion**. Neural impulses from cortical and subcortical pathways integrate motor and sensory data to the muscles of the oral cavity and the pharyngeal and laryngeal structures. The facial, glossopharyngeal, and vagus nerves provide the primary messaging system to the muscles of the oral, pharyngeal, and esophageal regions of the body.

> *A safe, normal swallow entails the timely interaction of the muscles of mastication, which are innervated by the trigeminal nerve, and the pharyngeal and laryngeal muscles, which are controlled by the efferent and afferent fibers of the glossopharyngeal and vagus nerves, respectively.*

Additional muscular innervation of the strap muscles of the swallowing mechanism by the ansa hypoglossis and ansa cervicalis aids in the complex motion of swallowing. A more detailed description of the muscular actions and neuromuscular control of these actions can be found in Ludlow.[4,5]

Damage to any of the nerves involved in swallowing or to the corresponding areas of the central nervous system (brainstem, medulla, and cortex) has a deleterious effect on normal swallowing. Thus, swallowing involves an intact nervous system, which drives the biomechanical events of the swallow.

Many conditions can disrupt the neuromuscular actions of a normal swallow at any point along the pathway leading to the stomach. In addition, conditions of the bolus in the stomach may affect the transit of the boluses that have not yet arrived in the stomach or that cause food to regurgitate back up from the stomach into the esophagus, or above.

Prior to reaching the stomach, the bolus must pass along a lumen that is shared with the respiratory/phonatory pathway. Each normal swallow involves the interruption of breathing (an apneic event) and the protection of the airway, and then the return of respiration once the bolus is safely beyond the laryngeal inlet. Airway protection during normal swallowing is brought about by the 3-tier closure of the laryngeal sphincter. This is composed of the closure of the true vocal folds, including the arytenoids and the false vocal folds, the aryepiglottic folds, and the tilting of the epiglottis (ie, supraglottis). The superior and anterior motion of the larynx caused by the contraction of the suprahyoid muscles opens the posterior cricoid space and moves the larynx superiorly to a protected position beneath the base of the tongue. Following the swallow, normal subjects usually resume respiration activities with exhalation as we described in the previous chapter.[6] When airway protection is incomplete or delayed, penetration of the bolus and even aspiration of the bolus may occur. Kendall et al[7] have shown that in most subjects, the arytenoids/epiglottis approximation occurs before the bolus reaches the upper esophageal sphincter, but in some cases it may occur after; however, the delay is never greater than 0.1 second. They also noted no delay of the supraglottic closure in normal elderly patients. Previously, others have found that following radiation therapy to the head or neck regions, these delays may extend beyond normal times. Fibrosis and stenosis of the tongue, pharynx, and esophagus as well as pharyngeal constriction contribute to the delays in oral pharyngeal transit, leading to delays in closure of vocal folds, which may result in penetration and aspiration.[8,9] It is clear that any condition that results in failure of the glottic sphincter to close timely and appropriately may allow the entry of food or liquid into the airway.

Although the neuromuscular pathogenesis is beyond the scope of this book, we outline the common conditions as well as rare conditions associated with disordered swallowing in adults. In this chapter, we introduce the terms of penetration, aspiration, and aspiration pneumonia, as their understanding is important to the remainder of the chapters in this book.

Penetration

Penetration is defined as the entry of bolus contents into the larynx to a level that does not extend beyond the true vocal folds. Figure 3–1 shows an example of penetration obtained during transnasal flexible endoscopy. Note the material below the epiglottis and above the vocal folds. See Video 3–1.

Aspiration

Aspiration is the entry of material into the airway below the true vocal cords. Aspiration can occur before, during, or after the swallow. **Prandial aspiration** is the result of food or liquid entering the airway.

Table 3–1 summarizes and updates Mendelsohn's classic review of the nature of prandial aspiration.[10] Figure 3–2 shows a portion of a food bolus at the level of the vocal folds. In this patient, sensory loss to the vagus nerve is apparent, as the bolus remained on the vocal folds and the patient did not expel the bolus.

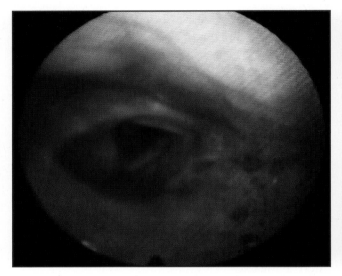

FIGURE 3–1. An example of penetration found during transnasal flexible endoscopy.

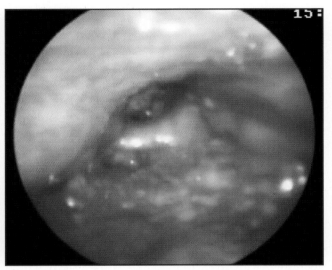

FIGURE 3–2. A portion of the bolus is shown at the vocal folds before the patient expels it.

TABLE 3–1. Classification of Prandial Aspiration[a]

Aspiration Before the Pharyngeal Stage
• Most common type in central neurological diseases
• Due to loss of bolus control during oral phase or to delayed pharyngeal swallow
• Conservative management: thicken the diet, neck flexion during deglutition, supraglottic swallow, effortful swallow, thermal stimulation
• Surgical management: horizontal epiglottoplasty, tongue base flaps, laryngeal suspension

Aspiration During the Pharyngeal Phase
• Least common type of aspiration
• Due to vocal palsy, paresis, or incoordination
• Conservative management: vocal adduction exercises, chin tuck, bolus modification
• Surgical management: augment the paralyzed vocal cord

Aspiration After the Pharyngeal Phase
• Due to inhalation of uncleared residue at the laryngeal inlet
• Conservative management: thinning the diet, alternating liquids, Mendelsohn maneuver, head rotation, reduce bolus size
• Surgical management: translaryngeal resection of the cricoid lamina, cricopharyngeal myotomy, laryngeal elevation
• Medical management: botulinum toxin injection to the superior pharyngeal constrictor muscle

[a]Adapted and expanded from Mendelsohn.[10(p9)]

Factors that influence the tolerance to aspiration include amount, frequency, and type of the aspirate, oral hygiene, pulmonary conditions, and the immune function of the host. These factors and their interaction with the neuromuscular system of the host are extremely variable. Thus, the definition of what constitutes "significant" aspiration should be individualized.

Pulmonary syndromes may be responsible for aspiration. Patients with compromised pulmonary problems that occur acutely or over a long period of time such as with cigarette smoking may lead to aspiration without other notable conditions. The most common pulmonary syndromes leading to aspiration pneumonia are shown in Table 3–2.[11]

Aspiration Pneumonia

Aspiration pneumonia is a condition resulting from the entrance of foreign materials, usually foods, liquids, or vomit, into the bronchi of the lungs with resultant infection. Aspiration syndromes occur in 3 ways based on pathophysiology. **Chemical pneumonitis** is a condition referring to chemical injury caused by inhalation of sterile gastric contents from the stomach or esophagus. **Bacterial infection** occurs as a result of an increased volume of oropharyngeal secretions coupled with impaired defense mechanisms. Oral, pharyngeal, or vocal fold weakness increase the risk of aspiration. These conditions are found in many patients following a recent stroke or in patients with paralysis to one or both vocal folds. **Acute airway obstruction** is the third path to aspiration pneumonia. The severity of aspiration depends on multiple factors that include the amount, nature, acidity of the aspirate, consistency, cough reflex, and host immune defense. Aspiration, shown in Video 3–2, occurred after multiple attempts to trigger the swallow due to inability to elevate the larynx.

Silent aspiration is defined as aspiration occurring without elicitation of a cough reflex. Liquid aspirates may disseminate into the lung fields by rapid inspiration or deep inspiration that allows spread to the peripheral alveoli of the lungs. Infil-

TABLE 3–2. Pulmonary Syndromes Related to Aspiration[a]

Acute respiratory distress syndrome (ARDS)	Interstitial and/or alveolar edema and hemorrhage, as well as perivascular lung edema. It may be caused by aspiration of acid refluxate.
Lipid (lipoid) pneumonia	Aspiration of oil-based liquids such as mineral oil given as a laxative, oil-based nasal sprays, or contrast material. In unconscious patients, especially those requiring mechanical ventilation, fever, hypoxia, and excessive tracheal secretions may suggest pneumonia. For patients requiring mechanical ventilation, placement in a semirecumbent position and active suction of the hypopharynx may reduce the risk of aspiration.
Aspiration pneumonia	Aspiration pneumonia is usually polybacterial and is associated with a high morbidity and mortality. It is usually found in dependent pulmonary lobes.
Chronic pneumonia	Some patients do not develop a radiographic consolidate that could be diagnosed as a pneumonia, but present with purulent, foul-smelling bronchorrhea, low-grade spiking fever, and varying degrees of respiratory compromise. A prominent bronchial pattern may be present in the chest radiogram.
Chronic obstructive pulmonary disease	A slowly progressive condition resulting from ongoing damage to the alveoli of the lungs either from cigarette smoking or exposure to inhaling hazardous materials such as those who work in coal or other underground mines.

[a]Modified from Krishna.[11]

tration of the posterior segments of upper and lower lobes, especially with patients in the supine position for long periods, increases the risk of aspiration simply due to gravity.

Bacterial infections that lead to aspiration pneumonia are either community acquired or hospital acquired. Community-acquired infections emanate from poor hand hygiene or other substandard hygiene preventions. Hospital-acquired aspiration pneumonia are potentially caused by organisms that are resistant to antibiotics. Patients may present with a wide spectrum of severity of aspiration syndromes prior to aspiration pneumonia. Multiple risk factors for aspiration are listed in Table 3–3.[12] Video 3–3 shows a flexible endoscopic evaluation of swallowing (FEES) with aspiration and no cough and the bolus at the level of the larynx. The patient will aspirate the bolus due to lack of sensation. Video 3–4 shows a videofluoroscopic swallowing study (VFSS) with silent aspiration.

Three distinct types of aspiration pneumonia also known as bronchopneumonia are generally recognized. **Anaerobic pneumonia,** in its early stages, results in a low-grade fever. However, extended periods of aspiration, such as fatigue, cough, and unconsciousness secondary to hypoxia, lead to more severe symptoms. **Lung abscess** is an accumulation of pus that has been contained by a surrounding inflammatory process. Radiologically, it appears as a spherical-looking area with an air fluid level often resembling a lung mass. **Empyema** is pus in the pleural space. If left untreated, empyema produces destructive changes resulting in rupture of the pleural walls.

Aspiration pneumonia may be initially difficult to identify and diagnose even with invasive studies. In stroke patients, the overall debilitation, malnutrition, dehydration, and other systemic problems that accompany the stroke or that precede the stroke increase the risk of aspiration and aspiration pneumonia after the stroke. Other risk factors that are often present in patients with a stroke, as well as with head and neck cancer, include poor oral hygiene with bacterial overgrowth, loss of sensory awareness that may occur after other prolonged illness, or degradation in pulmonary function even after an acute event has been stabilized medically or surgically.

The following conditions include the most important groups of patients that are predisposed to aspiration pneumonia.

TABLE 3–3. Aspiration: Risk Factors[a]

Altered level of consciousness
Head trauma
Coma
Cerebrovascular accident (CVA), acute stage
Metabolic encephalopathy
Seizure disorders
General anesthesia
Alcohol intoxication
Altered drug states
Elicit drug status
Excessive sedation
Cardiopulmonary arrest
Gastrointestinal dysfunction
Scleroderma
Esophageal spasm
Esophageal stricture
Gastroesophageal reflux
Laryngopharyngeal reflux
Erosive esophagitis
Zenker diverticulum
Tracheoesophageal fistula
Esophageal cancer
Hiatal hernia
Pyloric stenosis/gastric outlet obstruction
Enteral feeding
Pregnancy
Anorexia/bulimia
Iatrogenic
Prolonged mechanical ventilator support
Tracheotomy
Anticholinergic drugs
Miscellaneous
Obesity
Neck malignances
Medication overdose
Various underlying diseases
Postsurgical
Vocal fold paralysis
Certain skull base surgical procedures
Head and neck
Thyroid carcinoma
Supraglottic laryngectomy
Major oropharyngeal resection
Carotid endarterectomy
Anterior spinal fusion

[a]Adapted and revised from Falestiny and Yu.[12]

Altered mental status: Nearly 70% of patients with altered mental status, regardless of the underlying disease, aspirate. Leder et al found that the odds of liquid aspiration were 31% greater for patients not oriented to person, place, and time. The odds of liquid aspiration, puree aspiration, and being deemed unsafe for any oral intake, respectively, were 57%, 48%, and 69%. They were even greater for patients unable to follow single-step verbal commands.[13]

Factors such as the inability to protect the airways and/or the incoordination between breathing and swallowing generally affect those with altered mental status. Common conditions of altered mental status include diabetic coma, seizure, and medication overdose.

Prolonged mechanical ventilation: Patients requiring prolonged mechanical ventilation and patients with a tracheostomy are especially at risk for aspiration. Aspiration pneumonia can occur after only 2 weeks on mechanical ventilation and nearly 85% of these patients fail FEES or swallow testing using fluoroscopy for detection of aspiration.[14]

Gastroesophageal reflux (GER): Acute findings in acid aspiration–induced lung injury include mucosal edema, hemorrhage, and focal ulceration, followed by the development of focal necrosis and diffuse alveolar hyaline membrane formation. Prolonged (24-hour) esophageal pH monitoring is a test to diagnose gastroesophageal reflux disease **(GERD)**. In addition, ambulatory monitoring devices permit evaluation of the temporal relationship between reflux episodes and atypical symptoms. Monitoring of the acid (pH monitoring) is especially important in the diagnostic evaluation of patients with atypical presentations of GERD. The identification of lesions that may be caused by GERD requires direct examination (ie, laryngoscopy, esophagoscopy), whereas pH monitoring identifies and quantifies the gastroesophageal reflux.

Figure 3–3 shows a partial examination of the esophagus with evidence of GERD. Note the inflammation at the level of the larynx (upper right) and in the esophagus (lower right and left).

Dual-probe 24-hour pH monitoring (the use of 2 catheters) is now an accepted protocol for identifying esophageal and gastroesophageal reflux. The use of 24-hour pH monitoring is usually done

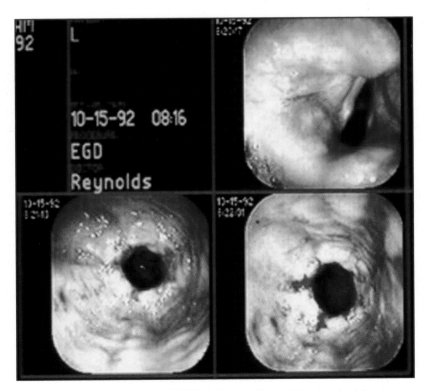

FIGURE 3–3. Evidence of GERD. Inflammation at the level of the larynx (*upper right*) and in the esophagus (*lower left and right*).

following an overnight fast. The pH catheter is inserted transnasally into the esophagus. Standard placement of the distal probe is at a position that is approximately 5 cm above the proximal border of the lower esophageal sphincter (LES). The proximal probe is located in the upper esophagus just below the esophageal inlet. The probes are attached to a recording device. Patients are asked to note in a diary, or in the recording device, the times that they eat, sleep, or perform any other activities. More importantly, patients will be asked to record any type of discomfort that they have, including heartburn, chest pain, wheezing, and coughing, and to record the time that these symptoms occurred. The most valuable discriminator between physiological and pathological reflux is the percentage of total time that the pH is less than 4. Normal values for the proximal probe have not yet been established. Dual-probe 24-hour pH monitoring is considered to be a sensitive and specific method of making a diagnosis of reflux disease. The difficulty with pH monitoring is the patient's need to maintain a "routine daily schedule" for 24 hours while wearing a nasal probe. Many patients do not tolerate the probe or alter their daily schedule, which renders the data suspect. Alternatives to the 24-hour pH probe test have been developed. These alternatives involve inserting a small pill-like camera into the esophagus that then travels through the digestive system and out after 48 hours while sending information back to a small, battery-operated device that is worn on a belt. These devices are more easily tolerated than wearing the nasal probe. Gastroesophageal reflux is discussed in greater detail in Chapter 6.

A controlled study was carried out to examine the relationship between dual-probe 24-hour pH testing, laryngopharyngeal sensory testing, and transnasal flexible laryngoscope (TFL) findings.[15] Seventy-six patients were enrolled in a tightly controlled study. All patients underwent dual-probe 24-hour pH testing 7 days after PPI treatment, laryngopharyngeal sensory testing, and TFL by otolaryngologists who were blinded to pH status and laryngopharyngeal sensory testing results. There were 3 patient groups: Group A—patients with GERD who had laryngopharyngeal reflux disease (LPRD) symptoms (study group); Group B—patients with GERD but no LPRD symptoms (GERD control group); and Group C—patients with no GERD or LPR symptoms (normal group).

Patients with GERD and LPRD symptoms (Group A) had significantly higher posterior laryngopharyngeal sensory thresholds than both patients with GERD but no LPRD symptoms and patients with no GERD or LPRD symptoms. Sensitivity of blinded TFL findings versus dual-probe 24-hour pH testing was 50%, and specificity was 83%. However, adding laryngopharyngeal sensory thresholds greater than 5 mm Hg air pulse pressure to the TFL findings increased the sensitivity of TFL versus dual-probe 24-hour pH testing from 50% to 88%, and specificity from 83% to 88%. This study showed that LPRD is associated with a posterior laryngeal sensory neuropathy with impairment of the laryngeal adductor response (LAR). The investigators reasoned that because greater air pulse strength was required to elicit the LAR in the patients with documented acid reflux compared to the patients without acid reflux, it effectively represented an alteration in laryngeal sensory nerve function—hence their use of the term "neuropathy." Furthermore, adding sensory testing, specifically a sensory deficit greater than 5 mm Hg air pulse pressure, to the TFL findings was essentially as sensitive and specific as dual-probe 24-hour pH testing to diagnose reflux disease.

Neuromuscular disorders: These patients lose motor and sensory function of the upper aerodigestive tract, leading to a variety of disorders affecting cognition, coordination of reflexive actions, and loss of sphincteric and propulsive mechanisms. Patients with advanced stages of Parkinson's disease generally show early evidence of dysphagia and eventually many will be diagnosed with aspiration pneumonia. Also, patients with diabetes mellitus succumb to aspiration pneumonia as the neuropathic symptoms spread to the muscles of swallowing. Regardless of comorbidities, Huang et al found pulmonary infection to be the second most common risk factor for aspiration in adults with type 2 diabetes mellitus.[16]

Upper aerodigestive tract tumors: Most of these patients experience some swallowing difficulty, from the mechanical effects of the tumor, its interference with the sphincteric mechanism of the larynx, or due to the anatomical and functional changes produced by surgery, radiation therapy, and chemotherapy. Their swallowing problems are not limited to the time of treatment or shortly after treatment. Surgery, radiation, and/or chemotherapy can result in long-term changes in bolus propulsion, ability to close the airway, and motility disorders of the esophagus.

The remainder of this chapter reviews the most common conditions and diseases that may require assessment and treatment of a swallowing disorder.

NEUROLOGICAL DISORDERS

Cerebrovascular accident is the most prevalent neurological condition associated with dysphagia in hospitalized adults.[17]

Dysphagia caused by neurological injuries and neuromuscular diseases is usually the end result of an impairment of the sensorimotor components of the oral and pharyngeal phases of swallowing. The onset and progression and severity of the disease, as well as the symptoms, may occur suddenly or may result in a slow progressive degeneration of neuromuscular systems.

Altman et al reported on the prevalence of dysphagia in people 75 years of age and older.[17] They found that dysphagia was more than twice the national average. Those with dysphagia had a 41% longer length of hospital stay than patients with the same diagnoses who did not have dysphagia. Eighty-nine percent of patients with dysphagia had at least 5 co-occurring medical diagnoses and 65% had 7, many of these other neurological conditions. Patients with dysphagia were 4.5 to 5 times more likely to have been hospitalized with Parkinson's disease or stroke, respectively. Among patients undergoing rehabilitation, those with dysphagia were 14 times more likely to die in hospital than those without dysphagia.

Not only swallowing but other neuromuscular systems (phonation, locomotion, etc) may also be affected and reduce the opportunity to treat the swallowing disorder effectively.

Reviews of the advances in sensorimotor control of the swallowing mechanisms suggest that brainstem mechanisms control many of the reflexive laryngeal functions associated with swallowing. These functions are thought to control the integration of respiration and swallowing.[18,19] Table 3–4 lists the more common neurological disorders associated with dysphagia, as identified by Perlman and Shultze-Delrieu[20] and by Coyle et al.[21]

For a quick review of the anatomy and physiology of the brain, the reader is directed to https://www .youtube.com/watch?v=kMKc8nfPATI.

Other sites of brain anatomy and physiology can also be found.

Evaluation of the cause of unexplained dysphagia should include a careful history, referral for neurological examination if not current, including possible magnetic resonance imaging (MRI) of the brain, blood tests (routine studies plus muscle enzymes, thyroid screening, vitamin B12 and anti-acetylcholine receptor antibodies), electromyography nerve conduction studies, and, in certain cases, muscle biopsy or cerebrospinal fluid examination. The following pages describe neurogenic conditions that have a significant incidence of swallowing disorders.

Amyotrophic Lateral Sclerosis (ALS)

Amyotrophic lateral sclerosis (ALS) is a progressive disease involving degeneration of the upper and lower motor neurons. It has an incidence around 2 per 100,000. Men are affected slightly more frequently than women, with onset around age 60, although it may present earlier. The progression is rapid and usually leads to death within 3 years. The changes in upper motor neuron disorders include a variety of symptoms such as muscle weakness, decreased motor control including a loss of the ability to perform fine movements, decreased threshold of spinal reflexes resulting in including spasticity, and extensor plantar response known as the Babinski reflex. Lower motor neuron disease is characterized

TABLE 3–4. Neurologic Disorders Associated With Dysphagia[a]

Parkinson's disease and other neurogenic disorders
Amyotrophic lateral sclerosis
Myasthenia gravis
Polymyositis/dermatomyositis
Guillain-Barré syndrome
Dystonia/tardive dyskinesia
Vocal fold paralysis
Progressive muscular dystrophy
Meningitis
Traumatic brain injury
Cerebral palsy
Progressive supranuclear palsy
Olivopontocerebellar atrophy
Huntington disease
Wilson disease
Torticollis
Alzheimer disease and other dementias
Motor neuron disease (amyotrophic lateral sclerosis)
Neoplasms and other structural disorders
Primary brain tumors
Intrinsic and extrinsic brainstem tumors
Base of skull tumors
Syringobulbia
Arnold-Chiari malformation
Neoplastic meningitis
Multiple sclerosis
Postpolio syndrome
Infectious disorders
Chronic infectious meningitis
Syphilis and Lyme disease
Diphtheria
Botulism
Viral encephalitis, including rabies
Myopathy
Polymyositis, dermatomyositis, including body myositis and sarcoidosis
Myotonic and oculopharyngeal muscular dystrophy
Hyper- and hypothyroidism
Cushing syndrome

[a]Adapted from Perlman and Schulze-Delrieu.[20]

by paralysis accompanied by loss of muscle tone (hypotonia). This is in contrast to an upper motor neuron lesion, which often presents with spastic paralysis.[22] An updated overview of ALS diagnosis and its effects on swallowing can be found in Siddique and Doonkevert.[23]

Diagnosis of ALS requires the **presence and progression** of lower motor neuron and upper motor neuron deficiency. Upper limb muscles are affected more frequently than lower limb muscles, and bulbar muscles may be affected, leading to significant prominent dysarthria and dysphagia. Bulbar involvement in ALS is associated with a worse prognosis because of the higher risk of pulmonary aspiration and malnutrition.

> It is important to monitor the weight and nutrition status of dysphagic patients with ALS and to begin discussions of **percutaneous endogastrostomy (PEG)** before the patient becomes severely deteriorated.

Lower motor neuron signs result from damage to the motor nuclei in the spinal cord (anterior horn cells) and brainstem motor nuclei. Upper motor neuron symptoms are due to damage to the corticospinal and corticobulbar tracts. Atrophy with or without fasciculations may be observed in the tongue and face. Spasticity or flaccidity may also be detected throughout affected regions. Patients with bulbar involvement are likely to show early lingual and labial weakness. The weakness progresses to the muscles of mastication and the intrinsic/extrinsic laryngeal muscle. The progressive loss of muscle function in patients with bulbar involvement produces difficulty controlling oral contents, including secretions, food, and liquids, which may be observed as drooling, early spillage of the bolus into the pharynx, or pooling of residue in the gingivobuccal gutters.

Some patients are aware of these problems and respond to aspiration by clearing their throat or coughing when eating or drinking, suggesting a degree of preserved sensory functions. Others, however, may have minimal or absent sensory response, or the effectiveness of the reflexive cough may be weak and eventually ineffective, resulting in considerable penetration and aspiration of liquids and foods.

Dysphagia in the ALS patient leads to secondary complications such as nutritional deficiencies and dehydration, which can compound the deteriorating effects of the disease, and therefore requires careful monitoring such as a severity scale like that proposed by Yorkston et al.[24] Table 3–5 offers an outline to assess severity of swallowing not only in ALS patients but in others with progressive neuropathy.

At least 73% of ALS patients have dysphagia before they require ventilator support, and even a higher percentage experience swallowing difficulty subsequently. Patients have more problems with liq-

uids and large pieces of food. For the ALS patient, pureed or soft foods are much easier to swallow. An investigation by Higo et al[25] reported the progression of dysphagia in 50 patients with ALS using videofluoroscopy (VF) and the ALS swallowing severity scale (ALSSS). The authors found delayed bolus transport from the oral cavity to the pharynx and bolus stasis at the piriform sinus (PS) in about half of the patients with no bulbar complaints. In contrast, upper esophageal sphincter (UES) opening was relatively well maintained in the late stage of dysphagia. Other parameters, such as bolus holding in the oral cavity, constriction of the pharynx, and elevation of the larynx, became worse over time

TABLE 3–5. Swallowing Severity Scale[a]

Normal Eating Habits	
10	**Normal Swallowing:** Patient denies any difficulty chewing or swallowing. Examination demonstrated no abnormality.
9	**Nominal Abnormality:** Only patient notices slight indicators such as food lodging in the recesses of the mouth or sticking in the throat.

Early Eating Problems	
8	**Minor Swallowing Problems:** Complains of some swallowing difficulties. Maintains an essentially regular diet. Isolated choking episodes.
7	**Prolonged Time or Smaller Bite Size:** Mealtime has significantly lengthened and smaller bite sizes are necessary. Patient must concentrate on swallowing liquids.

Dietary Consistency Changes	
6	**Soft Diet:** Diet is limited primarily to soft foods. Requires some special meal preparation.
5	**Liquefied Diet:** Oral (PO) intake is adequate. Nutrition is limited primarily to a liquefied diet. Patient may force self to eat. Adequate thin liquid intake is usually a problem.

Needs Tube Feeding	
4	**Supplemental Tube Feeding:** PO intake alone is no longer adequate. Patient uses or needs a tube to supplement intake. Patient continues to take significant amount (greater than 50%) of nutrition PO.
3	**Tube Feeding With Occasional PO Nutrition:** Primary nutrition and hydration are accomplished by tube. Patient receives less than 50% of nutrition PO.

NPO	
2	**Secretions Managed With Aspirator/Medication:** Patient cannot safely manage any PO intake. Patient swallows reflexively. An aspirator, medications, or both manage secretions.
1	**Aspiration of Secretions:** Secretions cannot be managed noninvasively. Patient rarely swallows.

[a]Adapted from Yorkston, Strand, Miller, Hillel, and Smith.[24]

following bulbar symptom onset and as the disease advanced. ALS patients in a group with normal eating habits showed disturbed bolus transport from the mouth to the pharynx, weak constriction of the pharynx, and bolus stasis at the pyriform sinus.[25] Similar results were reported in Leder et al[26] using FEES. They suggested that serial FEES evaluations prior to implementing diet changes or therapeutic strategies provide safe treatment.

Drooling can be an early and disturbing symptom of bulbar ALS, often leading to social isolation. Many therapeutic approaches have been suggested over the years to reduce salivary production, including the tricyclic amitriptyline. Some ALS patients benefit from treatment with beta antagonists to help control and thicken secretions.

In patients with prominent bulbar weakness, a palatal lift (see the discussion about prosthodontics in Chapter 12) is sometimes useful to improve the velopharyngeal sphincter. Spasticity may complicate the bulbar contribution to dysarthria and dysphagia in the ALS patient. In occasional patients, Baclofen can be effective in relieving some of the upper motor neuron (UMN) impairment. Diazepam can occasionally be useful, but sedation and increased weakness limit its use.

Cerebrovascular Accident

Stroke is the third most common cause of death in the United States each year. Cerebrovascular disease is the most common cause of neurogenic oral and pharyngeal dysphagia. About 30% to 40% of stroke victims will demonstrate symptoms of significant dysphagia. Twenty percent of stroke victims die of aspiration pneumonia in the first year following a stroke. In addition, 10% to 15% of stroke victims who die in the years following the stroke will die of aspiration pneumonia. Video 3–5 is of a 64-year-old patient with left CVA, right vocal fold paralysis, poor cough, and poor laryngeal elevation.

Dysphagia, aspiration, and aspiration pneumonia are devastating sequelae of stroke, accounting for nearly 40,000 deaths from aspiration pneumonia each year in the United States.

Although the correlation of site and size of the stroke with subsequent dysphagia is variable, the trend is that the larger the area of infarction, the greater the impairment of swallowing. In general, brainstem strokes produce dysphagia more frequently and more severely than cortical strokes. Robbins et al[27] suggest that the severity of dysphagia in patients with left hemisphere strokes seem to correlate with the presence of apraxia and the reported deficits are more significant during the oral stage of swallowing. Right hemisphere patients have more pharyngeal dysfunction, including aspiration and pharyngeal pooling.

Infarct size and distribution define the clinical presentation of the CVA and are dependent on the degree and site of interrupted arterial blood supply. Arterial supply to the brainstem is based in the vertebra-basilar complex. The bilateral internal carotid arteries give rise to the majority of the anterior and middle cerebral blood supply. Each anterior cerebral artery supplies the ipsilateral orbital and medial frontal lobe and the medial parietal lobe. Each middle cerebral artery supplies the ipsilateral orbital and medial frontal lobe and the medial parietal lobe. Branches to the middle cerebral artery also penetrate the brain and supply the ipsilateral basal nuclei, internal capsule region, and most of the thalamus and adjacent structures. Each posterior cerebral artery supplies portions of the ipsilateral brainstem and cerebellum and the inferior temporal and medial occipital lobes. Spinal arteries supply branches to the medulla. Robbins et al also noted that patients with only small vessel infarcts had a significantly lower occurrence of aspiration compared to those with both large and small vessel infarcts.[27]

Dysphagia after unilateral hemispheric stroke is related to the magnitude of pharyngeal motor representation in the affected hemisphere. Patients with right hemisphere stroke show longer pharyngeal transit and higher incidences of laryngeal penetration and aspiration of liquid, as compared to patients with left-sided strokes. Lesions in the left middle cerebral artery territory are known to produce aphasia, motor and verbal apraxia, hemiparesis, and dysphagia. More than half of patients with bilateral strokes aspirate. However, dysphagia, with its attendant risk of aspiration, decreases over time in most patients.

Dysarthria and dysphagia, when associated with emotional lability, is suggestive of pseudobulbar palsy, a condition characterized by weakness of muscles innervated by the medulla (tongue, palate, pharynx, and larynx) because of interruption of corticobulbar fibers, as may be seen with multiple bilateral strokes.

Patients with posterior circulation strokes are more likely to aspirate and show an abnormal cough, abnormal gag, and dysphonia. Lateral medullary syndrome (Wallenberg syndrome) is due to thrombosis of the posteroinferior cerebellar artery, which results in ischemia of the lateral medullary region of the brainstem. It differs from many other types of dysphagia in that the tongue driving force and oropharyngeal propulsion pump force are greatly increased, in part due to the failure of pharyngoesophageal sphincter opening during swallowing.

Early screening and management of dysphagia in patients with acute stroke has been shown to reduce the risk of aspiration pneumonia, is cost-effective, and assures quality care with optimal outcome.

The Burke Dysphagia Screening Test (BDST) is a highly regarded screening test to identify stroke patients at risk for developing pneumonia and recurrent upper airway obstruction.[28] The BDST and other tests of screening for swallowing disorders are discussed in Chapter 5. Direct therapy programs for chronic neurogenic dysphagia resulting from brainstem stroke show that functional benefits are long lasting without related health complications.

Parkinson's Disease

Parkinson's disease is a progressive degenerative neuromuscular disorder characterized by loss of striatal dopamine. Pneumonia is one of the most prevalent causes of death in patients with Parkinson's disease. Parkinson's disease is characterized by a release of subcortical inhibitory centers within the extrapyramidal motor system, which modulate motor function. This is thought to occur due to the degeneration and depigmentation of dopamine-containing neurons found in the substantia nigra and its connections to the basal nuclei. The result is depletion of dopamine in the caudate nucleus and putamen, causing a motor disturbance that includes, among other signs, rigidity and resting tremor.

Oral and pharyngeal dysphagia in Parkinson's disease is multifactorial. Conditions of Parkinson's disease including cognitive impairment, head and neck posture during meals, generalized upper extremity dysmotility, impulsive feeding behavior, and retention of food in the oral cavity are common in patients with advanced disease.

As Parkinson's disease progresses the dysphagia team must remain aware of signs of aspiration and reduced nutrition.

Pharyngoesophageal motor abnormalities also play a role in dysphagia in Parkinson's disease. Because of muscle weakness, patients also have limited pharyngeal contraction, abnormal pharyngeal wall motion, impaired pharyngeal bolus transport, and often show incomplete upper esophageal sphincter relaxation. Dysfunction of the lower esophageal sphincter (LES) includes an open LES or a delayed opening of the LES and gastroesophageal reflux. Other esophageal abnormalities include delayed transport, stasis, bolus redirection, and tertiary contractions of the esophagus. Video 3–6 shows a patient with mid-stage Parkinson's diseases working to achieve a swallow.

Disorders of the oral phase of swallowing, especially for solid foods, are common in Parkinson's disease. Excessive lingual rocking or pumping, incomplete transfer of a bolus from oral to pharyngeal cavity, preswallow loss of bolus containment with spillage into the pharynx and/or larynx (and sometimes our of the mouth) and swallow hesitation are seen. Deficits during the pharyngeal phase include pooling of residue within the pharyngeal recesses and delayed onset of the pharyngeal response, predisposing the patient to aspiration before the swallow. Figure 3–4 shows the result of pooling after the swallow in a patient with Parkinson's disease.

Reduced lingual range of motion and rigidity contribute to diminished hyolaryngeal excursion.

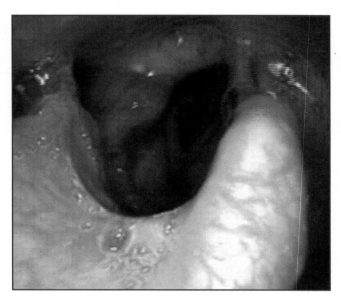

FIGURE 3–4. Puree pooling (*green matter*) after the swallow in patient with Parkinson's disease.

This results in an inadequate or incomplete distension of the upper esophageal segment and incomplete airway protection, which is often followed by aspiration. Esophageal motor abnormalities are also commonly detected in Parkinson's patients.

Data by Sapir et al[29] and by Plowman-Prime et al[30] suggest that patients with Parkinson's disease develop multiple neuromuscular deficiencies and that many of them may exhibit some improvement when given exercises, medications, and/or a medication adjustment. In addition, Parkinson's disease impacts other aspects related to swallowing such as depression, limitations in activities of daily living, communication abilities, and disorders related to body movement.[29,31] Over the past 15 years, Parkinson's patients have benefitted from Lee Silverman Voice Training (LSVT). Although the treatment was initially directed at improving voice and communication, it has been shown to have positive effects on swallowing for these patients.[32] Since the treatment is directed at improving vocal fold closure, this feature helps to prevent choking and aspiration of foods and liquids.

Miller et al[33] summarized the neurological functioning of Parkinson's disease with implications for swallowing disorders. They report that the challenges in treating the Parkinson's patient related to the progressive nature of the disease combined with the nonmotor aspects related to quality of life. They suggest that the rehabilitation team must continually reassess the patient's status and his or her medications and adjust the treatment according to the patient's functional level.

Myasthenia Gravis

Adult-onset **myasthenia gravis** is an acquired autoimmune disorder of neuromuscular transmission in which acetylcholine receptor antibodies attack the postsynaptic membrane of the neuromuscular junction. This reaction reduces the available muscle-activating neurotransmitter, producing rapid fatigability of all muscles. Myasthenia gravis is the most common of the diseases of the neuromuscular junction. Others include **Eaton-Lambert syndrome**, **botulism**, and extensive use of aminoglycosides.

Swallowing problems occur in approximately one-third of patients with myasthenia gravis. Choking and regurgitation are the usual presenting signs in neonates and in 6% to 15% of adult patients. Bulbar and facial muscles are frequently affected, causing dysphagia, dysarthria, nasal regurgitation, and weakness of mastication.[34] Examination may show masseter weakness, bifacial weakness, poor gag reflex and palate elevation, dysarthria, or dysphonia. In addition, most patients have **ptosis, diplopia**, dysarthria, and dysphagia.

> *Tongue weakness is very common when the bulbar musculature is involved and the oropharyngeal transit time (posterior tongue) is especially affected.*

Liquids may be swallowed more easily than solids and patients may fatigue with chewing because of masseter weakness. Patients typically do well at the beginning of a meal but tire at the end. Some patients deteriorate to a point where there is total loss of the ability to chew and swallow, causing aspiration. Patients should take meals when muscle strength is best, possibly 1 hour after medication. In the past, Mestinon was the primary medication. Other medications such as rituximab, a monoclonal antibody, have been found to aid in treating patients with myasthenia gravis. The specific effects on swallowing remain to be evaluated. Compensatory training involves posture modification, alteration of food consistencies, frequent smaller meals, and other voluntary maneuvers designed to circumvent the health consequences of the oropharyngeal deficit.

Myopathies

Duchenne Dystrophy

Duchenne dystrophy is the most common childhood form of muscular dystrophy, with a usual age of onset at 2 to 6 years. The inheritance is X-linked and, thus, only males are affected.

Virtually all patients with Duchenne dystrophy have severe dysphagia by 12 years of age. Episodes of aspiration pneumonia are common by age 18. For individuals with Duchenne dystrophy, deficits of oral preparatory and oral phases of swallowing, including increased mandibular angle and weakness of masticatory muscles, contribute to dysphagia.

Pharyngeal impairment in Duchenne dystrophy is associated with the appearance of macroglossia and weakness of the pterygoid and superior constrictor muscles. Weakness of lip and cheek muscles and tongue elevators may become more pronounced as the disease progresses. Pharyngeal swallowing reflexes are eventually delayed because of impaired elevation and retraction of the tongue. Aspiration of food and saliva, weight loss, and pulmonary complications ultimately occur as dysphagia progresses.

Facioscapulohumeral Muscular Dystrophy

Facioscapulohumeral muscular dystrophy is a slowly progressive, autosomal dominant neuromuscular disorder, with onset in adolescence or early adulthood. Less than 10% of individuals with facioscapulohumeral muscular dystrophy have dysphagia.

Inflammatory Myopathies

Inflammatory myopathies involve the inflammation and degeneration of skeletal muscle tissues. Inflammatory cells surround, invade, and destroy normal muscle fibers, eventually resulting in muscle weakness.

Dermatomyositis

Dermatomyositis usually presents with a rash characterized by patchy, bluish-purple discolorations on the face, neck, shoulders, upper chest, elbows, knees, knuckles, and back, accompanying, or more often preceding, muscle weakness. Dysphagia occurs in at least one-third of dermatomyositis patients, who typically present with oral dryness, delayed pharyngeal transit, and even aspiration.

High-dose prednisone is an effective treatment for many patients. In addition, other nonsteroidal immunosuppressants such as azathioprine and methotrexate are often used, and even intravenous administration of immunoglobulins (Ig) has also proven effective.

Inclusion Body Myositis

Inclusion body myositis is an inflammatory muscle disease characterized by slow and relentlessly progressive muscle weakness and atrophy, similar to polymyositis. Indeed, inclusion body myositis is often the correct diagnosis in cases of polymyositis that are unresponsive to therapy.

Unfortunately, there is as yet no known treatment for inclusion body myositis. The disease is unresponsive to corticosteroids and other immunosuppressive drugs. Intravenous immunoglobulins have shown some preliminary evidence for a slight beneficial effect in a small number of cases.

Polymyositis

Polymyositis does not have the characteristic rash of dermatomyositis. As with dermatomyositis, dysphagia is common in polymyositis and its symptoms also include dryness of the mouth and prolonged pharyngeal transit. Treatment is also similar to that of dermatomyositis and other autoimmune diseases with medications such as prednisone, azathioprine, methotrexate, and Ig.

Limb-Girdle Muscular Dystrophy

Limb-girdle muscular dystrophy is a slowly progressive form of muscular dystrophy with both autosomal recessive and dominant forms. Males and females are equally affected, with onset usually in adolescence or early adulthood. Swallowing abnormalities are demonstrated in up to one-third of patients, who show dysfunction of the pharyngeal muscles.

Myotonic Dystrophy

Myotonic dystrophy is an autosomal dominant disorder that results in skeletal muscle weakness and wasting, myotonia, and numerous nonmuscular manifestations including frontal balding, cataracts, gonadal dysfunction, cardiac conduction abnormalities, respiratory insufficiency, and hypersomnolence.

Radiological features of dysphagia in myotonic dystrophy include a marked reduction in resting tone of both the upper and lower esophageal sphincters, and a reduction in contraction pressure in the pharynx and throughout the esophagus. Contrast radiography shows hypotonic pharynx with stasis and a hypomotility, and often esophageal dilation and gastroesophageal reflux disease.

Oculopharyngeal Dystrophy

Oculopharyngeal dystrophy is a progressive neurological disorder characterized by gradual onset of dysphagia, ptosis, and facial weakness. Oculopharyngeal dystrophy is an autosomal dominant disorder that affects both males and females, with onset of symptoms in the fourth or fifth decade. Dysphagia is slowly progressive and may be a presenting symptom before a diagnosis is made.

Both striated skeletal and smooth muscles are affected, leading to very low pharyngeal manometric pressures, cricopharyngeal bar, and lower esophageal sphincter pressure. Cricopharyngeal myotomy is an effective treatment of dysphagia secondary to cricopharyngeal achalasia. However, a cricopharyngeal myotomy does not modify the final prognosis and is contraindicated in cases with weak pharyngeal propulsion.

Spinal Muscular Atrophies

Spinal muscular atrophies constitute a group of neuromuscular disorders defined pathologically by degeneration of the anterior horn cells in the spinal cord. Swallowing difficulties occur in over one-third of patients with spinal muscular atrophies. Bulbar and respiratory involvement is a prominent feature only in early onset, more severely affected patients, with respiratory insufficiency, difficulty sucking and swallowing, accumulation of secretions, and a weak cry.

Progressive Supranuclear Palsy

Progressive supranuclear palsy (PSP) is a progressive, degenerative extrapyramidal disease that often masquerades as Parkinson's disease.

Almost all patients with progressive supranuclear palsy show multiple abnormalities in swallowing, including uncoordinated lingual movements, absent velar retraction or elevation, impaired posterior lingual displacement, and copious pharyngeal secretions.

Tongue-assisted mastication, noncohesive lingual transfer, excessive spillage of the oral bolus into the pharynx prior to active transfer, valleculae bolus retention, abnormal epiglottis positioning, and hiatal hernias are also noted in about one-half of PSP patients. Unfortunately, patients with PSP do not respond to dopaminergic pharmacological treatment as well as patients with Parkinson's disease do. Likewise, their dysphagia is more life threatening and resistant to treatment. Early and aggressive swallowing evaluation and treatment are mandatory in PSP patients.

Traumatic Brain Injury

Following a traumatic brain injury (TBI), swallowing disorders generally consist of delayed or absent pharyngeal response, reduced lingual control, reduced pharyngeal clearance, and aspiration during and after the swallow. Due to its sudden onset, swallowing function may change rapidly after the initial traumatic event and may require repeated assessment with each change of neurological status. Cranial nerves can be affected due to skull base fractures and/or acceleration-deceleration injuries.

Concussions are the mildest form of TBI. They can occur in workplace settings, sports activities, fighting, and falling. Mild traumatic brain injury (mTBI) accounts for 75% of the TBI every year. Webb et al examined a large cohort of airmen subjected to concussions and found that men exposed to mTBI had a higher incidence of epilepsy, seizure disorders, and pain compared to those who had no history of mTBI.[35] Effects of concussion may not be seen until long after the incident(s).

Cognitive deficits in this population that may impact upon safe oral intake are disorders of attention, impulsivity, agitation, memory deficits, and reduced higher level reasoning skills.

Children are especially affected by repeated mTBI. Their heads are disproportionately large compared to their bodies and their level of activity (sports injury, falling, fighting, etc) makes them especially vulnerable to mTBI.

CONDITIONS FOUND IN CRITICAL CARE PATIENTS

Patients in critical care units often exhibit a variety of swallowing disorders. Macht et al recently reviewed the epidemiology of patients seen in critical care units.[36] They report that approximately 15% of all patients seen in an intensive care unit and 20% of all patients following cardiac surgery will have a swallowing problem. In addition, they found that patients seen with pneumonia and those recently extubated following acute respiratory failure all have a significant risk of dysphagia.

The minimum requirements for a patient to actively participate in the dysphagia treatment process include the ability to maintain alertness, follow basic commands, and ideally be 24 hours postextubation or 48 hours posttracheotomy.

Critical care patients are often elderly and may have multiple medical conditions. They are frequently debilitated and deconditioned. The medical staff monitors patients in surgical intensive care units continuously and a close communication between the medical staff and the swallowing rehabilitation staff must be maintained to ensure that a swallowing disorder does not adversely affect the recovery from surgery. Patients in both medical and surgical intensive care units often need nasogastric or endotracheal intubation and/or mechanical ventilation, which contribute to the swallowing difficulty and to aspiration or aspiration pneumonia.

Nasogastric tubes reduce pharyngeal sensitivity, predispose the patient to gastroesophageal reflux, and may produce inflammation and pain, which interfere with laryngeal elevation and increase the risk for swallowing difficulties.

Swallowing evaluation in orally or nasally intubated patients is usually deferred, although possible in selected cases (eg, young patients with normal upper aerodigestive tract). If swallowing evaluation is done using transnasal flexible endoscopy, it may be easier to pass the endoscope on the side of the nasogastric tube. Simonian and Goldberg[37] listed an extensive number of signs of dysphagia in this group (see Chapter 2, Table 2–3).

ESOPHAGEAL DISORDERS

The esophagus is a muscular, mucosal-lined tube that is considered to begin at the caudal end of the pharynx inferior to the cricopharyngeus (CPM) which functions as physiologically as the upper esophageal sphincter. The esophagus extends through the thoracic cavity in the posterior mediastinum, dorsal to the tracheobronchial tree, the heart, and most of the great vessels. It then pierces and enters the peritoneal cavity to join with the stomach. The esophagus serves as a conduit to pass food through the thoracic cavity into the abdominal cavity for digestion and absorption.

The muscular wall of the esophagus consists of two types of muscle tissue, smooth muscle fibers in the alimentary canal and striated fibers at the junction of the pharynx and esophagus. The muscles are arranged in circular and longitudinal bundles, with the longitudinal muscles located exteriorly. When a bolus enters the esophagus, a peristaltic wave travels at a relatively constant velocity due to the combination of constricting forces behind the bolus mediated by contraction of the circular muscles and shortening of the esophagus from contraction of the longitudinal muscle groups. Transit time through the upper esophagus is less than 1 second in normal individuals. In the smooth muscle lower two-thirds of the esophagus, transit time is approximately 3 seconds. Position changes impact esophageal transit time minimally because gravity plays only a minor role in normal swallowing.

Disorders of muscular coordination are manifested by weak or failure of peristalsis. Peristaltic activity changes and uncoordinated peristaltic activity increases with the normal aging process. Many neuromuscular diseases and others such as diabetes mellitus that are associated with peripheral neuropathy are frequently associated with esophageal dysfunction due to loss of an intact coordinating function.

Because of the tissue changes in the esophagus and also the coordination of the circular and long muscles of the upper and lower esophagus, respectively, a wide variety of diseases and injuries may affect the esophagus. For ease of understanding, we have divided esophageal swallowing disorders into those disorders resulting from esophageal cancer and its treatments or from other esophageal disorders. In many cases such as inflammatory esophageal disorders, the latter may lead to the former.

Esophageal Cancer

The most common manifestation of esophageal cancer is progressive dysphagia. Other symptoms include odynophagia, regurgitation, weight loss, and aspiration pneumonia. The barium swallow esophagram is the preferred diagnostic tool and serves as a "road map" of the esophagus, providing diagnostic information on the site of luminal narrowing, the degree and length of obstruction, and the presence of concomitant tracheoesophageal fistula. The modified barium swallow (as discussed in Chapter 5) provides functional information for the clinician in managing dysphagia in the patient with a diagnosis of esophageal disease.

Clinicians should be especially aware of the need for a barium esophagram when the modified barium swallow examination or FEES examination finds a normal oropharyngeal exam but the patient reports difficulty swallowing.

It is important for the clinicians treating swallowing disorders of the esophagus to understand the conditions under which the esophageal cancer is identified and treated. The primary methods for palliating dysphagia involve endoscopic techniques. Endoscopic modalities include the ablation of the tumor using Nd:YAG laser or bipolar electrocautery, photodynamic therapy, pulsed-dye laser (PDL), balloon dilatation, placement of expandable metal stents, and endoesophageal brachytherapy.

One of the simplest, but least effective, methods of endoscopic palliation is balloon dilatation. Dilatation is simple, relatively inexpensive, and easy to perform. However, it involves the risk of perforation, and the benefits are usually short-lived. Dilatation to the esophagus must be done carefully so as not to perforate the esophagus. Reports of esophageal perforation have suggested that the risk/benefit of this procedure must be assessed carefully as the treatment of esophageal perforation may require extensive treatment and slow down the treatment for the primary disease.[38]

In one large study, Nd:YAG was used as a palliative treatment for malignant dysphagia in 224 patients over a period of 8 years. The esophageal lumen was successfully reopened in 98.2% of patients, and 93.7% were able to ingest at least semisolids following the therapy.[39] Photodynamic therapy (PDT) is an alternative modality approved by the US Food and Drug Administration for palliation of obstructive esophageal carcinoma.[40] External beam radiation therapy (EBRT) has been one of the most common approaches in the management of obstructing esophageal cancer. More recently, intensity modulated radiation therapy (IMRT), an advanced type of radiation therapy that uses advanced technology to manipulate photon and proton beams of radiation to conform to the shape of a tumor has been used to treat cancerous diseases of the esophagus.[41] Brachytherapy, which involves inserting a radioactive source close to the tumor to maximize the delivery of radiation while minimizing its side effects, has also been used to treat cancerous diseases of the esophagus. In almost all cases, swallowing disorders following these treatments will result.

Esophageal cancer is rapidly rising in Western civilization, and explanations for this have been offered by numerous sources, from nonmedical websites to advertisements for esophageal health foods to pathological studies of tissues from patients deceased from esophageal cancer. The answers leave the reader with more questions than in the past. Suffice to say that esophageal phase dysphagia may remain persistent despite medications, swallowing exercises, and/or further surgery.[42] The treatment of swallowing disorders associated with esophageal cancer is reviewed in Chapters 7 and 8.

Other Esophageal Disorders

Motility Disorders

Achalasia. **Achalasia** means "failure to relax." The normal resting tone of the lower esophageal sphincter (LES) is maintained in part by the sphincteric function of the circular muscular fibers of the esophagus and in part by its position within the crural folds in the diaphragmatic muscle. Failure of this sphincter to relax when the bolus approaches results in inability of the bolus to move through into the stomach and is termed *achalasia.* Figure 3–5 shows a patient with achalasia after a swallow.

Achalasia is characterized by the degeneration of neural elements in the wall of the esophagus, particularly at the LES. The distal segment of the esophagus tapers, giving the appearance of a "bird's beak."

Achalasia may be suspected in patients who complain of the sensation of food remaining in the throat that they cannot clear on repetitive swallowing. If the esophagus ultimately relaxes, the food is passed. The common treatments for this are balloon dilation or injection of botulinum toxin to the cricopharyngeus muscle. The diagnosis of achalasia, however, is con-

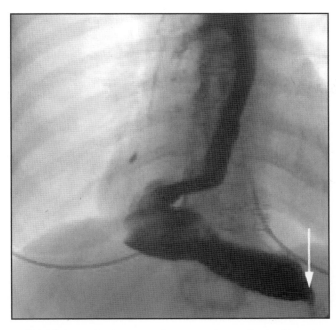

FIGURE 3–5. Barium esophagram of a patient with achalasia showing the distal segment of the esophagus tapering into a "bird's beak."

firmed with manometry with esophageal manometry studies, which are discussed in Chapter 5.

Curling. Curling is an alteration in esophageal motility frequently seen in elderly individuals. Curling represents tertiary contractions, which are nonpropulsive. This condition may occur as a result of scarring in the esophagus following surgery or bleeding.

Diffuse Esophageal Spasm. Diffuse esophageal spasm (DES) / is characterized by intermittent dysphagia, chest pain, and repetitive contractions of the esophagus. Dysphagia is present in 30% to 60% of patients with DES. Clinically, dysphagia is intermittent, with severity varying from mild to severe.

The distorted radiographic appearance of the esophagus is that of a "corkscrew" or of a "rosary bead." Figure 3–6 shows an esophagram with the classic corkscrew esophagus created by tertiary contractions.

Nonperistaltic or simultaneous contractions following a majority of the swallows are the most reliable criteria in the identification of diffuse esophageal spasm.

Diverticula. Esophageal **diverticula** are outpouchings of one or more layers of the esophageal wall. These diverticula occur in several places. Many are small and are of no consequence in swallowing. A traction diverticulum occurs near the midpoint of the esophagus. An epiphrenic diverticulum can form immediately above the lower esophageal sphincter or at the gastroesophageal junction. However, Zenker diverticulum that occurs immediately above the upper esophageal sphincter will always lead to swallowing problems once it enlarges. Patients often report that they feel the food coming back up, and indeed, the food or liquid that flows into the Zenker pouch does reflux back up into the larynx and can be seen on examination. The outpouching seen in Figure 3–7 shows folds of tissue commonly known as a hiatal hernia found near the lower esophageal sphincter near the location of the gastroesophageal junction. The hiatal hernia is a common finding on a barium esophagram and is often treated medically or if it is small, observed for future changes in swallowing.

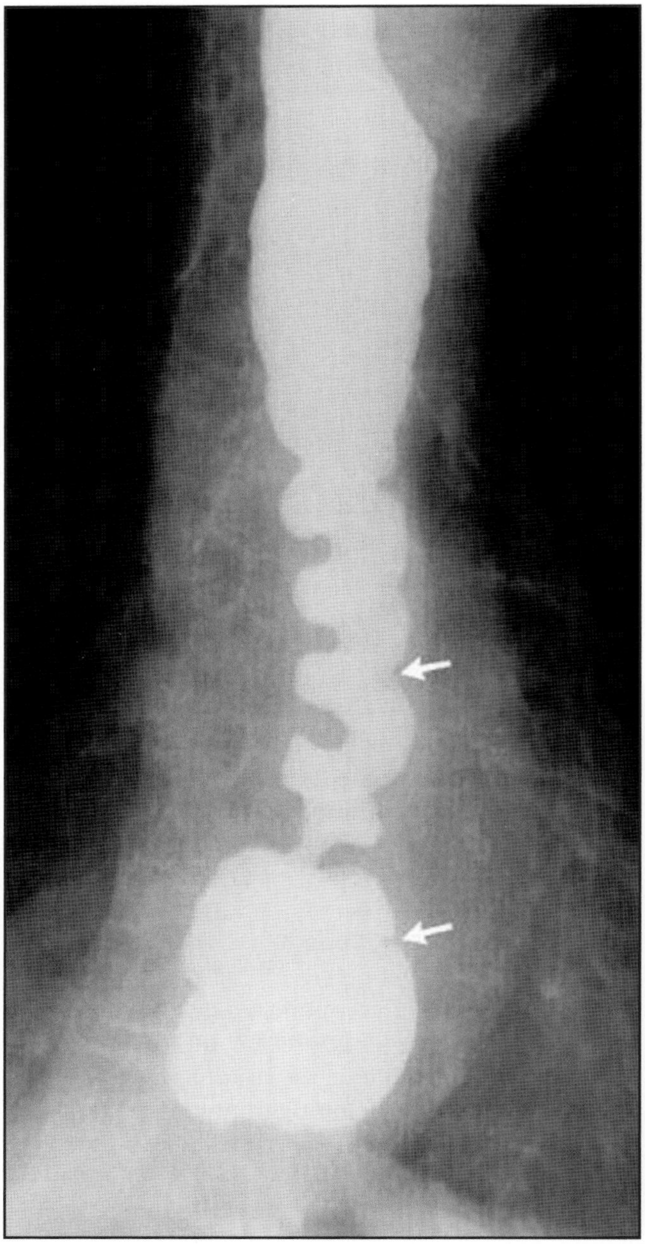

Webs/Rings. Patients with intermittent dysphagia for solids may have esophageal webs or rings. Esophageal webs are reported in 7% of the patients presenting with dysphagia. A **Schatzki ring** is a lower

FIGURE 3–6. Corkscrew esophagus (tertiary contractions). Oblique view of the thoracic esophagus shows irregularly spaced contractions (*arrows*) causing indentations of the thoracic esophagus. At fluoroscopy, this was transient but recurred and the bolus was ineffectively propelled through the thoracic esophagus. Adapted from Weissman.[43]

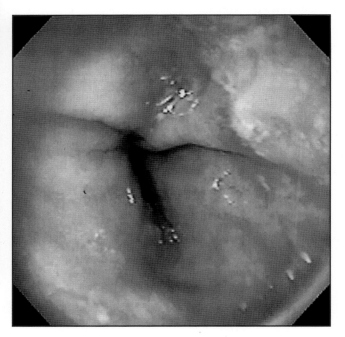

FIGURE 3–7. Hiatal hernia seen on esophagram. Patient with Zenker diverticulum was examined for hiatal hernia. The outpouching is near the upper esophageal sphincter.

esophageal mucosal ring that is located at the level of the squamous-columnar junction. (Figure 3–8 shows a Schatzki ring in the distal esophagus.)

Nonspecific esophageal motility disorders may be found during esophageal manometry in patients with dysphagia who have no evidence of other systemic diseases. Patients with nonspecific esophageal motility disorders constitute approximately 25% to 50% of the abnormal motility studies performed during the evaluation of chest pain.

Systemic diseases such as diabetes mellitus, amyloidosis, and most notably progressive systemic sclerosis (PSS), can produce esophageal dysmotility and dysphagia. An estimated 50% to 90% of patients with PSS have esophageal involvement.

Esophageal Inflammatory Disorders

Gastroesophageal Reflux Disease. Gastroesophageal reflux disease (GERD) is defined as the retrograde movement of gastric contents from the stomach through the lower esophageal sphincter and into the esophagus. The most common symptom is "heartburn." A study that surveyed presumably normal hospital staff and employees found that 7% of the people interviewed experience daily heartburn. The prevalence of monthly heartburn was estimated to be 36% to 44%. A randomized study of 2000 subjects demonstrated a prevalence of 58.1% of white patients with symptoms of heartburn and/or acid regurgitation. The prevalence of weekly or more frequent episodes of heartburn or acid regurgitation was 19.4%.[42]

Persons with GERD frequently complain of noncardiac chest pain, regurgitation of gastric contents, water brash (stimulated salivary secretion by esophageal acid), dysphagia, and sometimes **odynophagia** (pain upon swallowing).

> *GERD has also been associated with numerous extraesophageal symptoms including pharyngitis, laryngitis, hoarseness, chronic cough, asthma, and pulmonary aspiration.*

Acid reflux–induced symptoms referable to the oropharyngeal, laryngeal, and respiratory tracts are termed "extraesophageal reflux" or "atypical reflux" or, more commonly, laryngopharyngeal reflux disease and are discussed below.

Some investigators and clinicians feel that GERD may be the underlying etiology of **globus** (sensation of a lump in the throat). Gastroesophageal reflux disease was reported in 64% of patients reporting globus who were studied by ambulatory pH monitoring. GERD has also been implicated in the etiology of oropharyngeal dysphagia, the difficulty in passing a food bolus from the oropharynx into the upper esophagus. Cervical dysphagia is often linked to inflammation of the esophagus.

GERD occurs through one of three mechanisms:

1. Inappropriate or transient lower esophageal sphincter relaxation
2. Increased abdominal pressure or stress-induced reflux
3. Incompetent or reduced lower esophageal sphincter pressures or spontaneous free reflux

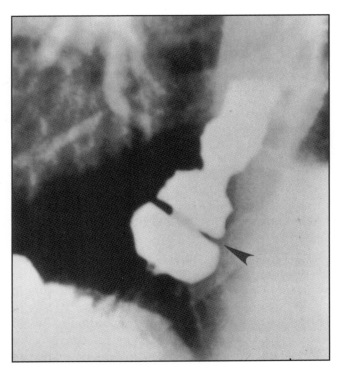

FIGURE 3–8. This barium esophagram shows a typical Schatzki ring (*arrow*) in the distal esophagus. Adapted from Padda and Young.[44]

Lower esophageal sphincter competence is the most important barrier to esophageal reflux. Transient relaxation of the lower esophageal sphincter is probably the most important cause of GERD, both in healthy individuals and in patients with **esophagitis**.[45] Table 3–6 lists the protective and injurious determinants of esophageal function as it relates to inflammation and control of inflammation.

Acid, **pepsin**, and **bile** are the active components of the refluxate contributing to GERD, as they are potentially damaging to the esophageal mucosa and submucosa. Table 3–7 lists the substances that influence the pressures in the lower esophagus and affect lower esophageal pressure. Figure 3–9 shows the vocal folds in a patient with GERD. The vocal folds are edematous due to the acid rising up to the level of the larynx.

The degree of mucosal damage by hydrogen seems to be potentiated by adding pepsin to the reflux material. The amount of time that the refluxed material is in contact with the esophageal mucosa might be a determining factor in the formation of esophagitis.

Upper esophageal dysfunction may contribute to GERD. The cricopharyngeus muscle has been implicated in the development of **Zenker diverticu-lum**, which is formed by the protrusion of the posterior hypopharyngeal mucosa between fibers of the inferior constrictor and cricopharyngeus muscles. Figure 3–10 shows x-ray images of the upper esophageal sphincter prior to and following the surgery for Zenker diverticulum.

The surgery to close the Zenker pouch may be done endoscopically or through an open surgical procedure. When the barium esophagram shows no evidence of Zenker diverticulum, the tight cricopharyngeus may be relaxed temporarily with injection of **botulinum toxin**.[46]

Laryngopharyngeal Reflux Disease. Laryngopharyngeal reflux disease (LPRD) is actually an inflammatory disease of the larynx, but it originates in the stomach like other reflux disorders. Acid from the stomach rises up to the level of the larynx and targets the laryngeal tissues to cause a number of disorders such as hoarseness, vocal process granulomas, and coughing. Reflux of acid into the hypopharynx is a very common and potentially debilitating disease. A healthy person complaining of hoarseness, throat clearing, and excess phlegm in the throat is typically describing the common symptoms of laryngopharyngeal reflux disease. In more severe cases, the symptoms might also include excessive coughing, occasional choking of liquids or foods, and globus. It differs from GERD in that it is an upright disease, occurring in the daytime and presenting with the common symptoms noted above and usually without the specific complaint of heartburn. GERD, on the other hand, usually results in complaints of heartburn, abdominal pain, and regurgitation.

The most common symptoms of LPRD have been identified by Belafsky et al[47] From a list of symptoms, they developed the Reflux Symptom Index (RSI; see Appendix 1), a patient self-assessment questionnaire of the severity of common symptoms of reflux. Heartburn and regurgitation, the classic symptoms of GERD, are unusual symptoms in patients with LPRD, occurring in as few as 10% of patients with LPRD symptoms, according to Belafsky et al.[47] Although the reasons for this are not completely understood, most investigators suspect that it relates to the lack of acid-clearing mechanisms in the laryngopharynx.

TABLE 3–6. Determinants of Reflux Protection and Injury[a]

Protective
Competency of antireflux barrier:
LES
UES
Esophageal acid clearance
Esophageal motility
Saliva
Epithelial tissue resistance
Injurious
Zenker diverticulum
Reflux constituents
Acid
Pepsin
Bile

[a]Adapted from Levy and Young.[49]

TABLE 3–7. Substances Influencing Lower Esophageal Sphincter Pressure[a]

	Increase LES Pressure	Decrease LES Pressure
Hormones	Gastrin	Secretin
	Norepinephrine	Cholecystokinin
	Acetylcholine	Glucagon
	Motilin	Nitric oxide
		Pancreatic polypeptide
		Intestinal polypeptide
		Substance P
		Progesterone
		Cholinergic agonists
		Cholinergic antagonists
		Alpha adrenergic agonists
		Alpha adrenergic antagonists
		Beta adrenergic antagonists
		Beta adrenergic agonists
		Antacids
		Barbiturates
Pharmacological Agents	Metoclopramide	Diazepam
	Cisapride	Calcium channel blockers
	Domperidone	Theophylline
	Prostaglandin F2	Morphine
		Dopamine
		Prostaglandin E2, I2
Diet	Protein	Fat
		Chocolate
		Caffeine
		Peppermint
		Spearmint
		Ethanol

[a]Adapted from Levy and Young.[49(p180)]

The physical exam findings of LPRD have also been quantified by Belafsky et al[47] and are referred to as the Reflux Finding Score (RFS; see Appendix 2). A clinician determines the RFS after the transnasal flexible laryngoscope (TFL) examination. A score of 9 or greater is significant and strongly suggests LPRD. Rarely are the signs of LPRD seen in isolation, meaning it would be very unusual for a patient to have only a pseudosulcus vocalis as the sole manifestation of their LPRD. Typically, the patient with LPRD has multiple laryngeal indicators. Edema of the larynx, not erythema, is the clinical hallmark of LPRD.

Traditionally, the diagnosis of LPR is made by a combination of patient history, physical examination of the larynx, and diagnostic instrumental testing. The test may consist of a 24-hour pH test or an in-office sensory test that takes minutes to perform and may be much more appealing to a patient.[48] Table 3–8 summarizes the salient differences between GERD and LPRD, as reported by Levy and Young.[49]

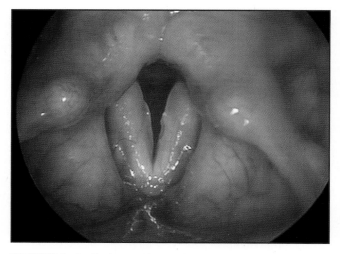

FIGURE 3–9. Patient with significant edema at the level of the larynx and vocal folds.

Barrett Esophagus. **Barrett esophagus** (sometimes referred to as Barrett metaplasia) is a compensatory change in the esophageal mucosa from squamous to specialized intestinal epithelium, and it occurs in up to 15% of patients with atypical presentations of GERD. This disease often presents as a swallowing problem with nonspecific complaints of heartburn and dyspepsia. Moreover, there is evidence that the condition predisposes one to esophageal adenocarcinoma, cancer of the lower esophagus, which is rapidly increasing in the Western world. Treatment is by medication for GERD and diet modification. Since this metaplastic condition may evolve into esophageal cancer, routine endoscopic follow-up examinations are recommended for patients identified with Barrett esophagus.

Burns

Esophageal burns come from injection of caustic substances, gasses, or hot liquids that are swallowed

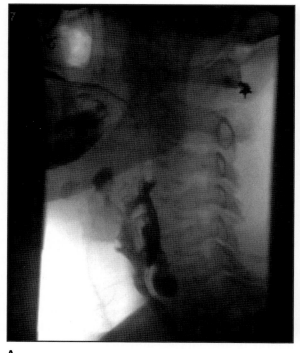

A

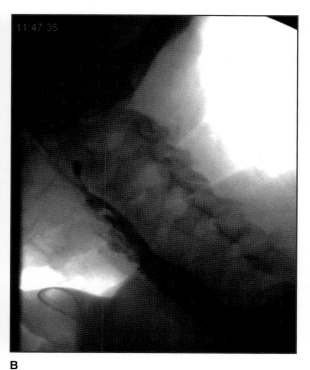

B

FIGURE 3–10. This barium esophagram allows easy delineation of the dilated esophagus. **A.** The Zenker diverticulum prior to surgery. **B.** The same esophageal segment following successful surgery.

Table 3–8. Symptoms of Gastroesophageal Reflux (GERD) and Laryngopharyngeal Reflux Disease (LPRD)

Esophageal (GERD)	Laryngopharyngeal (LPRD)
Heartburn	Pharyngitis
Acid regurgitation	Laryngitis
Water brash	Hoarseness
Dysphagia	Globus
Odynophagia	Daytime cough/throat clearing
Esophageal spasm	Shortness of breath
Nighttime cough	Air hunger
	Pulmonary aspiration

too quickly. Esophageal burns of lead to scarring or strictures in the esophagus resulting in food not going into the stomach or feeling "stuck" in the esophagus, may be as high as the cricopharyngeus muscle.[50] Emergency treatment includes prednisolone or other corticosteroids. Many burns result in esophageal strictures that are treated with esophageal stenting or with balloon dilation.[51] The role of the SLP comes at the chronic stage when there is a need to manage diet consistencies in order to reduce the effects of food lodging or the feeling of food lodged in the esophagus. Instrumental examination of the esophagus is necessary to identify the cause of the problem. Careful case history should always precede the instrumental exam.

INFECTIOUS DISEASES

Oral Cavity/Oropharynx

Bacterial infections of the oropharynx that result in dysphagia include tonsillitis, pharyngitis, and abscesses that may be associated with primary mucosal or lymphoid inflammation that causes pain and odynophagia. **Candidiasis** may also involve the oral cavity and the oropharynx in both immunocompetent and immunocompromised individuals. It is more common, however, in the latter group of patients and in those who require prolonged treatment with antibiotics.

Esophagitis

Primary esophageal infections are unusual in the general population. When they arise, these are typically due to **candidiasis** or **herpes simplex virus (HSV)**. Esophagitis, however, is a major cause of morbidity in individuals with impaired immunity caused by **human immunodeficiency virus (HIV)** infection, chemotherapy, or solid organ or bone marrow transplantation.

Eosinophilic Esophagitis

Eosinophilic esophagitis is an inflammation that builds up in a type of white blood cells in the esophagus. This buildup results in an inflammation that is often thought to be a reaction to foods, allergens, or acid reflux.[52] Damage through inflammation in the esophagus can lead to difficulty swallowing or cause food to get caught when you swallow. Eosinophilic esophagitis has been identified only recently but now is considered a chronic immune disease of the digestive system. Symptoms include chest or abdominal pain, possible vomiting in children, discomfort in swallowing, and regurgitation of foods or liquids.

Chagas Disease

Chagas disease is a parasitic infectious disease that leads to achalasia. Chagas disease, endemic in the Amazon basin, is caused by *Trypanosoma cruzi*, a parasite. It can lead to achalasia that, in severe cases, results in mega-esophagus as a result of destruction of the parasympathetic innervation.

Deep Neck Infections

Deep neck infections are typically the result of polymicrobial infections. In addition to symptoms of the primary infection site, patients may present with dysphagia, odynophagia, drooling, fever, chills, neck stiffness, and swelling. Treatment includes empiric therapy with broad spectrum agents, airway protection, and, often, surgical intervention.

Laryngeal Infections

Adult **epiglottitis** may cause life-threatening supraglottic edema that can progress to a delay in diagnosis and treatment. Common symptoms of supraglottic infection include a sore throat that is out of proportion to the findings of a pharyngeal examination, dysphagia, odynophagia, and dysarthria. Epiglottitis is diagnosed via endoscopic examination.

MEDICATIONS

The effects of medications are influenced by sex, age, body size, metabolic status, individual biological response, and concurrent use of other medications. A variety of medications, including those obtained over the counter and those medically prescribed, affect swallowing, impairing consciousness, coordination, motor and sensitivity functions, and the lubrication of the upper aerodigestive tract (Table 3–9).

Analgesics

Salicylates (aspirin) and nonsteroidal anti-inflammatory agents cause ulceration of the mouth, throat burning, mucosal hemorrhage, glossitis, and dry mouth.

Antibiotics

Side effects such as **glossitis**, **stomatitis**, and **esophagitis** have been described for penicillin, erythromycin, chloramphenicol, and the tetracyclines. Sulfa can cause a Stevens-Johnson syndrome-type reaction resulting in extensive mucosal ulceration and glossitis. Aminoglycosides can increase parkinsonian symptoms of weakness.

Antituberculous medications such as isoniazid, rifampin, ethambutol, and cycloserine can cause confusion, disorientation, and dysarthria. Antiviral agents such as acyclovir, amantadine, ganciclovir, and vidarabine can indirectly cause dysphagia with confusion, asthenia, and lingual facial dyskinesia. Amantadine can cause severe xerostomia and xero-

phonia in some patients. Zidovudine (AZT), an antiviral drug, causes dysphagia in approximately 5% to 10% of patients and tongue edema in 5% of patients. Chloroquine (Plaquenil), mostly used for treating malaria, can cause stomatitis.

Antihistamines

Antihistamines (H$_1$-receptor antagonists) are commonly used to treat allergies. However, because of their anticholinergic side effects, this class of medications commonly exerts a drying effect on the aerodigestive tract mucosa, causing difficulty in gastrointestinal motility during the swallowing process. Other side effects include sedation, disturbed coordination, and gastric distress. Central nervous system effects include ataxia, incoordination, convulsions, dystonia, and bruxism, which can lead to poor oral intake.

Antimuscarinics, Anticholinergics, and Antispasmodics

Antimuscarinics and antispasmodics, used for a variety of reasons such as bradycardia, excessive oral secretions, motion sickness, and diarrhea, diminish the production of saliva and mucus. Salivary secretion is particularly sensitive to inhibition by antimuscarinic agents, which can completely abolish the copious water secretions induced by the parasympathetic system. The mouth becomes dry, and swallowing and talking become difficult.

Prokinetic agents improve motility and speed gastric emptying. The two major drugs in this category are metoclopramide (Reglan) and cisapride (Propulsid); however, the latter is no longer available in the United States. The former is associated with greater antihistamine-like side effects and must be taken carefully to avoid confounding the swallowing disorder.

Mucolytic Agents

Mucolytic agents can be used to counter the effects of drying agents such as antihistamines. However,

TABLE 3–9. Common Medications Affecting Swallowing

Product Category	Examples	Common Indications	Possible Effects
Neuroleptics			
Antidepressants	Elavil (tricyclic) Gabapentin Amitriptyline Mirtazapine Remeron Lexapro Effexor Zoloft Celexa Wellbutrin Paxil Prozac Cymbalta	Relief of endogenous depression	Drying of mucosa, drowsiness Possible weight gain
Antipsychotics	Haldol Thorazine Clozapine Risperidone	Management of patients with chronic psychosis	Tardive dyskinesia
Sedatives			
Barbiturates	Phenobarbital Nembutal	Treatment of insomnia	CNS depressant (drowsiness causing decompensation of patients with cognitive deficits)
Antihistamines	Cold and cough preparations	Relief of nasal congestion and cough	Drying mucosa, sedative effects
Diuretics	Lasix Hydrochlorothiazide Spironolactone Aldosterone	Treatment of edema (eg, associated with congestive heart failure)	Signs of chronic dehydration (dryness of mouth, thirst, weakness, drowsiness)
Mucosal anesthetics	Hurricaine Benzocaine	Topical anesthetic used to aid passage of fiberoptic nasopharyngoscopes, control of dental pain	Suppresses gag and cough reflex
Anticholinergics	Cogentin Atrovent Oxivent Spireva	Bronchodilator Help to open the lungs	Dry mouth and reduced appetite

[a]Adapted and modified from Perlman and Schulze-Delrieu.[20]

no medications, including mucolytic agents, are a substitute for adequate hydration and, indeed, these medications are dependent on adequate water intake.

Antihypertensives

Almost all of the antihypertensive agents have some degree of parasympathetic effects and thus dry the mucous membranes. Hydration is the first step to improve swallowing when taking these medications.

Antineoplastic Agents

These agents affect swallowing mainly through the mechanism of inflammation, sloughing, and occasionally causing infection of the aerodigestive tract mucosa. This effect results in mucositis, stomatitis, pharyngitis, esophagitis, and esophageal ulceration. Common antineoplastic agents are cisplatin and tamoxifen, both used in chemotherapy protocols to treat cancer in various organs.

Vitamins

An overdose of vitamin A causes hypervitaminosis, a condition that includes dermatological, gastric, skeletal, and cerebral and optic nerve edema. Fissures of the lips, dry mouth, and abdominal discomfort can result. A similar stomatitis can result with vitamin E overdose.

Neurological Medications

Anticonvulsants

Phenobarbital is a sedative and anticonvulsant with side effects similar to the tricyclic antidepressants: dry mouth, sweating, hypotension, and tremor. Phenytoin's (Dilantin) adverse effects include central nervous system signs such as ataxia, slurred speech, incoordination, and dystonia. Carbamazepine (Tegretol) is an anticonvulsant used primarily for seizures. Digestive symptoms can also be serious, such as glossitis, stomatitis, and dryness of the mouth.

Anti-Parkinson's Disease Agents

Levodopa may improve all symptoms of Parkinson's disease, including swallowing, but it can cause gastrointestinal discomfort, dyskinesia, and oral dryness.

Antipsychotics

Antipsychotic medications primarily work by dopamine antagonism. Commonly used drugs in this class include haloperidol (Haldol), aripiprazole lauroxil, chlorpromazine (Thorazine), thioridazine (Mellaril), and prochlorperazine (Compazine). These medications can have anticholinergic effects, such as dry mouth, nasal congestion, and hypotension. Patients receiving long-term antipsychotic medications will develop tardive dyskinesia, with symptoms ranging from tongue restlessness, disfiguring choreiform, and/or athetoid movements, leading to significant swallowing and feeding problems.

Life-threatening dysphagia can occur after prolonged neuroleptic therapy. Neuroleptic drugs can induce extrapyramidal symptoms such as **dystonia**, **akathisia**, and **tardive dyskinesia**. Contrast radiography has revealed poor contractions in the upper esophagus, a hypertonic esophageal sphincter, and hypokinesia of the pharyngeal muscles.

Anxiolytics

Significant dysphagia can result from chronic use of benzodiazepines. Reported effects include hypopharyngeal retention, cricopharyngeal incoordination, aspiration, and drooling. Benzodiazepines can inhibit discharges from interneurons in the nucleus of the tractus solitarius or nucleus ambiguus, both of which are critical to the pharyngeal phase of swallowing.

SWALLOWING DISORDERS FOLLOWING RADIATION THERAPY

Dysphagia is a major side effect of treatment for head and neck cancers. The head and neck areas include numerous structures, each with an inherent response to radiation that is largely governed by the presence or absence of mucosa, salivary glands, or specialized organs within that site. Irradiated mucocutaneous tissues demonstrate increased vascular permeability that leads to fibrin deposition, subsequent collagen formation, and eventual fibrosis.

Dysphagia is a common side effect of radiation therapy for all cancers of the upper aerodigestive tract and the head and neck regions. It is further complicated by the effect of surgical procedures that may be done prior to radiation. The etiology of dysphagia following radiation therapy is multifactorial and can be divided into acute and late effects.

> *Acute adverse effects of chemoradiation therapy include dermatitis, pain, loss of energy, xerostomia, mucositis, soft tissue edema, weight loss, impaired taste, voice changes, muscle fibrosis, trismus, and dysphagia. The most common and problematic long-term side effects of chemoradiation therapy include xerostomia, muscle fibrosis, trismus, and dysphagia.*

Due to the impact of long-term dysphagia on quality of life, malnutrition, aspiration, and death, early identification of a swallowing impairment and appropriate intervention is critical.

Irradiation produces mitotic death of the basal cells of the mucosa, as this is a rapidly renewing system. With a standard course of radiation therapy (180–200 cGy/fraction; 5 daily fractions per week for approximately 6 weeks), there is a 2-week delay from the start of therapy before the onset of mucositis.

The acute phase of dysphagia is primarily due to radiation effects on mucosa (erythema, pseudomembranous mucositis, ulceration), taste buds (decreased, altered, or loss of taste acuity), and salivary glands (thickened saliva secondary to decreased serous secretions). These conditions tend to last for several months after the completion of radiation, especially if the dosage exceeds 60 cGy. Acute effects present during and immediately following a course of irradiation, and late effects manifest themselves from several months to as many as 5 to 10 years after completion of radiation therapy.

Late effects of radiation to the head and neck have been examined by Lazarus et al[53] and by Jensen et al.[54] The long-term effects of external beam radiation therapy (XRT) include loss of tongue strength and disruption of the timing of the swallow. Late effects also include injury to salivary glands resulting in **xerostomia** and damage to connective tissue (fibrosis) resulting in **trismus** and poor pharyngeal motility. Video 3–7 shows the effects of inflammation and mucositis several years after XRT.

Late complications involving the mucosa of the upper aerodigestive tract are primarily related to atrophy, manifested by pallor and thinning, submucosal fibrosis, manifested as induration and diminished pliability, and occasionally chronic ulceration and necrosis with resultant exposure of the underlying bone/soft tissue.

In humans, the parotid glands are purely serous, the submandibular glands are made of serous and mucous **acini**, and the minor salivary glands are predominantly mucous secreting. The normal human salivary glands produce approximately 1000 to 1500 cc of saliva per day. The parotid gland accounts for about 60% to 65% of the salivary flow; the submandibular gland contributes 20% to 30% and sublingual glands 2% to 5%. Standard radiotherapy treatment results primarily in injury to the serous acini; thus, patients complain of dry mouth and tongue.

A decrease in the salivary flow can be detected 24 to 48 hours after initiation of standard fractionated irradiation and it continues to decline through the course of therapy. In addition to the decrease in flow, there is increase in viscosity and decreased pH and IgA in saliva. Because the serous acini are primarily affected, the saliva becomes thick, sticky, and ropy, resulting in dry mouth, difficulty with mastication, and swallowing. Most patients are unable to clear these thick secretions. These changes allow for an increased yeast flora of the oral cavity.

Irradiated salivary tissue degenerates after relatively small doses, leading to markedly diminished salivary output. This, in turn, affects the teeth by promoting dental decay, which in turn affects the integrity of the mandible. Details of these changes, including their pathophysiology, clinical syndromes, and potential treatment, are presented by Cooper et al.[55] The dose at which 50% of patients develop xerostomia at 5 years after irradiation was 7000 cGy.[56] Figure 3–11 shows the larynx following XRT for laryngeal cancer. Note the heavy white secretions.

Xerostomia results from permanent injury to the salivary glands. The most effective treatment for

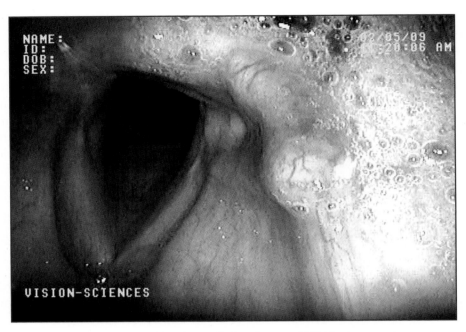

FIGURE 3–11. The larynx following radiation therapy (XRT) for laryngeal cancer.

xerostomia is prevention. Once xerostomia develops, its treatment primarily consists of saliva substitute (water and glycerin mixture) and salivary gland stimulants such as pilocarpine hydrochloride, bromohexine, and anethole-trithione.

Pilocarpine is a cholinergic agonist that simulates the smooth muscle and exocrine glands; it affects the postganglionic cells. This results in increased excretion of saliva and sweat.

Intensity modulated radiation therapy (IMRT) is a method of delivering the radiation dose to specific structures while preserving surrounding structures, specifically the parotid gland. Currently, there is an increase in the use of chemotherapy combined with IMRT to treat head and neck cancers. Evidence now exists that suggests as many as 50% of those treated with IMRT and chemotherapy will have long-term swallowing problems.[57] Of course, the degree of dysphagia is related to dosage and size and location of tumor. Caudell et al identified concurrent chemotherapy, primary tumor site (larynx, hypopharynx, base-of-tongue, or pharyngeal wall), and elderly age as significant clinical factors associated with long-term dysphagia.[58] They defined gastrostomy tube dependence at 12 months, aspiration (trace or frank) seen by modified barium swallow, and/or pharyngo-esophageal stricture with subsequent need for dilation as the primary as the primary causes. They suggest limiting the IMRT dosage to less than 40 cGy for the glottic and supraglottic regions and to less than 55 cGy for the pharyngeal constrictor regions should help to reduce the long-term swallowing problems. Huang et al investigated two groups of patients treated with either standard radiotherapy or IMRT and found late toxicity was significantly less in the IMRT group.[59] They suggest careful monitoring of patients prior to, during, and after treatment to maintain adequate diet in view of the effects of either treatment method.

AUTOIMMUNE DISORDERS AND DISEASES

The diagnosis and treatment of swallowing disorders in patients with autoimmune disorders and diseases is complex and commonly limited by their primary condition or by the other treatments or medications that they may be receiving. Autoimmune conditions often result in dryness, inability to swallow certain types of foods, symptoms of reflux disease, and lack of taste. The role of the speech-language pathologist is to work with the team to manage safe swallowing, support the need to be alert to conditions that have a negative effect on swallowing such as rapid eating and poor bolus preparation, and assure patients that with the correct diet they can remain healthy. Since reflux is a common condition of patients with autoimmune diseases, dietary support should always be part of the treatment plan.

Autoimmune Diseases

Autoimmune diseases are characterized by the production of antibodies that react with host tissue or immune effector T cells that react to self-peptides. Autoimmune diseases may affect swallowing by causing intrinsic obstruction, external compression, abnormal motility, or inadequate lubrication.

Crohn Disease

Crohn disease produces lesions throughout the digestive tract that vary in appearance, often resembling aphthous ulcers or cheilitis. Dysphagia is the most common presenting symptom of esophageal Crohn disease.

Epidermolysis Bullosa

Epidermolysis bullosa is a rare disorder characterized by blistering of the mucosal lining, often elicited by minimal trauma. It has a variable onset and no racial or gender predilection. The oral cavity, pharynx, larynx, and esophagus may be severely affected, resulting in severe dysphagia. Pharyngeal and esophageal webs and/or scarring may be severe, necessitating a gastrostomy or jejunostomy. The disease is often refractory to standard therapy using corticosteroids.

Giant Cell Arteritis

Giant cell arteritis, also known as temporal arteritis, is an inflammatory disorder affecting large- and medium-size vessels. The arteries that originate from the arch of the aorta are the most affected. Pharyn-

geal, tongue, or jaw claudication may occur when the ascending pharyngeal, lingual, deep temporal, or mesenteric arteries are affected. Systemic corticosteroids often resolve these all within 1 to 2 weeks.

Mixed Connective-Tissue Disease

Mixed connective-tissue disease **(MCTD)** is characterized by clinical findings that may be found in progressive systemic sclerosis, systemic lupus erythematous, and polymyositis/dermatomyositis. Similarly, the swallowing disorders described under each of these disorders can be part of MCTD.

Esophageal motility is severely affected and the majority of the patients have little or no peristalsis, or they have low amplitude peristalsis contributing to gastroesophageal reflux disease. Heartburn and dysphagia are present in up to 50% of the patients with MCTD. The treatment of GERD in these patients may reduce the dysphagia.

Myositis

Polymyositis and dermatomyositis are characterized by inflammation of the skeletal muscle. Thus, muscles of the pharynx are often affected while the esophageal smooth muscle is spared. Endoscopic evaluation of swallowing with transnasal flexible laryngoscopy (TFL) may reveal prominence of the cricopharyngeus muscle, decreased epiglottis tilt, and moderate to severe residue in the pharynx, which fails to pass into the esophageal inlet even with multiple swallows. Two-thirds of these patients have demonstrable delayed esophageal transit. Polymyositis and dermatomyositis are treated with corticosteroids.

Pemphigus Vulgaris

Pemphigus vulgaris is a rare, chronic intraepidermal bullous disease. Blisters most commonly develop on the soft palate but can occur anywhere on the oral cavity. Painful ulcerations that can become infected follow the ruptured blisters. Ulcerations heal by secondary intention, often leading to scarring. Distal involvement of the pharynx, larynx, and esophagus is possible and may account for the dysphagia noted by some patients.

Ocular Cicatricial Pemphigoid

Ocular cicatricial pemphigoid is a chronic blistering disease that affects the oral mucosa in almost all cases. Typical lesions are characterized by erosion of the gingiva and buccal mucosa that usually are not as painful as those associated with pemphigus vulgaris. As the targeted proteins are found in the basement-membrane zone, the lesions heal with submucosa scarring. Treatment of ocular cicatricial pemphigoid is primarily with corticosteroids.

Rheumatoid Arthritis

Rheumatoid arthritis (RA) is a chronic, relapsing inflammatory arthritis, usually affecting multiple diarthrodial joints with a varying degree of systemic involvement. The female-to-male ratio is 3:1.

Rheumatoid arthritis is associated with xerostomia, temporomandibular joint (TMJ) syndrome, a decrease in the amplitude of the peristaltic pressure complex in the proximal, striated part of the esophagus, as well as from cervical spine arthritic disease, all of which cause or contribute to swallowing problems. Rheumatic laryngeal involvement can result in cricoarytenoid joint fixation. Objective functional testing is necessary to determine the contributions of the oral phase and pharyngeal phase to the swallowing disorder. Patients may benefit from a modified barium swallow to identify the oral phase components amenable to therapeutic exercises.

Treatment of the dysphagia is focused on hydration and artificial saliva and/or pilocarpine for the xerostomia. TMJ dysfunction (ie, trismus, mastication problems) is treated with nonsteroidal anti-inflammatory agents and exercises with mechanical devices. Laryngeal closure exercises may also be useful. These are further described in Chapter 6.

Sarcoidosis

Sarcoidosis is a chronic systemic disorder presumed to have an autoimmune pathogenesis. Sarcoidosis may cause laryngeal lesions, extrinsic compression of the esophagus by mediastina adenopathy, and esophageal dysmotility due to myopathy, infiltration of Auerbach plexus, or granulomatous infiltration of the esophageal wall, which may produce long esophageal strictures.

Scleroderma

Systemic sclerosis (**scleroderma**) is a disorder characterized by progressive fibrosis and vascular changes. The most common and the earliest symptom in people with progressive systemic sclerosis is Raynaud disease, characterized by pallor and sweating of the fingers or hands that progresses to cyanosis and pain. Dysphagia, which is the second most common symptom of this disorder, is usually first noticed while swallowing solids.

Dysphagia is most often due to poor motility through the inferior two-thirds of the esophagus. The process starts affecting the Auerbach plexus, which coordinates the smooth muscle. This is followed by a myopathy, which is then followed by fibrosis and strictures secondary to the effects of gastroesophageal reflux.

The dysphagia can be minimized by adequate chewing and by reducing the bolus size. Esophageal motility can be improved by prokinetic agents, which, other than Reglan, were taken off the market several years ago.

Sjögren Disease

Sjögren disease includes dry eyes and mouth. Xerostomia, oral pain, **glossodynia**, and **dysgusia** are prominent features of the syndromes. Xerostomia also increases the incidence of GERD, because it decreases the ability of the esophagus to clear gastric refluxate, and the bicarbonate antacid effect of saliva is diminished.

Treatment of xerostomia is often palliative and includes saliva preparations, pilocarpine, antacids, and H_2 blockers. Diet modification to a mixed thickened and slippery combination of foods also is helpful.

Systemic Lupus Erythematous

Systemic lupus erythematous is an inflammatory disorder that is associated with a variety of autoantibodies against many different tissue components.

The vast majority of patients with systemic lupus erythematous do not experience dysphagia and have normal esophageal transit studies. Dysphagia and/or chest pain is most often attributed to esophageal dysmotility associated with lower esophageal sphincter insufficiency and thus gastroesophageal reflux disease (GERD).

Wegener Granulomatosis

Wegener granulomatosis is characterized by a granulomatous arteritis involving the upper and lower respiratory tracts, a progressive glomerulonephritis, and extra respiratory symptoms attributable to systemic small-vessel arteritis. Wegener granulomatosis often affects the hard and soft palate and may lead to extensive ulceration, oronasal fistulas, and velopharyngeal insufficiency.

SUMMARY

A brief summary of the phases of swallowing along with the critical cranial nerve involvement at these phases is summarized here:

Oral Phase

Retention and Mastication—retention of the bolus in the mouth (CN VII)

Sensation—feel, taste, temperature (CN VII, CN IX)

Salivation—needed to form the bolus (CN VII, CN IX)

Oral and Lingual Transit—Cranial nerves operating motorically (CN X, CN XII)

Pharyngeal Phase

Sensation—perception of bolus at posterior pharyngeal wall (CN IX)

Transit—oral cavity to pharynx (CN IX, CN X, CN XII)

Transit—pharynx to esophagus (CN X, CN XII)

Esophageal Phase

Sensation—perception of bolus at or below the cricopharyngeus muscle (CN X)

Transit—to lower esophagus (CN X)

Reverse Transit (regurgitation)—UES and LES pressure irregularities

The conditions and diseases encountered by the members of the swallowing rehabilitation team extend from occasional coughing or choking while eating to obvious debilitating diseases such as esophageal cancer or Parkinson's disease. The clinician should not be fooled, however, into thinking that a patient complaining of occasional choking does not have a significant swallowing disorder or a disease or disorder that is being reflected in its early stages. In this chapter, conditions and diseases that give rise to swallowing disorders or that foretell future dysphagia are reviewed. It should be pointed out that causal relationships are not the hallmark of many swallowing disorders. Rather, the swallowing disorder may develop shortly after the disease or disorder or may develop long after a condition, such as a swallowing disorder years after radiation therapy to the larynx or pharynx. The astute clinician, regardless of his or her medical or paramedical specialty, should work as a team member with other clinicians who are also treating the patient. In some cases, this may be the general practitioner, whereas in other cases, the team may include an entire surgical or neurological group.

DISCUSSION QUESTIONS

1. Discuss the possible complications of treating a patient with a swallowing disorder who has (a) advanced Parkinson's disease or (b) advanced ALS. What are some of the differences in these patients that affect treatment?
2. The current literature on reflux disease suggests that both GERD and LPRD may contribute to swallowing disorders. Why

is it important for the speech-language pathologist to understand the importance of GERD and LPRD as they relate to the treatment of swallowing disorders? See, for example, Fletcher KC, Goutte M, Slaughter JC, Garrett CG, Vaezi MF. Significance and degree of reflux in patients with primary extraesophageal symptoms. *Laryngoscope.* 2011 Dec;121(12):2561–2565; and Altman KW, Prufer N, Vaezi MF. The challenge of protocols for reflux disease: a review and development of a critical pathway. *Otolaryngol Head Neck Surg.* 2011 Jul;145(1):7–14 or Milan, MR. Belafsky, PC. Cough and swallowing dysfunction. *Otolaryngol Clin North Am.* 2010;43(1):35–42.

STUDY QUESTIONS

1. Aspiration occurs when
   A. Food or liquid remains at the entrance to the laryngeal inlet
   B. Food or liquid is regurgitated up from the esophagus into the oral cavity
   C. Food or liquid enters the airway below the vocal folds
   D. The patient coughs following drinking or eating

2. Aspiration pneumonia
   A. Is a swallowing disorder resulting from food or liquid residing in the trachea or lungs
   B. Is a condition of the elderly who recently had a CVA and continued to be fed orally without assessment of his or her swallowing status
   C. Is a condition in which a chemical inflammation or bacterial infection results in entry of foreign materials into the bronchi of the lungs
   D. Is diagnosed with a modified barium swallow or fiberoptic endoscopic evaluation of swallowing test (FEEST)

3. The swallowing problems associated with cerebrovascular accidents (CVAs)
   A. Usually end shortly after the acute period has passed
   B. May occur during the first 24 hours after a CVA or may develop weeks or even months after the occurrence
   C. Are generally not life threatening if the CVA is on the right side of the brain
   D. Are primarily dangerous if the patient is also elderly

4. Autoimmune disorders of swallowing are generally due to
   A. Obstruction along the passageway of food or liquid
   B. Inflammation within the esophagus causing regurgitation or choking
   C. Inadequate lubrication for the normal passage of food or liquid from the oropharynx to the hypopharynx
   D. All of the above

5. Gastroesophageal reflux disease and laryngo-pharyngeal reflux disease are
   A. Inflammatory disorders of the lower esophagus
   B. Inflammatory disorders of the esophagus that affect structures within and above the esophagus
   C. Not true swallowing disorders because they rarely cause aspiration or aspiration pneumonia
   D. Usually exist in patients with dysphagia but rarely require specialized treatment

REFERENCES

1. Barczi SR, Sullivan PA, Robbins J. How should dysphagia care of older adults differ? Establishing optimal practice patterns. *Semin Speech Lang.* 2000;21:347–361.
2. World Health Organization (WHO). Ageing and life course. 2013. http://www.who.int/ageing/en.
3. Wang X, You G, Chen H, Cai X. Clinical course and cause of death in elderly patients with idiopathic Parkinson's disease. *Chinese Medical Journal (English ed.).* 2002;115:1409–1411.

4. Ludlow CL. Central nervous system control of voice and swallowing. *J Clin Neurophysiol.* 2015 Aug;32(4):294–230.

5. Ludlow CL. Central nervous system control of interactions between vocalization and respiration in mammals. *Head Neck.* 2011 Oct; 33(suppl 1):S21–S25.

6. Martin-Harris B, Brodsky MB, Michel Y, Ford CL, Walters B, Heffner J. Breathing and swallowing dynamics across the adult lifespan. *Arch Otolaryngol Head Neck Surg.* 2005;131(9):762–770.

7. Kendall KA, Leonard RJ, McKenzie S. Airway protection: evaluation with videofluoroscopy. *Dysphagia.* 2004;19:65–70.

8. Vu KN, Day TA, Gillespie MB, et al. Proximal esophageal stenosis in head and neck cancer patients after total laryngectomy and radiation. *ORL.* 2008;70:229–235.

9. Nguyen NP, Frank C, Moltz CC, et al. Long term aspiration following treatment for head and neck cancer. *Oncology.* 2008;74:25–30.

10. Mendelsohn N. New concepts in dysphagia management. *J Otolaryngol.* 1993;22 (suppl 1):9–10.

11. Krishna P. Aspiration pneumonia. Ch. 53. In: Carrau RL, Murry T, Howell R, eds. *Comprehensive Management of Swallowing Disorders.* San Diego, CA: Plural Publishing; 2015:499–508.

12. Falestiny MN, Yu VL. Aspiration pneumonia. Ch. 55. In: Carrau RL, Murry T, eds. *Comprehensive Management of Swallowing Disorders.* San Diego, CA: Plural Publishing; 2006:383–387.

13. Leder SB, Suiter DM, Lisitano Warner H. Answering orientation questions and following single-step verbal commands: effect on aspiration status. *Dysphagia.* 2009 Sep;24(3):290–295.

14. White AC, O'Connor HH, Kirby K. Prolonged mechanical ventilation: review of care settings and an update on professional reimbursement. *Chest.* 2008;133:539–545.

15. Botoman VA, Hanft KL, Breno SM, et al. Prospective controlled evaluation of pH testing, laryngoscopy and laryngopharyngeal sensory testing (LPST) shows a specific post inter-arytenoid neuropathy in proximal GERD (P-GERD). LPST improves laryngoscopy diagnostic yield in P-GERD. *Am J Gastroenterol.* 2002;97(9 suppl):S11–S12.

16. Huang CH, Tsai JS, Chen IW, Hsu BR, Huang MJ, Huang YY. Risk factors for in-hospital mortality in patients with type 2 diabetes complicated by community-acquired *Klebsiella pneumoniae* bacteremia. *J Formos Med Assoc.* 2015 Aug 24. doi:10.1016/j.jfma.2015.07.011.

17. Altman KW, Yu G, Schaefer SD. Consequence of dysphagia in the hospitalized patient: impact on prognosis and hospital resources. *Arch Otolaryngol Head Neck Surg.* 2010;136(8):784–789.

18. Ludlow C. Recent advances in laryngeal sensorimotor control for voice, speech and swallowing. *Curr Opin Otolaryngol Head Neck Surg.* 2004;12:160–165.

19. Kunibi I, Nonaka S, Katada A. The neuronal circuit of augmenting effects on intrinsic laryngeal muscle activities induced by nasal air jet stimulation in de-cerebrate cats. *Brain Res.* 2003;978:83–90.

20. Perlman A, Shultze-Delrieu K. *Deglutition and Its Disorders.* San Diego, CA: Singular Publishing; 1997:352–359.

21. Coyle JL, Rosenbek JC, Chignell KA. Pathophysiology of neurogenic oropharyngeal dysphagia. In: Carrau RL, Murry T, eds. *Comprehensive Management of Swallowing Disorders.* 2nd ed. San Diego, CA: Plural Publishing; 2015:93–108.

22. Ruoppolo G, Schettino I, Frasca V, et al. Dysphagia in amyotrophic lateral sclerosis: prevalence and clinical findings. *Acta Neurol Scand.* 2013;128:397–401.

23. Siddique T, Donkervoort S. Amyotrophic lateral sclerosis overview. In: Pagon RA, Bird TC, Dolan CR, Stephens K. *GeneReviews* [Internet]. Seattle: University of Washington. Updated July 28, 2007.

24. Yorkston KM, Strand E, Miller R, Hillel A, Smith K. Speech deterioration in amyotrophic lateral sclerosis: implications for the timing of intervention. *J Med Speech-Lang Pathol.* 1993;1:35–46.

25. Higo R, Tayama N, Nito T. Longitudinal analysis of progression of dysphagia in amyotrophic lateral sclerosis. *Auris Nasus Larynx.* 2004 Sep;31(3):247–254.

26. Leder SB, Novella S, Patwa H. Use of fiberoptic endoscopic evaluation of swallowing in patients with amyotrophic lateral sclerosis. *Dysphagia.* 2004;19:177–181.

27. Robbins J, Levine RL, Maser A, Rosenbek JC, Kempster JB. Swallowing after unilateral stroke of the cerebral cortex. *Arch Phys Med Rehabil.* 1993;74:1295–1300.

28. DePippo KL, Holas MA, Reding MJ. The Burke Dysphagia Screening Test: validation of its use in patients with stroke. *Arch Phys Med Rehabil.* 1994;75:1284–1286.

29. Sapir S, Ramig L, Fox C. Speech and swallowing disorders in Parkinson's disease. *Curr Opin Otolaryngol Head Neck Surg.* 2008 Jun;16(3):205–210.

30. Plowman-Prine EK, Sapienza CM, Okun MS, et al. The relationship between quality of life and swallowing in Parkinson's disease. *Mov Disord.* 2009 Jul 15;24(9):1352–1358.

31. Santos-García D, de la Fuente-Fernández R. Impact of non-motor symptoms on health-related and perceived quality of life in Parkinson's disease. *J Neurol Sci.* 2013 Sep 15;332(1-2):136–140.

32. Mahler LA, Ramig LO, Fox C. Evidence-based treatment of voice and speech disorders in Parkinson's disease. *Curr Opin Otolaryngol Head Neck Surg.* 2015 Jun;23(3):209–215.

33. Miller N, Noble E, Jones D, Burn D. Hard to swallow: dysphagia in Parkinson's disease. *Age Aging.* 2006;35:6614–6618.

34. Sebastian S, Nair PG, Thomas P, Tyagi AK. Oropharyngeal dysphagia: neurogenic etiology and manifestation. *Indian J Otolaryngol Head Neck Surg.* 2015 Mar;67(suppl 1):119–123. doi:10.1007/s12070-014-0794-3. Epub 2014 Nov 9.

35. Webb TS, Whitehead CR, Wells T, Gore K, Otte N. Neurologically-related sequaelae associated with mild traumatic brain injury. *Informa Healthcare.* 2014; Dec 26. doi:10.3 3109/02699052.2014.989904.

36. Macht M, White SD, Moss M. Swallowing dysfunction after critical illness. *Chest.* 2014;146(6):1681–1689.

37. Simonian MA, Goldbert AN. Swallowing disorders in the critical care patient. In: Carrau RL, Murry T, Howell R, eds. *Comprehensive Management of Swallowing Disorders.* 2nd ed. San Diego, CA: Singular Publishing; 2015: 363–369.

38. Ferri L, Lee JK, Law S, Wong KH, Kwok KF, Wong J. Management of spontaneous perforation of esophageal cancer with covered self expanding metallic stents. *Dis Esophagus.* 2005;18(1):67–69.

39. Houghton A, Mason R, Allen A, McColl I. Nd:YAG laser treatment in the palliation of advanced oesophageal malignancy. *Br J Surg.* 1989 Sep;76(9):912–913.

40. Mognissi K, Dixon K. Photodynamic therapy (PDT) in esophageal cancer: a surgical view of its indications based on 14 years experience. *Technol Cancer Res Treat.* 2003 Aug;2(4):319–326.

41. http://www.mayoclinic.org/tests-procedures/imrt/

42. Belafsky P, Rees CJ. Esophageal phase dysphagia. In: Leonard R, Kendall K, eds. *Dysphagia Assessment and Treatment Planning: A Team Approach.* 2nd ed. San Diego, CA: Plural Publishing; 1997:63–65.

43. Weissman JL. Chapter 11. In: Carrau RL, Murry T, eds. *Comprehensive Management of Swallowing Disorders.* San Diego, CA: Singular Publishing; 1999:73, Figure 11–12.

44. Padda S, Young MA. The radiographic evaluation of dysphagia. In: Carrau R, Murry T, eds. *Comprehensive Management of Swallowing Disorders.* San Diego, CA: Plural Publishing; 1999:192, Figure 27–4.

45. Aviv JE, Liu H, Parides M, Kaplan ST, Close LG. Laryngopharyngeal sensory deficits in patients with laryngopharyngeal reflux and dysphagia. *Ann Otol Rhinol Laryngol.* 2000;109:1000–1006.

46. Murry T, Wasserman T, Carrau RL, Castillo B. Injection of botulinum toxin A for the treatment of dysfunction of the upper esophageal sphincter. *Am J Otolaryngol.* 2005; 26:157–162.

47. Belafsky P, Postma GN, Amin MR, Koufman JA. Symptoms and findings of laryngopharyngeal reflux. *Ear Nose Throat J.* 2002; 81(9 suppl 2):10–13.

48. Belafsky PC, Postma GN, Koufman JA. The validity and reliability of the reflux finding score (RFS). *Laryngoscope.* 2001;111:1313–1317.

49. Levy B, Young MA. Pathophysiology of swallowing and gastroesophageal reflux. In: Carrau RL, Murry T, eds. *Comprehensive Management of Swallowing Disorders.* San Diego, CA: Singular Publishing; 1999:175–186.

50. Contini S, Scarpignato C. Caustic injury of the upper gastrointestinal tract: a comprehensive review. *World J Gastroenterol.* 2013 Jul 7;19(25):3918–3930.

51. Cabral C, Chirica M, de Chaisemartin C, et al. Caustic injuries of the upper digestive tract: a population observational study. *Surg Endosc.* 2012 Jan;26(1):214–221.

52. Kochar B, Dellon ES. Management of proton pup inhibitor responsive-esophageal eosinophilia and eosinophilic esophagitis: controversies in treatment approaches. *Expert Rev Gastroenterol Hepatol.* 2015;9:1359–1369.

53. Lazarus C, Logemann JA, Pauloski BR, et al. Effects of radiotherapy with or without chemotherapy on tongue strength and swallowing in patients with oral cancer. *Head Neck.* 2007;29:632–637.

54. Jensen K, Lambertsen K, Grau C. Late swallowing dysfunction and dysphagia after radiotherapy for pharynx cancer; frequency, intensity and correlation with dose and volume parameters. *Radiother Oncol.* 2007;85(1):74–82.

55. Cooper JS, Fu K, Marks J, Silverman S. Late effects of radiation therapy in the head and neck. *Int J Radiat Oncol Biol Phys.* 1995;31(5):1141–1164.

56. Schindler A, Denaro N, Russi EG, et al. Dysphagia in head and neck cancer patients treated with radiotherapy and systemic therapies: literature review and consensus. *Crit Rev Oncol Hematol.* 2015;9(2):372–384.

57. Forastiere AA, Goepfert H, Maor M, et al. Concurrent chemotherapy and radiotherapy for organ preservation in advanced laryngeal cancer. *N Engl J Med.* 2003;349: 2091–2098.

58. Caudell JJ, Schaner PE, Meredith RF, et al. Factors associated with long-term dysphagia after definitive radiotherapy for locally advanced head-and-neck cancer. *Int J Radiat Oncol Biol Phys.* 2009;73:410–415.

59. Huang TL, Chien CY, Tsai WL, et al. Long-term late toxicities and quality of life for survivors of nasopharyngeal carcinoma treated with intensity-modulated radiotherapy versus non-intensity-modulated radiotherapy. *Head Neck.* 2015 Jun 3. doi:10.1002/hed.24150.

Swallowing Disorders Following Surgical Treatments

A Look at Chapter 4

In this chapter, we look at the conditions and diseases of the head and neck that require surgery and that leave the patient with a swallowing disability. Conditions such as anterior spine surgery initially limit the patient's ability to use certain postures to aid swallowing. Other conditions such as head and neck cancers require organs or parts of organs to be removed or treated with radiation or chemotherapy. All of these conditions may affect the ability to swallow normally and some involve nerve damage as a result of treating the disease. Clinicians must be aware of the surgical changes that take place in treating this conditions and disease, know the function of the remaining organs following surgery, and appreciate the neurological changes accompanying surgery and medical treatments.

INTRODUCTION

Virtually all patients requiring surgery for treatment of diseases and disorders in the region of the head and neck or other disorders of the upper respiratory tract and the esophagus will experience some degree of dysphagia in the perioperative or postoperative recovery process. Dysphagia may be short term, requiring neither special tests nor the implementation of diet modifications, or long term due to severe nerve damage or tissue destruction, requiring the involvement of the entire dysphagia rehabilitation team. For all patients being treated for a disease involving organs of swallowing, even those who are deemed safe to swallow, a clinical bedside assessment should be done and documented. The finding of a delayed swallow or the patient reporting difficulty swallowing certain foods or liquids should be noted and further evaluation should be planned. A report of the CSE should be part of the discharge planning, and when in doubt, a follow-up assessment should be arranged.

When any one or more of the swallowing valves does not work due to injury or proper innervation,

swallowing will be affected. Surgery, radiation, or a combination of the two can lead to minor swallowing difficulty or life-threatening aspiration. This chapter reviews the major swallowing problems after surgery to the head and neck regions.

ANTERIOR CERVICAL SPINAL SURGERY (ACSS)

Anterior cervical spine surgery (ACSS) is becoming more common with dysphagia as both a short-term and long-term side effect. This surgery is done for patients who have undergone some type of trauma such as spinal cord compression or for other conditions such as arthritis. Prior to the surgery, the patient often reports numbness in the hands and/ or feet. The surgical preference for treating these conditions is an anterior approach to the spinal cord to avoid further damage to the spinal cord. Surgeons approach the spinal cord anteriorly, using a cervical incision to mobilize the laryngotracheal complex away from the great vessels of the neck to reach the prevertebral space to allow inspection and repair of the cervical spine.

Postoperative dysphagia is found in almost all patients who undergo ACSS.[1] The dysphagia is often of short duration, but it can persist beyond 1 year in as many as 23% of patients.[2] A report by Hart et al[3] found that dysphagia was the most frequent complication of surgical spine surgery, accounting for 46% of the postoperative complications. Many of the complications reported were minor; however, percutaneous endogastrostomy (PEG) feeding was required in 15% of patients. Long-term vocal fold paralysis requiring surgical correction was found in 7% of the patients.

There are several possible etiologies for dysphagia following ACSS in addition to vocal fold paralysis. These are shown in Table 4–1. First, the patient may have dysphagia preoperatively, which may worsen after the surgery. Thus, many surgeons are now seeing that there is a need for assessment of the swallow function prior to ACSS.

Second, because of postoperative swelling, the patient may become more aware of symptoms immediately after the surgery, leading to fear of swallow-

TABLE 4–1. Etiological Factors for Postoperative Dysphagia After Anterior Cervical Spine Surgery

Pain	Muscles of Tongue, Pharynx/Larynx (post-ET)
Edema	Tongue, pharynx, larynx, neck
Hematoma	Retropharyngeal space
Infection/abscess	Retropharyngeal space
Interruption of motor innervations	Ansa cervicalis RLN Pharyngeal plexus
Interruption of neuromuscular function	Anterior tongue Base of tongue
Injury to sensory innervations	SLN Pharyngeal plexus
Mechanical factors	Perforation Bulky reconstruction plate Adhesions—posterior pharyngeal wall
Velopharyngeal incompetence	Palatal shortening Wound breakdown

Abbreviations: ET, endotracheal tube; RLN, recurrent laryngeal nerve; SLN, superior laryngeal nerve.

ing/choking. Additionally, neurological damage may result from direct trauma or retraction trauma to the recurrent laryngeal nerve, superior laryngeal nerve, or glossopharyngeal nerve.

> *A major complication is airway edema, reducing sensation and the ability to manage the bolus in the oral or oropharyngeal stage of swallowing.[4]*

A list of common complications identified by Dornbos et al[5] found 100% of ACSS patients experience at least 1 month of dysphagia following surgery and as many as 11% with dysphagia lasting up to 1 year. These are summarized in Table 4–2.

A host of surgical complications, side effects, and sequalae that may affect deglutition include

TABLE 4–2. Complications of Anterior Cervical Spine Surgery Approach[a]

Early dysphagia (≤1 month): 100%
Prolonged dysphagia (≥12 months): 5%–11%
Hematoma: 1%–3%
RLN injury: 1%–16%
SLN injury: 1%
Esophageal perforation: 0.2%–0.9%

Abbreviations: RLN, recurrent laryngeal nerve; SLN, superior laryngeal nerve.

[a]Adapted from Dornbos, Seim, and Mendel.[5]

edema, hematoma formation, infection, and denervation. The following are the most common:

1. Prevertebral soft tissue swelling and associated reduced epiglottis inversion may result in dysphagia following ACSS. Swelling of the posterior pharyngeal wall or a prevertebral **hematoma** may cause displacement of the pharyngeal wall toward the epiglottis, preventing the epiglottis from inverting. This causes a transient obstruction that traps the bolus, resulting in residue at the valleculae and piriform sinuses.

2. Hypertonicity of the upper esophageal sphincter (UES), as diagnosed by manometry, results in dysphagia following ACSS. Hypertonicity of the UES may prevent passage of the bolus into the esophagus, resulting in pharyngeal residue. It may be caused by direct inflammation to the muscle caused by retraction or dissection or by parasympathetic (vagal) denervation. Hypertonicity of the UES may be secondary to gastroesophageal reflux disease (GERD). This should also be ruled out prior to surgery or treated with medication and an anti-reflux diet.

3. Esophageal perforation is a rare but serious cause of dysphagia following ACSS (approximately 1 in 500). A perforation often is not recognized until the patient develops an abscess or tracheoesophageal fistula in the immediate postoperative period.

4. Size and positioning of the bone graft and/or plate during ACSS must be optimal so there is not impingement on or compression of the posterior pharyngeal wall. Use of bone grafts or plates that produce a bulge of the posterior pharyngeal wall may lead to dysphagia or to the sensation that the bolus is not passing into the lower esophagus but remaining in the laryngopharynx or upper esophagus.

5. Screw or plate displacement or extrusion following ACSS also may result in dysphagia. This may not be readily noticed if the screw loosens slowly. When dysphagia occurs some time after surgery, a loose or loosening screw must be considered. Repeating the surgical procedure and removing or replacing the screw corrects this.

In some cases, dysphagia after ACSS can be addressed immediately with diet modification, and no long-term treatment is necessary. The assessment process ultimately may lead to long-term treatments, which are discussed in Chapter 6. Wang et al reported a detailed analysis of complications and mortality associated with cervical spine surgery in the United States in 2008.[6]

> *Wang et al found that complications increased according to age of the patient, posterior fusion, surgery related to cervical spondylosis and other spine degenerative diseases, and combined anterior/posterior procedures.*

Short-term effects were seen in almost all of the 932,000 patients whose hospital discharge records were reviewed by Wang et al.[6] The highest morbidity and mortality were found immediately following posterior procedures. Dysphagia was the most common short-term and long-term complication, regardless of the patient's age, type of surgery, or preoperative diagnosis.

A recent study by Joaquim et al reviewed the potential preventative measures for dysphagia following ACSS.[2] Speech-language pathologists (SLPs) working with patients following ACSS must be aware that certain postural adjustments like the chin tuck maneuver or the head turned to one side to facilitate a swallow may not be possible. The SLP should review the operative report and x-rays if available to know what postures or maneuvers must be avoided.

NEOPLASMS

Neoplasia causes distortion, obstruction, reduced mobility, or neuromuscular and sensory dysfunction of the passageways in upper aerodigestive tract and can affect swallowing at any place along the way.

Consider the act of swallowing as a bolus passing through a series of valves. The valves in this order are

Lip closure

Anterior tongue

Posterior tongue

Palate

Velopharyngeal contact

Larynx

Cricopharyngeus sphincter

Each valve can be the sole basis of the swallowing problem or the valves may fail to interact appropriately or timely to cause the problem to be complex.

Exophytic Tumors

Exophytic tumors interfere with swallowing principally by distorting or obstructing the aerodigestive tract. Tumors with an infiltrating growth pattern may cause reduced mobility or fixation of the tongue, soft palate, pharynx, or larynx. Extrinsic tumors may lead to obstruction or fixation and with that may impinge on various cranial nerves. Intrinsic tumors are primarily compressive; however, they may also lead to disruption of the swallow by restricting blouse flow. Table 4–3 lists the common physiologic changes that occur following intrinsic and extrinsic tumors.

Tumors also affect swallowing by interfering with the afferent fibers (sensory input) from the

TABLE 4–3. Pathophysiology of Swallowing in Accordance With Tumor Origin and Growth Pattern

Tumor	Swallowing Pathophysiology
Intrinsic tumor	
Exophytic growth	Obstruction
	Distortion
	Anesthesia/hypesthesia
Infiltrating growth	Fixation
	Pain
	Trismus
	Cranial nerve deficits
Extrinsic tumor	
	Compression
	☐ Obstruction
	☐ Distortion
	Cranial nerve deficits
	Fixation

mucosa of the upper aerodigestive tract by invasion and destruction of mucosal nerve endings, or sensory nerves such as the trigeminal (V), glossopharyngeal (IX), and vagus (X) cranial nerves and their branches.

Neoplasms of the floor of the mouth, tongue, or buccal mucosa may by mass effect or by restricting mobility of the tongue and floor of the mouth impair a patient's ability to interpose food between the teeth. Tumor invasion of the dorsum of the tongue or involvement of the lingual nerve (CN V) may affect sensory input causing premature spillage of the bolus into the pharynx and, consequently, aspiration.

Tumors of the pharynx may cause an adynamic segment that interferes with peristalsis or laryngeal elevation or may cause mechanical obstruction. Tumor invading or destroying the larynx may cause either an incompetent laryngeal sphincter or sensory denervation of the larynx.

HEAD AND NECK SURGERY

Improved head and neck surgery combined with radiotherapy and/or chemotherapy for cancers in the head and neck organs have improved the rate and length of survival. Treatments combined with chemotherapy are intense, and with these treatments, there is an increase of early and late toxicities leading to reduction in tissue mobility. In the past, dysphagia was an underestimated symptom in head and neck patients. However, in the past 20 years, there is increasing interest in treating dysphagia following medical and surgical cancer treatment to improve quality of life, nutrition status, and early discharge from surgery. When dysphagia is a complication of the treatment for head and neck cancer, there is generally increased malnutrition, dehydration, aspiration, and pneumonia.

Issues contributing to the dysphagia include loss of or partial loss of swallowing organs, scar formation, and loss of motor control and sensation. All these factors contribute to the presence of dysphagia in the postoperative period. In addition, many of these patients require reconstruction with insensate tissue flaps that can result in incoordination of the swallowing mechanism or even cause mechanical obstruction or diversion of the bolus into the airway. In general, aspiration for liquids varies from 12% to 50%, and is higher after oropharyngeal resection. Postoperative radiotherapy increases swallow function in the groups reviewed.[2,5,7] In Chapter 7 various swallowing problems and treatment options will be outlined.

Lip Surgery and Floor of the Mouth Surgery

Table 4–4 lists the causes of abnormal oral phase swallowing related specifically to surgical resection of the lip, floor of the mouth, palate, or mandible. It should be kept in mind that there is not a direct correlation between surgery in one area and a specific dysphagia problem as evidenced from the information seen in Table 4–4. However, identification of dysphagia after surgery must begin with the assessment of the site affected by surgery. It should be noted that two-thirds of patients with head and neck cancer have dysphagia at the time of their diagnosis. Table 4–5 summarizes the common findings of dysphagia after oropharyngeal resection.

TABLE 4–4. Causes of Abnormal Oral Phase Swallowing After Head and Neck Surgery

Loss of oral sphincter
  a. Resection of lip
  b. Poor reapproximation of orbicularis oris
  c. Marginal mandibular and lingual nerve section

Dental extractions

Floor of mouth resection
  a. Loss of glossoalveolar sulcus
  b. Tethering of anterior tongue

Tongue resection   a. Improper bolus preparation

Hard palate resection
  a. Loss of oronasal separation
  b. Nasal regurgitation

Mandibulectomy
  a. Loss of dentition
  b. Altered oral sphincter

TABLE 4–5. Dysphagia After Oropharyngeal Resection

Soft palate
  a. Loss of oropharyngeal suction pump
  b. Velopharyngeal insufficiency

Tonsil   a. Altered mobility of lateral pharyngeal wall

Tongue base
  a. Loss of laryngeal protection
  b. Loss of sensation
  c. Loss of laryngeal elevation

In 2009, Kreech et al reported on a systematic review of the speech and swallowing problems following oral and oropharyngeal cancer.[7]

> *Kreech et al found that speech production in patients 1 year after treatment (surgery) was impaired. Swallowing, which was often found to be abnormal before surgery, was even more severely compromised after treatment.*

Lip Surgery

The orbicularisoris muscle is crucial to the sphincteric function of the lips. This muscle is divided during lip-splitting procedures and must be carefully reapproximated during closure to restore function. The loss of lower lip sensation secondary to mental nerve injury makes sphincteric control difficult if not impossible. Lip resection may hinder swallowing by creating difficulty in getting food into the mouth. Motor denervation of the lower lip secondary to sacrifice of the marginal mandibular nerve often manifests itself as loss of sphincteric control, resulting in drooling.

Floor of the Mouth Surgery

The floor of the mouth acts as a sulcus for saliva and food particles that aids in the preparation and direction of the bolus. When obliterated by surgery, the lack of this sulcus and the loss of mobility of the anterior tongue become a major impairment during the preparation of the food bolus. To preserve sensation in the tongue, all efforts should be made to protect the lingual nerve. Video 4–1 shows a videofluoroscopic study with the residue of food in the mouth after each swallow. The patient is unaware of the bolus and moves on to the next one which also is a partial swallow with residue.

Few reports have provided specific long-term swallowing disorders other than loss of floor of the mouth or anterior tongue limit one's ability to transfer food posteriorly. Sessions et al[8] suggest that the patient be followed closely for 5 years for signs of metastatic disease since tumors in this area tend to spread to lymph nodes. The SLP who monitors the swallowing problem in these patients for 5 years may be the most appropriate for making significant observations from the periodic assessments.

Surgery of the Tongue

Following partial glossectomy surgery, near normal swallowing and normal speech can be predicted if the patient can protrude the tongue past the sublabial crease. Small defects of the mobile tongue are repaired primarily. Large defects, however, lead to the loss of tongue driving force and inability to propel the bolus posteriorly. The bolus is often improperly prepared and, due to the lack of proper control, may be presented to the oropharynx prematurely, or the patient may not be able to drive the bolus back effectively, requiring an extension of the head to move the bolus by gravity. Recently, Son et al[9] reported on the reasons for dysphagia in tongue cancer patients. These included:

Inadequate tongue control

Inadequate chewing

Delayed oral transit time

Aspiration

Penetration

Piriform residue

Inadequate laryngeal elevation

The major risk factors for aspiration in their group of 133 tongue cancer patients were male gender, extensive tumor resection, a high nodal stage at the time of surgery, and lymph node dissection. Video 4–2 shows a patient with partial glossectomy attempting to swallow with the bolus in the front of his mouth. Note the delayed attempts to move the bolus to the posterior tongue where the muscle mass remains.

Because of poor tongue mobility, the swallowing problem worsens if the oral sphincter (lips) has been altered or if the patient's lower lip has no feeling (anesthetic). Thus, both motor and sensory implications suggest careful and long-term management of the patients with tongue cancer.

Palate Surgery

Tumors of the hard palate that require partial or total maxillectomy affect both speech and swallowing. Resection results in loss of oronasal separation, which will cause leakage of food into the nose (nasal regurgitation) and hypernasal speech. Unilateral maxillectomy is usually best reconstructed with a dental prosthesis. Free microvascular flaps can be used to reconstruct large palatal defects in edentulous patients in whom prosthesis would not be retained. The reconstruction options, however, are limited and offer no sphincteric action. Defects in the soft palate are best managed by dental prostheses with extensions to close the nasopharyngeal isthmus. The swallowing problems facing the patient undergoing palatal surgery depend on the extent of the lesion and the need for radiation therapy following surgery. With small lesions, swallowing therapy follows bolus size and bolus texture management since the ability to form a pressure gradient to push the food posteriorly is usually limited.[10]

Mandibular Surgery

Mandibular defects of the midline arch cause problems with proper chewing, oral sphincter control, laryngeal suspension and elevation, and the driving force of the tongue. With appropriate exercises to maintain mandible motion, swallowing may improve. However, scarring and fibrosis may require long-term mandible exercises. Oral motor assessment at regular intervals by the SLP should be considered for these patients.

Oropharyngeal Surgery

Control of the liquid or food bolus into the oropharynx is critical to preventing aspiration. Problems affecting swallowing are dependent on several factors:

Extent of surgical excision

Preservation of salivary glands

Postoperative radiation treatment dose

Resection of the lateral pharyngeal wall leads to decreased pharyngeal wall mobility, which alters oropharyngeal propulsion. The muscles of the base of the tongue assist in elevation of the larynx and are essential for the oropharyngeal propulsion pump and for adequate oral cavity–pharyngeal separation. Although resection is usually well tolerated, large defects often cause dysphagia. Reconstruction of up to one-third of the base of the tongue is best accomplished with a sensate flap. Resection of even limited portions of the soft palate produces **velopharyngeal insufficiency**, alters the propulsion of the bolus, and can lead to poor oral cavity–pharyngeal separation, with early spillage of the bolus and aspiration before the pharyngeal swallow is initiated.

Hypopharyngeal Surgery

The hypopharynx is generally considered the inferior portion of the pharynx, between the epiglottis and the larynx. It corresponds to the height of the epiglottis. This area is critical to maintaining control of liquids during swallowing. Hypopharyngeal cancer usually requires extensive surgery plus radiation therapy. The resected tumor may require additional surgery to form a swallow tube. The radial forearm free-flap (RFFF) is one of the optimal choices for hypopharyngeal reconstruction.[11] Table 4–6 presents the common problems after surgery in the hypopharynx. Reports indicate that if the flap survives, oral swallow may follow.

Resection of hypopharyngeal tumors arising on the posterior pharyngeal wall poses several problems for swallowing rehabilitation. Small defects (less than 2 cm) can be closed primarily or the edges can be stitched to the prevertebral fascia. Reconstruction with a split-thickness skin graft or radial forearm free flap (RFFF) provides a satisfactory closure of larger defects. However, neither technique restores the gliding action of the posterior wall on the vertebral fascia, because of scarring of the posterior hypopharyngeal wall to the prevertebral fascia. Impairment of pharyngeal contraction leads to significant retention at the hypopharynx, leading to postprandial aspiration.

> *Reconstructive grafts and flaps are also almost always devoid of sensation, which further weakens laryngeal protection.*

Reconstruction using a RFFF or a split-thickness skin graft frequently results in scarring that forms horizontal "shelves" along the posterior pharyngeal wall. These shelves divert the food bolus anteriorly, into the larynx, and may retain secretions and ingested food.[12] When enough food or saliva accumulates, the material is dumped anteriorly into the entrance of the larynx. That may result in significant

TABLE 4–6. Dysphagia After Surgery of the Hypopharynx

Piriform Sinus
  a. Scarring of lateral pharyngeal wall
  b. Injury to superior laryngeal nerve and loss of sensation

Posterior Pharyngeal Wall
  a. A dynamic insensate flap reconstruction
  b. Scarring and aspiration

aspiration, especially if the patient lacks sensation due to injury or sacrifice of the sensory nerves during surgery. Commercial products may be used to thicken liquids and other thin foods so that the transit time is increased, possibly increasing the opportunity for laryngeal protection.

SKULL BASE SURGERY

Patients undergoing skull base surgery are at risk for injury to the lower cranial nerves, brainstem, brain parenchyma, and soft tissues of the upper aerodigestive tract, depending on the location and nature of the tumor. Injury to these vital structures can lead to dysfunction of speech, swallowing, and airway protection. In addition to these deficits, patients undergoing skull base surgery frequently need reconstruction with insensate soft tissue flaps, which may compound the motor and sensory deficits by the mechanical obstruction caused by their bulk. After skull base surgery, patients frequently need enteral tubes, prolonged intubation and ventilation, and tracheotomies that further compound the swallowing deficits. Lower cranial neuropathies are common sequalae and/or complications of skull base surgery or of the tumor itself.

> *A high vagal injury leads to ipsilateral laryngeal anesthesia and vocal fold paralysis. In addition, it produces paralysis of the ipsilateral soft palate, loss of vagus-mediated relaxation of the cricopharyngeus muscle, dis-coordination of the pharyngeal musculature, esophageal dysmotility, and gastroparesis.*

A high vagal lesion, in addition to other cranial nerve or neurological deficits, produces marked postoperative deglutition and airway morbidity. This can be compounded by injury to other lower cranial nerves such as IX or XII. Table 4–7 summarizes the clinical manifestations of cranial nerve deficits following head and neck and/or skull base surgery.[13] Changes in the anatomical structures and the neurological complications will affect the treatment of dysphagia. These patients will benefit from surgical procedures that optimize the compensatory mechanisms of the remaining function (see Chapter 11).

TRACHEOTOMY

A **tracheotomy** is an operation during which the surgeon makes a cut or opening in the trachea. A tube is then inserted into the opening to bypass a blockage, to remove secretions, or to allow air to pass into and out of the lungs. The indications for tracheotomy can be divided into 3 major categories: airway obstruction, ventilator support, and management of tracheobronchial secretions (known as pulmonary toilet).

A tracheotomy does not prevent aspiration nor does aspiration of secretions prevent tracheotomy.

Approximately 43% to 83% of patients with tracheotomy tubes will manifest signs of aspiration or aspiration pneumonia. Dysphagia is produced by the physiological changes associated with opening the trachea to atmospheric pressure, not merely the presence of the tube in the neck.[14] Table 4–8 summarizes the most common changes following tracheotomy.

Tracheotomy results in 5 well-known alterations to normal physiology:

Decreased subglottic pressures

Decreased laryngeal motion

Decreased glottis closure

Desensitization of the larynx

Loss of the protective reflex

TABLE 4–7. Clinical Manifestations of Cranial Nerve Deficits[a]

Dysfunctional Cranial Nerve	Clinical Manifestations
V	Impaired oral preparation and transport
VII	Drooling
	Impaired oral preparation
	Retention in gingivobuccal sulcus
IX and X	Delayed initiation of pharyngeal phase
	Nasal reflux
	Pharyngeal stasis and pooling
	Voice weakness or loss
	Aspiration
XII	Lack of awareness of food in mouth
	Impaired oral preparation
	Impaired oral transport

[a]Adapted from Crawley.[13]

TABLE 4–8. Changes Following Tracheotomy

Loss or change in airway resistance
Inability to generate subglottic air pressure during the swallow
Reduced ability to produce an effective cough
Loss of sense of smell
Loss of phonation
Reduced mucosal sensitivity
Reduced true vocal fold closure and coordination
Disruption of the respiration/swallowing cycle
Foreign body effect
Reduced laryngeal elevation during deglutition

Airway Pressure Changes

A major factor contributing to aspiration is that a tracheotomy results in a reduction of airway resistance. Expiratory resistance during respiration is provided by the vocal folds, with a constant resistance of about 8 to 10 cm H_2O/L/min. This "valving" helps maintain lung inflation through physiological prolongation of the expiratory phase. Pressure measurements during swallowing in patients with an occluded tracheotomy are similar to those of normal individuals and are significantly diminished with an open tracheotomy. This pressure is present in the trachea following glottic closure during swallowing, and peaks at about 8 to 10 cm H_2O. Subglottic air pressure seems to be critical to swallow function. Its restoration reverses, at least in part, the disordered swallowing function that accompanies tracheotomy. Care should be taken to monitor the patient with a tracheotomy as the need for suction may increase following the procedure.

Expiratory Speaking Valves

Removal of the tracheotomy tube known as **decannulation** will usually enhance swallowing function in the patient. However, this is not feasible in all patients. An alternative strategy is to place an expiratory speaking valve on the open tracheotomy tube, which restores subglottic air pressure during swallowing (Figure 4–1).

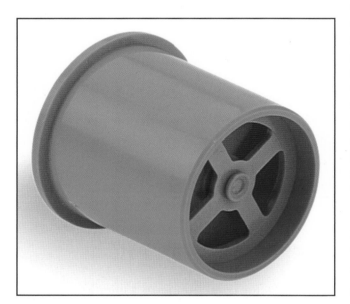

FIGURE 4–1. An expiratory speaking valve designed to fit over the open tracheostomy tube to restore subglottic air pressure during swallowing.

The beneficial effect of a valve strengthens the fact that subglottic air pressure is a critical factor in swallowing efficiency, probably through restoring proprioceptive cues. There are certain restrictions in using a speaking valve. Following are conditions where a speaking valve is not appropriate and should not be used[14]:

Unconscious/comatose patients

Severe behavior problems

Severe medical instability

Airway obstruction above the breathing tube that does not allow expiration through the glottis, such as bilateral vocal fold paralysis, glottic and tracheal stenosis

Persistent thick and copious secretions

Foam-filled tracheostomy cuffs

Total laryngectomy or laryngotracheal separation

Severely compromised respiratory system

Inability to maintain adequate ventilation with cuff deflation

Clinical use of a speaking valve in swallowing therapy, when appropriate, may provide better communication between the patient and the therapist when administering various swallowing trials. Verbal communication during trial swallows enhances the therapeutic activity. In addition, since the speaking valve may improve sensation, patients may initiate a cough sooner rather than later and thus prevent aspiration. The use of a speaking valve improves the buildup of subglottic air pressure and thus improves the patient's ability to adduct the vocal folds during voice exercises.

Laryngeal Elevation

The vertical motion of the larynx is dependent on the function of the suprahyoid musculature, and results in shortening of the pharynx and simultaneous active opening of the cricopharyngeal sphincter. Laryngeal elevation is reduced following tracheotomy, and probably plays a significant role in the dysphagia associated with the procedure.

Glottic Closure

Lung protection is provided by cessation of respiration and the maintenance of glottic closure. In the typical individual, swallowing is timed to occur during expiration. This relationship is lost in patients with severe respiratory disease and is probably also lost in the presence of a tracheotomy. Glottic closure during swallowing is an extremely basic reflex mediated by the superior laryngeal nerve (uncrossed) and requiring from approximately 18 to 40 msec.[15] The rapid response demonstrates that the reflex arc is located in the lower brainstem and does not require input from higher centers. The laryngeal surface of the epiglottis and the other supraglottic structures are richly endowed with receptors, including water receptors.

> *Interruption of this sensory input by superior laryngeal nerve or high vagal nerve interruption will limit reflexive glottic closure and contribute to aspiration.*[3]

Disruption of the integrity of the subglottic airway by the presence of a tracheotomy will also blunt or eliminate this reflex.

Pharyngeal Transit With Tracheostomy

Bolus transit from the tongue base to the esophagus typically requires less than a second in normal swallowing. Prolongation of bolus transit time, as well as disruption of the glottic closure, will result in food or liquid being in the pharynx while the glottis is open, thus placing the individual at risk for aspiration. It has been demonstrated that this transit time can be prolonged in the presence of a tracheotomy and that this effect is reversible. Restricted range of motion of pharyngeal structures due to the tethering of the larynx by the presence of a tracheotomy tube also affects transit time.

ZENKER DIVERTICULUM

Zenker diverticulum is a pulsion diverticulum that forms above the cricopharyngeal sphincter muscle through areas of lesser muscle strength, such as Killian triangle. The diverticulum (pouch) is created by failure of the upper esophageal sphincter to open before the propulsive wave, and by failure of active opening of the cricopharyngeal muscle due to weakness of the laryngeal elevators. Zenker diverticula are often seen in elderly men, and when they enlarge, surgery to close the pouch is recommended. Typical symptoms are summarized in Table 4–9.[16] As surgery is the only effective therapeutic option for Zenker diverticulum, the decision to operate is driven by the degree of the patient's symptoms. These include regurgitation of partially digested food, which may lead to a foul smell and halitosis, dysphagia, coughing, and choking on swallowing; malnutrition and weight loss; obstruction; and recurrent aspiration pneumonia. Symptomatic patients who desire excision and can tolerate anesthesia are candidates for excision.

The indications and contraindications are shown in Table 4–10. Surgical treatment options are many and include a range of options, from cricopharyngeal

TABLE 4–9. Symptoms of Zenker Diverticulum[a]

Symptom	Patients (%)
Dysphagia	48 (100)
Aspiration	20 (42)
Postdeglutitive cough	17 (35)
Regurgitation	14 (29)
Noisy swallowing	13 (27)
Weight loss (>4.5 kg)	13 (27)
Recumbent cough	10 (21)
Sore throat	8 (17)
Unable to swallow	8 (17)
Halitosis	2 (4)

[a]Adapted from Schmidt and Zuckerbraun.[16]

TABLE 4–10. Zenker Diverticulum: Surgical Indications and Contraindications

Indications	Contraindications
Coughing and choking during swallowing	Inability to withstand general anesthesia
Recurrent aspiration pneumonia	Carcinoma of the esophagus
Regurgitation/halitosis	Untreated severe GERD (relative)
Inanition/weight loss	
Dysphagia	
Esophageal obstruction	

myotomy to myotomy and excision of the pouch (diverticulectomy). Small diverticula may be found on endoscopic examination and can be observed if patient does not report symptoms of regurgitation or if signs of regurgitation are not observed during the examination. Absolute contraindications to surgery include inability to tolerate anesthesia (a significant consideration in the elderly population in which Zenker diverticula are found) and carcinoma of the esophagus (which has rarely been reported within the actual diverticular pouch). The presence of untreated severe gastroesophageal reflux disease (GERD) is a relative contraindication.

External surgical approaches to Zenker diverticulum have been used with considerable success since the beginning of the 20th century. Cricopharyngeal **myotomy** is performed sometimes prior to the removal, pexy, or imbrication of the diverticulum. Endoscopic approaches for the management of a Zenker diverticulum have been performed successfully for the last 40 years. During the endoscopic approach, the mucosa and muscle that make up the party wall between the diverticular pouch and the esophagus are divided with an electrocautery laser or an automatic stapler.[17] Prolonged follow-up of the patient is recommended, though no specific guidelines for reevaluation have been recommended. Yearly follow-up appears to be a logical interval.

SUMMARY

Surgery of the head and neck, skull base, and upper aerodigestive tract can have detrimental effects on the swallowing function. The role of the SLP is critical in the management of the swallowing changes following surgery. Removal or disruption of the soft tissues, including muscles and nerves, may lead to weakness, scarring, or incoordination of the swallowing apparatus. These problems are often predictable and their treatment should be included in the preoperative plan, as most patients will benefit from an early intervention.

DISCUSSION QUESTIONS

1. Anterior cervical spine surgery may result in dysphagia in up to 15% of patients undergoing the surgery. Given the complications and the etiological factors that are described in the chapter, discuss the possible assessment and treatment modifications that must be considered when seeing these patients shortly after surgery.

2. Interactions between the speech-language pathologist and the head and neck surgeon have multiple benefits for the patient. At what times should the speech-language pathologist and the surgeon interact when a patient is scheduled for surgery in the oral cavity or pharynx? Why are these points in time important?

STUDY QUESTIONS

1. Dysphagia after cervical spine surgery is
   A. Common in the early postoperative period
   B. Often self-limited
   C. Often due to injury to the recurrent laryngeal nerve
   D. All of the above
   E. A and B

2. Dysphagia after cervical spine surgery is due to
   A. Scarring of the retropharyngeal space
   B. Edema
   C. Disruption of the pharyngeal plexus
   D. Pain
   E. All of the above

3. After skull base surgery, patients may suffer aspiration due to
   A. Injury to the vagus nerve
   B. Injury to the trigeminal nerve
   C. Deconditioning
   D. All of the above
   E. A and C

4. Patients with a Zenker diverticulum often present
   A. Prandial aspiration
   B. Emotional lability
   C. Regurgitation
   D. Early onset of dysphagia to liquids
   E. All of the above

5. Dysphagia in patients with cancer of the upper aerodigestive tract is
   A. Often present at the time of diagnosis
   B. Often intractable
   C. Corrected with the successful treatment of the cancer
   D. A and C
   E. All of the above

REFERENCES

1. Anderson KK Arnold PM Oropharyngeal dysphagia after anterior cervical spine surgery: a review. *Global Spine J.* 2013;3(4):273–286.
2. Joaquim AF, Murar J, Savage JW, Patel AA. Dysphagia after anterior cervical spine surgery: a systematic review of potential preventative measures. *Spine J.* 2014; 14(9):2246–2260.
3. Hart RA, Tatsumi RL, Hiratzka JR, Yoo JU. Perioperative complications of combined anterior and posterior cervical decompression and fusion crossing the cervicothoracic junction. *Spine.* 2008;33(26):2887–2891.

4. Emery S, Smith MD, Bohlman HE. Upper airway obstruction after multilevel cervical corpectomy for myelopathy. *Spine.* 1991;16:544–550.
5. Dornbos D III, Seim NB, Mendel E. Swallowing disorders after cervical spine surgery. In: Carrau RL, Murry T, Howell, R, eds. *Comprehensive Management of Swallowing Disorders.* 2nd ed. San Diego, CA: Plural Publishing; 2016:251–260.
6. Wang MC, Chan L, Maiman DJ, Kreuter W, Deyo RA. Complications and mortality associated with cervical spine surgery for degenerative disease in the United States. *Spine.* 2007;32(3):342–347.
7. Kreeft AM, Van der Molen L, Hilgers FJ, Balm AJ. Speech and swallowing after surgical treatment of advanced oral and oropharyngeal carcinoma; a systematic review of the literature. *Eur Arch Otorhinolaryngol.* 2009;266: 1687–1698.
8. Sessions D, Spector G, Lenox J, et al. Analysis of treatment results for floor-of-mouth cancer. *Laryngoscope.* 2000;110:17774–17782.
9. Son Y, Choi K, Kim T. Dysphagia in tongue cancer patients. *Ann Rehabil Med.* 2015;39(2):210–217.
10. Yang X, Song X, Chu W, Li L, Ma L, Wu Y. Clinicopathological characteristics and outcome predictors in squamous cell carcinoma of the maxillary gingiva and hard palate. *J Oral Maxillofac Surg.* 2015 Jul;73(7):1429–1436.
11. Song M, Chen SW, Zhang Q, et al. External monitoring of buried radial forearm free flaps in hypopharyngeal reconstruction. *Acta Otolaryngol.* 2011;131:204–209 [Epub 2010 Oct 29].
12. Vainshtein JM, Moon DH, Feng FY, Chepeha DB, Eisbruch A, Stenmark MH. Long-term quality of life after swallowing and salivary-sparing chemo-intensity modulated radiation therapy in survivors of human papillomavirus-related oropharyngeal cancer. *Int J Radiat Oncol Biol Phys.* 2015;91(5):925–933.
13. Crawley B. Neoplasia of the upper aerodigestive tract: primary tumors and secondary involvement. In: Carrau RL, Murry T, Howell, R. eds. *Comprehensive Management of Swallowing Disorders.* 2nd ed. San Diego, CA: Plural Publishing; 2016:293–304.
14. Gross RD, Enloe LD, Reyes SE. Passy-Muir valve decannulation. In: Carrau RL, Murry T, Howell R, eds. *Comprehensive Management of Swallowing Disorders.* 2nd ed. San Diego, CA: Plural Publishing; 2016:355–365.
15. Sasaki CT, Hundal JS, Kim YH. Protective glottic closure: biomechanical effects of selective laryngeal denervation. *Ann Otol Rhinol Laryngol.* 2005;114(4):271–275.
16. Schmidt PJ, Zuckerbraun L. Treatment of Zenker's diverticula by cricopharyngeus myotomy under local anesthesia. *Ann Surg.* 1992;58:710–716.
17. Howell R. Pathophysiology of Zenker's diverticulum. In: Carrau RL, Murry T, Howell R, eds. *Comprehensive Management of Swallowing Disorders.* 2nd ed. San Diego, CA: Plural Publishing; 2016:269–275.

Clinical Evaluation of Swallowing Disorders

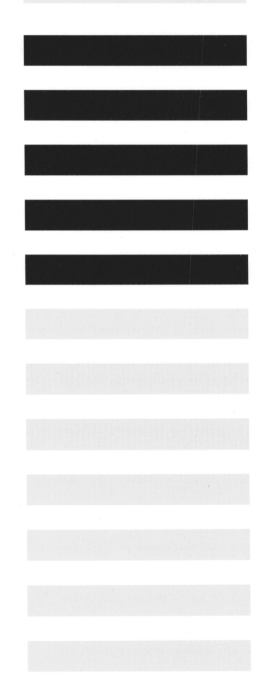

A Look at the Chapter

Patients who are suspected of having swallowing problems start with a swallowing assessment before management strategies can be proposed. The swallowing assessment is generally divided into a clinical or bedside screening and assessment, and an instrumental evaluation. This chapter will focus on the clinical swallow examination. The scope of clinical screening or assessment protocols will be discussed with reference to the World Health Organization's International Classification of Functioning, Disability and Health (ICF) framework.[1] The current available evidence in support of the clinical screening or assessment protocols will also be presented.

INTRODUCTION

A typical evaluation of swallowing encompasses a case history, a clinical or bedside swallow examination, and an instrumental evaluation. According to the ICF framework, the scope of assessment should include (1) body structures and functions that are related to swallowing, (2) body functions that may influence eating or drinking behaviors, (3) swallowing activities and participation, (4) activities and participation in events related to eating or drinking, and (5) personal and environmental factors that may affect swallowing.[1] The swallowing evaluation is designed to address the issues of

- Swallow safety
- Nutritional status
- Continuation or possible modification of present diet
- Need for specialized treatments
- Impact on the quality of life

Based on the swallow evaluation, referrals for additional tests may be requested.

MULTIDISCIPLINARY DYSPHAGIA TEAM

Given the complexity of the causes and impacts of dysphagia, dysphagia is best assessed and managed by a team of professionals to ensure patients can swallow safely and have adequate nutritional support. A speech-language pathologist (SLP) is often the leader of a **dysphagia team**. Other equally important team members may include dietitian, otolaryngologist, gastroenterologist, radiologist, pulmonologist, neurologist, dentist, occupational therapist, physiotherapist, nurse, and social worker. The members and roles of the dysphagia team are likely to differ for individual patients and for different settings.

The key to successful and efficient swallowing assessment and management relies on good communication, collaboration, and coordination among the team members.

DYSPHAGIA SCREENING

A clinician may want to conduct a brief dysphagia assessment to determine the need to perform a full evaluation and make further referrals. An effective "screening" test should allow clinicians to identify individuals who have dysphagia and are at risk of having aspiration (**high sensitivity**) and screen out individuals who do not have dysphagia (**high specificity**). These screening tools and tests should be easy to administer, be time- and cost-effective, and may be used by any member of the dysphagia team. When using a validated dysphagia screening test, it is important to remember that sometimes it is difficult to accurately detect the presence or absence of penetration and/or aspiration in patients who have the following conditions:

- Are severely ill
- Have significant communication impairments and cannot follow directions
- Lack sensitivity in parts of the swallowing organs and may aspirate without any observable signs

For these patients, it might be to their benefit to receive a full swallowing assessment instead. Some commonly used screening tests are outlined in Table 5–1, and the most common ones are presented in more detail below.

Toronto Bedside Swallowing Screening Test (TOR-BSST)

The Toronto Bedside Swallowing Screening Test (TOR-BSST) is a dysphagia screening test for stroke survivors in acute and rehabilitative settings.[15] The test consists of an oral exam and a water swallow. It can be administered by health care professionals who have completed a standardized training workshop from certified TOR-BSST trainers. The screening will be discontinued if the patient fails in any item of the test. The test takes approximately 10 minutes to complete. The test has high sensitivity and good reliability and validity. However, it has low specificity. The test is copyrighted, requiring online training and purchase before use.

TABLE 5–1. Characteristics of Selected Dysphagia Screening Tests

Test	Inclusion of Swallowing Items	Inclusion of Non-Swallowing Items	Who Administers	Psychometrics	Duration
Toronto Bedside Swallowing Screening Test (TOR-BSST)[2]	✓	✓[a]	Trained health care professionals	Sensitivity 91%; specificity 67%; reliability: intraclass correlation 92%	<10 minutes
3-oz Water Swallow Test (WST)[3,4]	✓	X	Discipline not stated (SLP in papers)	Sensitivity 97%; specificity 49%	<5 minutes
Bedside Swallowing Assessment[5–8]	✓	✓[a]	MD and SLP	Sensitivity 47% to 70%; specificity 66% to 86%; reliability: $k = 0.24$–0.79	~20 minutes
Standardized Swallowing Assessment[9–11]	✓	✓[a]	RN, SLP, and junior doctors (5 practice sessions)	Sensitivity 0.97; specificity 0.9	Not specified
Gugging Swallow Screen (GUSS)[12]	✓	✓[a]	RN or SLP	Sensitivity 100%; specificity 50% to 69%; reliability: 95% agreement	~15 minutes
Acute Stroke Dysphagia Screening (also called Barnes Jewish Hospital Stroke Dysphagia Screen)[13]	✓	✓[a]	RN	Sensitivity 91%; specificity 74%; reliability: k = 93.6	2 minutes
Modified Mann Assessment of Swallowing Ability (MMASA)[14]	X	✓	Stroke neurologists	Sensitivity 90%; specificity 85%; reliability: k = 0.76	5 minutes

[a]Discontinue if any item is positive/present.

Modified Mann Assessment of Swallowing Ability (MMASA)

The Modified Mann Assessment of Swallowing Ability (MMASA) is a 12-item assessment tool based on the Mann Assessment of Swallowing Ability.[14] The test was originally developed and validated to be used by physicians; however, the authors proposed that the test is simple enough to be used by other health care professionals. No swallowing tasks are involved in the MMASA. The test has high sensitivity, specificity, and good reliability. No formal training is involved, but the test has not been validated against instrumental swallowing examination.

3-oz Water Swallow Test (WST)

The WST[4,16] is a simple swallow test that involves drinking 3 oz (90 cc) of water without interruption. If the patient shows any signs of swallowing difficulties, such as inability to complete the task, coughing, choking or wet voice within one minute, the patient would require further swallowing assessment. The WST is commonly used as a dysphagia screening test alone or as part of a larger screening test.[17] It has high sensitivity but low specificity. The WST is only recommended for patients who are alert and can be seated upright.

Burke Dysphagia Screening Test (BDST)

The Burke Dysphagia Screening Test (BDST) reported by DePippo et al[18] was one of the first dysphagia screening tests available in the literature. It is a quick screening test that consists of 7 items, including a 3-oz water swallow test. If the patient has a positive response to one or more of the items in the test, he or she is considered to have failed and is referred for a complete clinical swallow evaluation (CSE). The reliability and validity of this test have not been as rigorously tested as the other screening tests. The form for BDST is shown in Appendix 3.

The Modified Blue Dye Test

The **modified blue dye test,** also known as the **Modified Evans Blue Dye Test** (MEBDT), may be used to determine the presence of aspiration in a tracheotomized patient. The general procedures for the MEBDT involve (1) deflating and suctioning the tracheostomy tube before the test; (2) conducting swallow trials of different food and liquid consistencies that are mixed with blue food coloring (with cuff on or off); (3) and again performing deep suction of the patient's tracheotomy tube, this time looking for evidence of dyed material in the airway (this procedure may be repeated over a period of time). Good sensitivity but low specificity was reported for the MEBDT.[19,20]

SELF-ASSESSMENTS

Validated tools are available to obtain information on swallowing from the patient's perspective.[21] Table 5–2 shows some examples of existing self-assessment tools and how they may be applied according to the ICF framework. Data from the patient's perspective provide the clinician with a guide as to what the specific problems the patient is facing, how severe they are, and what the impacts are on the patient's quality of life.

> *When valid and reliable self-assessment tools are used prior to intervention and following intervention, an additional avenue of outcome data is available.*

There are a number of self-report tools available in the literature. This chapter will highlight only those that are more commonly used.

The SWAL-QOL and SWAL-CARE

The SWAL-QOL and SWAL-CARE are two tools for assessing the swallowing quality of life and quality of care that are completed by the patient.[22–24] They can be used as outcome measures following treatment. There are 44 items in the SWAL-QOL and 15 items in the SWAL-CARE. The SWAL-QOL is divided into 10 scales that assess quality-of-life concepts, and the SWAL-CARE consists of 15 items

TABLE 5–2. Common Self-Assessment Tools That Address Different Components of the ICF Framework

Screening Tool	Body Functions and Structures	Activity and Participation: Swallowing (S) and Related to Eating and Drinking	Contextual Factors: Environmental (E) and Personal (P)
Eating Assessment Tool (EAT-10)	✓	✓	X
Swallowing Quality of Life (SWAL-QOL) Questionnaire	✓	✓	✓
Sydney Swallow Questionnaire (SSQ)	✓	X	✓
The Deglutition Handicap Index (DegHI)	✓	X ✓	X
The Dysphagia Handicap Index (DHI)	✓	✓	X
M.D. Anderson Dysphagia Inventory	✓	✓	X

that assess quality of care and patient satisfaction. Multiple scales are used in the two questionnaires. It takes approximately 20 minutes to complete both. The scoring of the SWAL-QOL and SWAL-CARE takes additional clinical time. Studies have shown that SWAL-QOL can differentiate individuals without swallowing problems from those with oropharyngeal swallowing disorders.[25–27] In addition, the scales are sensitive to the severity of dysphagia in those with a swallowing disorder. The SWAL-QOL and SWAL-CARE have been translated into a number of languages, including Dutch, French, Swedish, and Chinese.[28–31] Studies have used SWAL-QOL to assess treatment outcomes in a range of populations, including individuals with head and neck cancers, stroke,[32,33] and Parkinson's disease.[34] SWAL-QOL is one of the few questionnaires that fully address multiple ICF domains; however, the long administration time and complexity of the wording may limit its use clinically.[35]

The MD Anderson Dysphagia Inventory

The MD Anderson Dysphagia Inventory (MDADI) is a validated self-assessment tool developed specifically to evaluate the impact of dysphagia on the quality of life of patients with head and neck cancers.[36] The MDADI consists of 20 items that are divided into 4 subscales: (1) a global measure on the impact of swallowing ability on daily life and (2) emotional, (3) functional, and (4) physical statements related to swallowing. Each item is rated on a 5-point ordinal scale. It takes about 10 to 15 minutes to complete and score the questionnaire. The MDADI has been translated to and validated in a number of languages, including Italian,[37] Swedish, Korean, and Dutch.[38–40] MDADI has been extensively used as an outcome measurement tool in dysphagia studies. It is shown in Appendix 4.

Eating Assessment Tool (EAT-10)

The EAT-10 is a 10-item outcome measure of dysphagia symptom severity.[41] Each item is rated on a 5-point interval scale. The EAT-10 was validated on 7 groups of patients in various diagnostic categories. The instrument has excellent internal consistency, test-retest reproducibility, and criterion-based validity. The EAT-10 is shown in Appendix 5.

Dysphagia Handicap Index (DHI)

The Dysphagia Handicap Index (DHI) is a 25-item self-report questionnaire that evaluates the level of dysphagia handicap.[42] The items are divided into 3 scales: physical, functional, and emotional. Each item is rated on a 3-point ordinal scale. DHI has good internal consistency, reliability, and criterion and construct validity. The DHI is shown in Appendix 6.

The use of all of the above tests is restricted to patients who have the cognitive abilities to respond reliably to the statements in the assessments. Thus, the clinician must be aware of when to use these assessments and how to interpret the results in lieu of the patient's condition. Although self-assessment tools may provide a way of assessing current status or severity from the patient's perspective as well as for outcomes following intervention, the clinician must be aware of their limitations in neurologically disadvantaged patients, as well as in patients who demonstrate the need to want to swallow despite obvious safety concerns.

RELATED SELF-ASSESSMENTS TO DYSPHAGIA

The Reflux Symptom Index (RSI) and Reflux Finding Score (RFS)

The **Reflux Symptom Index (RSI)** is a 10-statement patient self-assessment measure that quantifies a patient's perception of his or her reflux symptoms.[41] The RSI has been validated using a 24-hour pH meter and has been found to be a valid index of reflux severity. Gastroesophageal reflux disease (GERD) or laryngopharyngeal reflux disease (LPRD) is often associated with dysphagia, and when treated maximally, the improvement of GERD and/or LPRD is usually related to an improvement in swallow function.

The RFS has been studied in relation to the reflux finding score (RSI), a clinician-based assessment tool used to score the severity of reflux symptoms as seen on laryngeal endoscopy. The RSI and RFS are shown in Appendices 1 and 2.

CLINICAL SWALLOW EVALUATION

A thorough clinical swallow examination should include case history; physical examination; oral, pharyngeal, and laryngeal examinations; and trial swallows (if appropriate). The **clinical swallow evaluation (CSE),** sometimes called the bedside swallow evaluation, provides a roadmap for the diagnosis and treatment of swallowing disorders. Nonetheless, the clinician must understand that the CSE has significant limitations, because it does not include an examination of the pharynx and larynx, nor does it accurately determine if the patient is aspirating silently. Moreover, depending on the status of the patient (eg, severe impairment from stroke or extensive trauma), a complete CSE is sometimes not possible.

Detecting the presence of penetration and aspiration is an important part of the CSE because the potential consequences of health status and recovery are dependent on nutrition and safe swallowing. Several investigators have examined the sensitivity and specificity of the CSE for predicting aspiration. McCullough, Wertz, and Rosenbek[43] examined 60 stroke patients and found that the CSE was not highly predictive of patients who subsequently aspirated during the modified barium swallow instrumental examination. Ramsey and colleagues[8] found that the CSE had highly variable specificity and sensitivity and also concluded that the CSE was poor at detecting silent aspiration. Peruzzi and colleagues[44] compared the use of a colored bedside dye test to the videofluoroscopic studies of swallowing and found that in 20 consecutive patients with tracheotomy, the videofluoroscopic exam was significantly better at detecting aspiration than the colored bedside dye test.

Although the majority of CSE reports in the literature focus on stroke patients, there are reports that relate findings from the CSE of swallowing to other patient groups. In general, these findings suggest that for surgical patients, the larger the surgical excision, the more likely the patient will exhibit a longer course of dysphagia. Patients in these categories will require more extensive evaluation and treatments.

Once the CSE is completed, the clinician will be able to establish a reasonable differential diagnosis and determine which other tests are needed (Table 5–3).

Case History

Prior to any assessment of the patient, the clinician should identify the chief complaint or define the current status of the patient. The detailed history should account for the current physical status, any recent surgeries, or conditions from previous surgeries that may contribute to the dysphagia. Time since oral food intake, anatomical changes to the swallowing mechanism, neurological status, and degree of alertness help to make those determinations. Table 5–4 summarizes the critical components of the case history.

Common clinical findings that are associated with dysphagia and/or aspiration are shown in Table 5–5. It should be pointed out that even when

TABLE 5–3. Differential Diagnosis[a]

Type	Possible Etiology
Congenital	Dysphagia lusoria Tracheoesophageal fistula Laryngeal clefts Other foregut abnormalities
Inflammatory	GERD Infections: • Lyme disease with neuropathies/encephalitis • Chagas disease • Candidiasis
Trauma	CNS Upper aerodigestive tract Spine Chest
Endocrine	Goiter • Hypothyroidism • Diabetic neuropathy/gastropathy
Neoplasia	Upper aerodigestive tract • Thyroid • Central nervous system
Systemic	Autoimmune • Dermatomyositis • Scleroderma • Sjögren's syndrome • Mixed connective tissue disorder • Myopathies Amyloidosis Sarcoidosis
Iatrogenic	Surgery Chemotherapy
Other	Medications Radiation therapy

[a]Adapted from Carrau, Murry, and Howell.[45]

TABLE 5–4. Critical Components of the Clinical Case History

The clinician should be prepared to answer the following questions as a result of conducting a thorough case history:

1. Is the patient currently eating by mouth or is he or she relying on nonoral feeding?
2. Is there a history of aspiration pneumonia?
3. Was the patient recently hospitalized, and if so, for what reasons?
4. Does the patient have other associated medical conditions (including past surgery and trauma)?
5. Is the patient thriving or maintaining his or her general health and nutrition status based on the current diet and method of eating?

The clinician should be prepared to answer the following questions as a result of completing a clinical swallow examination:

1. Is there a risk of aspiration given the present nutritional status and diet?
2. What is the anatomical and functional status of the oral mechanism?
3. Should the patient be referred for further evaluation of his or her swallowing based on the information gleaned at the CSE?
4. Is the patient cognitively capable of participating in instrumental testing and rehabilitation?
5. What changes in the treatment plan should be anticipated or planned given the outcome of the CSE?

TABLE 5–5. Common Clinical Findings in Dysphagic Patients

General Health Status
• Weight loss
• Bronchorrhea
• Fluctuating low fever
• Pulmonary infiltrates
• Increased or insufficient oral or pharyngeal secretions
• Edentulous (lacking teeth)
• Drooling
• Ineffective cough
Behaviors or Observations During Mealtimes
• Resistance to eating or drinking
• Increased time to consume meal
• Changes in taste
• Difficulty in swallowing foods of specific texture
• Complaints of food stuck in throat
• Oral residue
• Multiple swallow patterns
• Coughing or choking during or after swallow
• Wet vocal quality during or after mealtime

the majority of these symptoms are absent, swallow safety may still be an important issue.[21] Table 5–5 emphasizes that observing the patient, reviewing the case history, and acquiring information from caregivers are important aspects of the CSE.

The Physical Examination

The physical examination should include a basic head and neck and neurological examination, with assessment of gait, balance, sensory and motor function of the extremities, deep tendon reflexes, and full assessment of the cranial nerves. This may be done by an SLP, neurologist, otolaryngologist, gastroenterologist, or a combination of these professionals as a team. For those patients with a weak or breathy voice, a consultation with an otolaryngologist is recommended. The otolaryngologist may perform an examination of the larynx and vocal folds using a **flexible endoscope**.

The Oral, Pharyngeal, and Laryngeal Examination

A thorough examination of the oral, laryngeal, and pharyngeal structures should include an assessment of lip closure, tongue strength and mobility, facial symmetry, voice quality, and volitional cough strength. Table 5–6, modified from Daniels, McAdam, Brailey, and Foundas,[46] provides a comprehensive orderly approach to the oropharyngeal examination. Clinicians, even those with extensive experience in oral examination, may profit from this structure, as it provides an orderly approach to assessing muscular function related to the cranial nerves most important for swallowing.

> *Prior to the oropharyngeal examination, the clinician should have a general knowledge of the patient's characteristics that may interfere with parts of the examination.*

These include

A. Airway
B. Cognition/alertness/endurance
C. Ability to follow instructions
D. Body tone/size/posture/positioning
E. Self-feeding potential

Oral Examination

The oral examination should include assessment of the range of motion, strength, and sensory function of all oral structures. Prominent atrophy and **fasciculation** of the tongue not related to any previous medical conditions should raise the possibility of **amyotrophic lateral sclerosis (ALS)**.

1. *Reflexes and responses*
   ■ The **gag reflex** includes a head and jaw extension, rhythmical tongue protrusions, and pharyngeal contractions in response to stimulation at the posterior part of the oral cavity. Recent literature suggests that the gag reflex may not be important for normal swallowing to occur.

TABLE 5–6. The Oropharyngeal Examination for the Clinical Swallow Examination

Name _____ Date _____

Diagnosis _____

Mandible (CN V)

  Symmetry on Extension _____ Strength _____

Lips (CN VII)

  Symmetry: Rest _____ Retraction _____ Protrusion _____

  Strength _____

  Nonspeech Coordination: Repetitive Movement _____ Alternating Movement _____

  Speech Coordination: Repetitive (/p,w/) _____ Alternating (/p-w/) _____

Tongue (CN XII)

  Symmetry: Rest _____ Protrusion _____ Lateralization _____

  Elevation   Yes/No   Lateralization   Yes/No   Fasciculations   Yes/No

  Strength _____

  Nonspeech Coordination: Repetitive Movement _____ Alternating Movement _____

  Alternating Movement (/p^t^k^/) _____

  Multisyllabic Word Repetition (tip top, baseball player, several, caterpillar, emphasize) _____

  Conversation: (speech, voice, coordination characteristics) _____

  Laryngeal Function: Isolated Movement (/i-i-i/ on one breath) _____

  Alternating Movement (/u-i/) _____

  Buccofacial Apraxia: "Blow out the candle" _____ "Lick an ice cream cone" _____

  "Lick milk off your top lip" _____ "Sip through a straw" _____ "Kiss a baby" _____

Velum (CN IX, X XI)

  Symmetry: Rest _____ Elevation _____

  Coordination: Repetitive Movement (/a/) _____

  Appearance of Hard Palate _____

  Dentition _____

Reflexes (CN IX, X, XI)

  Gag (Abnormal: Yes/No) _____

  Swallow (Cough: Yes/No) _____

  Voice Change (Yes/No) _____

Additional Information

  c/o Facial Numbness or Tingling: Yes/No _____ Light Touch _____

  Dysphonia: Yes/No (mild, moderate, severe) _____

  Dysarthria: Yes/No (mild, moderate, severe) _____

  Breath Support _____

  Resonance _____

  Volitional Cough (Abnormal: Yes/No) _____

_____   _____

Clinician   Date

[a]Adapted with permission from Daniels, McAdam, Brailey, and Foundas.[46]

- The **bite reflex** is clamping of the teeth or up and down movement of the jaw in response to stimulation of the gum, molar, or other dental surfaces.
- The **transverse tongue response** is a lateral movement in response to tactile stimulation at the lateral border of the tongue.

2. *Sensation.* Assess by light touch of lips, tongue, and buccal cavity.
3. *Structural anatomy.* Look for abnormalities of lips and oral cavity.
4. *Range and coordination of movement*
   - Jaw—ability to open and close the jaw
   - Lips—labial closure and compression at rest and during swallowing
   - Tongue—anterior lingual movement may be assessed by having the patient extend, lateralize, elevate, and depress the tip and by having the patient sweep the tongue from front to back along the roof of the mouth
   - Velum—movement of the velum, or soft palate, may be assessed by having the patient open the mouth, and then observing palatal movement during production of a sustained /a/ sound
5. *Secretions.* Note location and amount.
6. *Articulation.* Screen with sentences or words containing tongue tip and posterior tongue consonants (p,t,b,d,th,k,g).
7. *Resonance.* Note presence of hypernasal quality.

Pharyngeal and Laryngeal Examinations

1. Vocal quality/changes—listen to patient talking before and after swallowing. Is there a difference in voice quality?
2. Pitch control/range—a voice without pitch changes may be indicative of sensory paralysis. Is the pitch of the voice appropriate and does the patient have variation in his or her pitch range?
3. Breathing—is the patient experiencing labored breathing or is there an audible noise associated with inhalation or exhalation?
4. Volitional cough/throat clear—lack of the ability to cough may suggest poor vocal fold closure. Can the patient produce a normal cough and clearing of the throat?

5. Saliva swallow: laryngeal management—does the patient continue to feel saliva or mucous in the throat? This may sometimes be a sign of reflux or a more serious problem called **Zenker diverticulum**.
6. Laryngeal elevation—lack of laryngeal elevation usually suggests a nerve injury at the laryngeal level. Place your finger on the thyroid cartilage, do you feel the larynx elevate when the patient is asked to swallow?

Trial Swallows

Based on the patient's input, family input, medical records, and the severity of the problem, clinicians will decide whether to proceed to trial swallows. The final portion of the CSE consists of trial swallows of water and different food textures. This can be combined with the measurement of oxygen saturation or auscultation. The clinician should be consistent in the amount of water to be swallowed. The majority of reports suggest that it is appropriate to begin with a 5-mL bolus.[27] Depending on the results, one can advance to 10- and 20-mL boluses. The fluid consistencies may be thickened or thinned according to the patient's performance. A selection of food textures should also be tested to determine if diet modification may be necessary for the patient. Laryngeal elevation, identified by palpation of the thyroid prominence, should be monitored for each swallow. After each swallow, the patient is asked to sustain the /a/ vowel for a few seconds or count from 1 to 5 to determine if there is wet hoarseness or other drainage in voice quality. Daniels and her associates[17] suggest that wet hoarseness and a weak cough are two signs of increased risk for aspiration. If aspiration is suspected, the patient should be referred for further instrumental swallow evaluation.

Cervical Auscultation (CA)

Cervical auscultation refers to placing a stethoscope gently on the lateral aspect of the larynx to listen to "swallowing sounds" and respiration. Cervical auscultation assesses swallowing-respiration coordination and detection of aspiration and penetration.[47,48] The sensitivity of using CA to detect aspiration is approximately 85%, with specificity ranging from

56% to 71% across studies.[49] The interrater reliability was considered to be poor to fair across studies. It is suggested that cervical auscultation should only be used in conjunction with other swallowing tests, instead of using this technique as a screening test to detect aspiration.

Trial Swallows with Pulse Oximetry

Pulse oximetry refers to the monitoring of peripheral blood oxygen saturation level while conducting trial swallows.[50,51] It aims to identify aspiration based on the principle that aspiration of food or liquids will lead to hypoxia and desaturation. Conflicting results have been reported in the literature. Some studies have reported that the use of pulse oximetry during trial swallows achieved excellent sensitivity and good specificity for detecting aspiration.[52] However, a number of other studies reported poor sensitivity and specificity and found no additional value in the use of oximetry during clinical swallow examination.[53,54]

Mann Assessment of Swallowing Ability

A noninvasive assessment protocol for quantifying the severity of swallowing impairment was developed by Mann.[55] This protocol, called the Mann Assessment of Swallowing Ability (MASA), is a comprehensive clinical examination of oropharyngeal dysphagia consisting of 24 items. The MASA is one clinical measure of dysphagia that has demonstrated strong reliability and has been validated against videofluoroscopic and videoendoscopic swallowing examinations in several populations. It provides a numerical score reflecting the severity of dysphagia symptoms, and is sensitive to change in patient performance over time. The 24 items in the MASA combine to provide a total score and cutoff criteria for dysphagia and aspiration severity. It is considered simple to use and score.

Silent Aspiration and the Clinical Swallow Examination

Silent aspiration is the penetration of food, liquid, or saliva to the subglottic area without the elicitation of a cough.

The clinician must always be aware of the possibility of silent aspiration. It has been estimated that silent aspiration may be as high as 40% in patients with dysphagia, and it is not generally identifiable during the CSE. However, a history of pneumonia, a weak or absent cough, changes in body temperature after eating, and a voice that has a "wet hoarse" quality suggest the possibility of silent aspiration. Additionally, the use of sensory testing provides an objective test of sensory awareness that may be the best indicator that the patient is a silent aspirator.[56,57]

SUMMARY

Normal swallowing consists of a series of well-coordinated neuromuscular movements beginning with placement of a bolus in the mouth. From that point, bolus transport and bolus awareness become an integrated neural process. Although originally thought to be a serial processing pattern, we now know that the 4 phases of swallowing (described in detail in Chapter 1) overlap considerably in a parallel processing paradigm. This chapter pointed out the importance of the clinical assessment and case history to guide further evaluation of the swallowing complaints. Depending on the types of patient complaints and by using self-assessment techniques and case history information, tests may be selected by one or more specialists involved in the patient's care. It should be noted that the diagnosis of swallowing disorders extends into many disciplines and that there is no single gold standard test for all swallow complaints. Different disciplines may opt for specific tests based on their initial evaluations. There is a significant growth in new screening and diagnostic clinical tools for dysphagia over the past decade. Some of them remain experimental or may be extremely costly to use on a regular basis. Nonetheless, clinicians should be aware of all of the possible tests for identifying the basis of the swallowing disorder and how the tests may aid in treating the problem.

DISCUSSION QUESTIONS

1. Which screening and self-assessment tool would you use for a patient with (a) physical

disability, (b) myasthenia gravis, (c) pain, and (d) stroke? Why?

2. If a patient cannot cooperate during the clinical swallow evaluation, what alternatives does the clinician have to assess patient's readiness to swallow?

STUDY QUESTIONS

1. Patient self-assessment in the management of swallowing disorders has limitations related to
   A. The number of tests now available
   B. The lack of construct validation of scales or charts now being used
   C. The cognitive condition of the patient when asked to complete the assessment
   D. The length of assessment scales

2. In conducting various clinical screenings of swallowing function, a false-positive test
   A. Is better because it will suggest conservative treatment procedures
   B. Indicates the patient is having problems that he really does not have
   C. Suggests that feeding or oral eating should be stopped due to aspiration
   D. Requires another test to verify the results

3. The prerequisites of conducting an oropharyngeal examination are
   A. Patient has self-reported swallowing problems
   B. Clinician is aware of patient's characteristics that may interfere with the examination
   C. The swallowing problems are because of neurological deficits
   D. Patient is on nonoral feeding

REFERENCES

1. Threats TT. Use of the ICF in dysphagia management. *Semin Speech Lang.* 2007;28(04):323–333.
2. Martino R, Silver F, Teasell R, et al. The Toronto Bedside Swallowing Screening Test (TOR-BSST): development and validation of a dysphagia screening tool for patients with stroke. *Stroke.* 2009;40(2):555–561.
3. Suiter DM, Leder SB. Clinical utility of the 3-ounce Water Swallow Test. *Dysphagia.* 2008;23(3):244–250.
4. DePippo KL, Holas MA, Reding MJ. Validation of the 3-oz Water Swallow Test for aspiration following stroke. *Arch Neurol.* 1992;49(12):1259–1261.
5. Smithard DG, O'Neill PA, Parks C, Morris J. Complications and outcome after acute stroke. Does dysphagia matter? *Stroke.* 1996;27:1200–1204.
6. Smithard DG, O'Neill PA, Park C, et al. Can bedside assessment reliably exclude aspiration following acute stroke? *Age Ageing.* 1998;27(2):99–106.
7. Smithard DG, O'Neill PA, England RE, et al. The natural history of dysphagia following a stroke. *Dysphagia.* 1997;12:188–193.
8. Ramsey DJ, Smithard DG, Kalra L. Early assessments of dysphagia and aspiration risk in acute stroke patients. *Stroke.* 2003;34(5):1252–1257.
9. Perry L. Screening swallowing function of patients with acute stroke. Part two: detailed evaluation of the tool used by nurses. *J Clin Nurs.* 2001;10(4):474–481.
10. Perry L. Screening swallowing function of patients with acute stroke. Part one: identification, implementation and initial evaluation of a screening tool for use by nurses. *J Clin Nurs.* 2001;10(4):463–473.
11. Perry L, Love CP. Screening for dysphagia and aspiration in acute stroke: a systematic review. *Dysphagia.* 2001;16(1):7–18.
12. Trapl M, Enderle P, Nowotny M, et al. Dysphagia bedside screening for acute-stroke patients The Gugging Swallowing Screen. *Stroke.* 2007;38(11):2948–2952.
13. Edmiaston J, Connor LT, Loehr L, Nassief A. Validation of a dysphagia screening tool in acute stroke patients. *Am J Crit Care.* 2010;19(4):357–364.
14. Antonios N, Carnaby-Mann G, Crary M, et al. Analysis of a physician tool for evaluating dysphagia on an inpatient stroke unit: The Modified Mann Assessment of Swallowing Ability. *J Stroke Cerebrovasc Dis.* 2010;19(1):49–57.
15. Martino R, Silver F, Teasell R, et al. The Toronto Bedside Swallowing Screening Test (TOR-BSST): development and validation of a dysphagia screening tool for patients with stroke. *Stroke.* 2009;40(2):555–561.
16. Suiter DM, Leder SB. Clinical utility of the 3-ounce water swallow test. *Dysphagia.* 2007;23(3):244–250.
17. Daniels SK, Anderson JA, Willson PC. Valid items for screening dysphagia risk in patients with stroke: a systematic review. *Stroke.* 2012;43(3):892–897.
18. DePippo KL, Holas MA, Reding MJ. The Burke dysphagia screening test: validation of its use in patients with stroke. *Arch Phys Med Rehabil.* 1994;75(12):1284–1286.
19. O'Neil-Pirozzi MT, Lisiecki JD, Jack Momose KD, Connors JJ, Milliner PM. Simultaneous modified barium swallow and blue dye tests: a determination of the accuracy of blue dye test aspiration findings. *Dysphagia.*18(1):32–38.

20. Belafsky PC, Blumenfeld L, Lepage A, Nahrstedt K. The accuracy of the Modified Evan's Blue Dye Test in predicting aspiration. *Laryngoscope.* 2003;113(11):1969–1972.

21. Timmerman AA, Speyer R, Heijnen BJ, Klijn-Zwijnenberg IR. Psychometric characteristics of health-related quality-of-life questionnaires in oropharyngeal dysphagia. *Dysphagia.* 2014;29(2):183–198.

22. McHorney CA, Bricker DE, Kramer AE, et al. The SWAL-QOL outcomes tool for oropharyngeal dysphagia in adults: I. conceptual foundation and item development. *Dysphagia.* 2000;15(3):115–121.

23. McHorney CA, Bricker DE, Robbins J, Kramer AE, Rosenbek JC, Chignell KA. The SWAL-QOL outcomes tool for oropharyngeal dysphagia in adults: II. item reduction and preliminary scaling. *Dysphagia.* 2000;15(3):122–133.

24. McHorney CA, Robbins J, Lomax K, et al. The SWAL-QOL and SWAL-CARE outcomes tool for oropharyngeal dysphagia in adults: III. documentation of reliability and validity. *Dysphagia.* 2002;17(2):97–114.

25. Lovell SJ, Wong HB, Loh KS, Ngo R, Wilson JA. Impact of dysphagia on quality-of-life in nasopharyngeal carcinoma. *Head Neck.* 2005;27(10):864–872.

26. dos Santos Queija D, Portas JG, Dedivitis RA, Lehn CN, Barros APB. Swallowing and quality of life after total laryngectomy and pharyngolaryngectomy. *Braz J Otorhinolaryngol.* 2009;75(4):556–564.

27. McHorney AC, Robbins J, Lomax K, et al. The SWAL-QOL and SWAL-CARE outcomes tool for oropharyngeal dysphagia in adults: III. documentation of reliability and validity. *Dysphagia.*17(2):97–114.

28. Bogaardt HCA, Speyer R, Baijens LWJ, Fokkens WJ. Cross-cultural adaptation and validation of the Dutch version of SWAL-QoL. *Dysphagia.* 2008;24(1):66–70.

29. Khaldoun E, Woisard V, Verin É. Validation in French of the SWAL-QOL scale in patients with oropharyngeal dysphagia. *Gastroentérol Clin Biol.* 2009;33(3):167–171.

30. Finizia C, Rudberg I, Bergqvist H, Rydén A. A cross-sectional validation study of the Swedish version of SWAL-QOL. *Dysphagia.* 2011;27(3):325–335.

31. Lam PM, Lai CKY. The Validation of the Chinese version of the Swallow Quality-of-Life Questionnaire (SWAL-QOL) using exploratory and confirmatory factor analysis. *Dysphagia.* 2010;26(2):117–124.

32. Bandeira AKC, Azevedo EH, Vartanian JG, Nishimoto IN, Kowalski LP, Carrara-de Angelis E. Quality of life related to swallowing after tongue cancer treatment. *Dysphagia.* 2008;23(2):183–192.

33. Robbins J, Kays SA, Gangnon RE, et al. The effects of lingual exercise in stroke patients with dysphagia. *Arch Phys Med Rehabil.* 2007;88(2):150–158.

34. Troche MS, Okun MS, Rosenbek JC, et al. Aspiration and swallowing in Parkinson disease and rehabilitation with EMST: a randomized trial. *Neurology.* 2010;75(21):1912–1919.

35. Keage M, Delatycki M, Corben L, Vogel A. A systematic review of self-reported swallowing assessments in progressive neurological disorders. *Dysphagia.* 2014;30(1):27–46.

36. Chen AY, Frankowski R, Bishop-Leone J, et al. The development and validation of a dysphagia-specific quality-of-life questionnaire for patients with head and neck cancer: The MD Anderson Dysphagia Inventory. *Arch Otolaryngol Head Neck Surg.* 2001;127(7):870–876.

37. Schindler A, Borghi E, Tiddia C, Ginocchio D, Felisati G, Ottaviani F. Adaptation and validation of the Italian MD Anderson Dysphagia Inventory (MDADI). *Rev Laryngol Otol Rhinol.* 2007;129(2):97–100.

38. Carlsson S, Rydén A, Rudberg I, Bove M, Bergquist H, Finizia C. Validation of the Swedish M.D. Anderson Dysphagia Inventory (MDADI) in patients with head and neck cancer and neurologic swallowing disturbances. *Dysphagia.* 2011;27(3):361–369.

39. Kwon C-H, Kim YH, Park JH, Oh B-M, Han TR. Validity and reliability of the Korean version of the MD Anderson Dysphagia Inventory for head and neck cancer patients. *Ann Rehabil Med.* 2013;37(4):479–487.

40. Speyer R, Heijnen BJ, Baijens LW, et al. Quality of life in oncological patients with oropharyngeal dysphagia: validity and reliability of the Dutch version of the MD Anderson Dysphagia Inventory and the Deglutition Handicap Index. *Dysphagia.* 2011;26(4):407–414.

41. Belafsky PC, Mouadeb DA, Rees CJ, et al. Validity and reliability of the Eating Assessment Tool (EAT-10). *Ann Otol Rhinol Laryngol.* 2008;117(12):919–924.

42. Silbergleit AK, Schultz L, Jacobson BH, Beardsley T, Johnson AF. The Dysphagia Handicap Index: development and validation. *Dysphagia.* 2011;27(1):46–52.

43. McCullough G, Wertz R, Rosenbek J. Sensitivity and specificity of clinical/bedside examination signs for detecting aspiration in adults subsequent to stroke. *J Commun Disord.* 2001;34(1):55–72.

44. Peruzzi WT, Logemann JA, Currie D, Moen SG. Assessment of aspiration in patients with tracheostomies: comparison of the bedside colored dye assessment with videofluoroscopic examination. *Respir Care.* 2001;46(3):243–247.

45. Carrau RL, Murry T, Howell RJ. *Comprehensive management of swallowing disorders.* San Diego, CA: Plural; 2016.

46. Daniels SK, McAdam CP, Brailey K, Foundas AL. Clinical assessment of swallowing and prediction of dysphagia severity. *Am J Speech Lang Pathol.* 1997;6(4):17–24.

47. Borr C, Hielscher-Fastabend M, Lücking A. Reliability and validity of cervical auscultation. *Dysphagia.* 2007;22(3):225–234.

48. Leslie P, Drinnan MJ, Finn P, Ford GA, Wilson JA. Reliability and validity of cervical auscultation: a controlled comparison using videofluoroscopy. *Dysphagia.* 2004;19(4):231–240.

49. Lagarde ML, Kamalski DM, van den Engel-Hoek L. The reliability and validity of cervical auscultation in the diagnosis of dysphagia: a systematic review. *Clin Rehabil.* 2016;30(2):199–207.

50. Collins MJ, Bakheit A. Does pulse oximetry reliably detect aspiration in dysphagic stroke patients? *Stroke.* 1997;28(9):1773–1775.

51. Smith HA, Lee SH, O'Neill PA, Connolly MJ. The combination of bedside swallowing assessment and oxygen saturation monitoring of swallowing in acute stroke: a safe and humane screening tool. *Age Ageing.* 2000;29(6): 495–499.

52. Lim SH, Lieu P, Phua S, et al. Accuracy of bedside clinical methods compared with fiberoptic endoscopic examination of swallowing (FEES) in determining the risk of aspiration in acute stroke patients. *Dysphagia.* 2001; 16(1):1–6.

53. Kolb G, Bröker M. State of the art in aspiration assessment and the idea of a new noninvasive predictive test for the risk of aspiration in stroke. *J Nutr Health Aging.* 2009;13(5):429–433.

54. Ramsey DJC, Smithard DG, Kalra L. Can pulse oximetry or a bedside swallowing assessment be used to detect aspiration after stroke? *Stroke.* 2006;37(12):2984–2988.

55. Mann G. *The Mann Assessment of Swallowing Ability: MASA.* Philadelphia, PA: Delmar Thomson Learning; 2002:5–39.

56. Splaingard M, Hutchins B, Sulton L, Chaudhuri G. Aspiration in rehabilitation patients: videofluoroscopy vs. bedside clinical assessment. *Arch Phys Med Rehabil.* 1988; 69(8):637–640.

57. Aviv JE, Martin JH, Debell M, Keen MS, Blitzer A. Air pulse quantification of supraglottic and pharyngeal sensation: a new technique. *Ann Otol Rhinol Laryngol.* 1993; 102(10):777–780.

Chapter

6

Instrumental Evaluation of Swallowing Disorders

A Look at the Chapter

Instrumental evaluation of swallowing disorders is important for detecting aspiration and penetration in patients with swallowing disorders. Instrumental evaluation also helps to determine the causes of swallowing problems and the effects of certain treatment procedures (such as posture and diet modifications). This chapter will introduce the common instrumental measurements for swallowing. Note that clinicians or student clinicians usually need to attend dedicated hands-on workshops for most instrumental measurements before they can be skillful in operating the instruments or interpreting the results. Other health professionals are also usually involved in conducting these instrumental measurements.

INTRODUCTION

Screening assessments of dysphagia, case histories, and clinical swallow examination are important steps in learning about the patient, his or her concerns regarding swallowing, his or her ability to follow instructions, and his or her ability to cooperate in more detailed examinations of the swallowing mechanisms. However, none of the procedures in these preliminary screening or clinical assessment measures offer direct information about the safety of swallowing—namely, if the patient aspirated on the bolus. For that reason, it is often necessary to do an instrumental evaluation of swallowing to verify the impressions of the clinical assessment and to offer direct guidance regarding the safety of oral nutrition. The American Speech-Language-Hearing Association (ASHA) published an official statement on "clinical indicators for instrumental assessment of dysphagia."[1] The guidelines were developed by a group of experts in swallowing based on available evidence. The guidelines indicated that the objectives of the instrumental examination should be to allow the speech-language pathologist to

- Visualize the swallowing and respiratory-related structures (from the oral cavity to the esophagus).

- Assess the physiologic functioning, sensation, coordination, and effectiveness of swallowing-related structures and muscles.
- Determine the presence, cause, and patterns of aspiration.
- Visualize the management of secretions in the hypopharyngeal and laryngeal area.
- Screen the anatomy and physiology of the esophageal area to assist in determining the cause and presence of dysphagia.
- Assist in determining whether oral or nonoral feeding is most suitable for the client.
- Determine the safety and efficiency of different swallowing management options (such as rate, volume, and consistency of foods and drinks; delivery methods; postures, positioning, and maneuvers during mealtimes).

Table 6–1[1] highlights some of the indications for and against conducting instrumental swallowing evaluation as proposed by ASHA.

New instruments or improvement on current instrumental measures for swallowing functions

TABLE 6–1. Indications for and Against Conducting Instrumental Swallowing Evaluation Proposed by the American Speech-Language-Hearing Association[a]

Indications
Instrumental evaluation is suggested when the following conditions occur: • Inconsistent findings from clinical swallow examination   • A need to confirm diagnosis or cause of dysphagia   • Past history of nutritional or pulmonary complications that may be a result of dysphagia   • A need to confirm swallow safety and efficiency   • Dysphagia is confirmed; further information needed to guide rehabilitation/management
Instrumental evaluation is *not* suggested when the following conditions occur: • Unstable medical conditions   • Inability to cooperate or participate in the instrumental evaluation   • Swallowing rehabilitation or management strategies will not be affected by the results of the instrumental evaluation

[a]Adapted from American Speech-Language-Hearing Association.[1]

are being developed rapidly. Clinicians should fully understand the rationale, requirements, operations, and interpretation of the instruments before implementing them in clinical practice. Table 6–2 highlights the characteristics of the more commonly used instrumental evaluations of swallowing. Some of these instruments require hands-on training before clinicians may use them.

FLEXIBLE ENDOSCOPIC EVALUATION OF SWALLOWING (FEES)

The **flexible endoscopic evaluation of swallowing (FEES)** assessment was first described by Langmore and colleagues in 1988.[2] FEES is an assessment that uses a transnasal flexible laryngoscope (TFL) to evaluate the swallow before and after the pharyngeal swallow (Figure 6–1). FEES may be conducted at the bedside, at the speech therapy clinic, or in an endoscopy suite. The assessment of swallowing using this technique requires the passage of a flexible laryngoscope into the nares, over the velum, and to a position above the epiglottis (Figure 6–2).

This procedure may be conducted either independently by a speech-language pathologist who has received the relevant training or as a team including an otolaryngologist and a speech-language pathologist.

Before the start of swallowing trials, the anatomy of the pharynx and larynx should be observed during quiet and forced respiration, coughing, speaking, and dry swallows. Attention is also given to the motion of the base of the tongue, pharyngeal walls, arytenoids, and other endolaryngeal structures. Symmetry, coordination, and range of movement between the 2 sides of the upper aerodigestive tract are also noted. Pooling of secretions or food residue in the vallecula or piriform sinuses is noted.

Specific amounts of liquids and food consistencies treated with food dye are viewed as they pass the pharynx and larynx. The speed of the pharyngeal swallow, premature flow of food or liquid into the pharyngeal and laryngeal areas, and residual amounts of the bolus can all be seen during this examination.

TABLE 6–2. Characteristics of Commonly Used Instrumental Measures

	"Visualize" Structures	Measures Physiologic Functioning	Detects Aspiration	Determine Etiology	Assist in Determining Safety of Intake Methods
FEES/FEEST	✓	✓	✓	✓	✓
MBS	✓	✓	✓	✓	✓
Ultrasound	✓	✓	X	X	X
(High-resolution) Manometry	X	✓	✓[a]	✓	X
Tongue strength/ endurance measurement	X	✓	X	X	X

Abbreviations: FEES, flexible endoscopic evaluation of swallowing; FEEST, flexible endoscopic examination of swallowing with sensory testing; MBS, modified barium swallow examination.

[a]Indirect detection of aspiration.

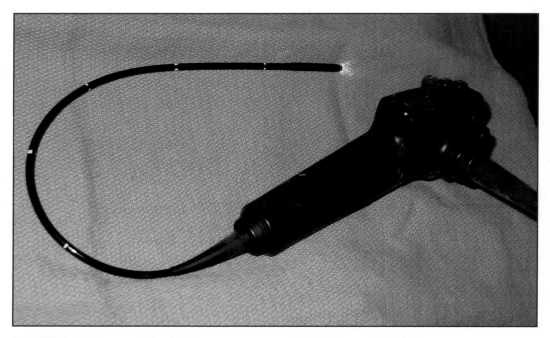

FIGURE 6–1. Transnasal flexible laryngoscope used for FEES and FEESST examinations.

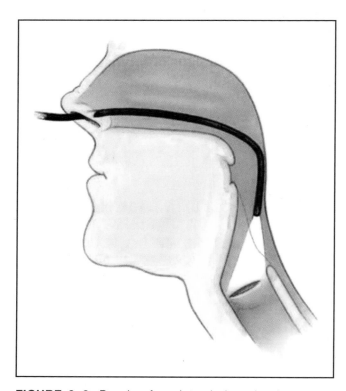

FIGURE 6–2. Drawing from lateral view showing proper placement of scope prior to feeding the patient. Note the scope is above the epiglottis.

*Note that during the time of airway closure, the swallow cannot be visualized, as the pharyngeal walls contract over the bolus, collapsing the lumen over the endoscope (**whiteout phase**).*

Monitoring of the bolus is only possible after the pharyngeal swallow. However, the bolus can be monitored as it enters into view from the oral cavity to the pharynx. The endoscope may remain in place for long periods to monitor the residual bolus and examine anatomical structures. Swallowing, using compensatory strategies and changes in neck position, is easily accomplished while the endoscope is in place.

Flexible endoscopic evaluation of swallowing with sensory testing (FEESST) is a sensory and motor test of swallowing developed by Aviv[3] to quantify the sensory and motor deficiencies in dysphagia. This protocol was developed to compensate for the lack of sensory test in the protocol originally proposed for FEES. Early research on transnasal flexible endoscopy for swallowing suggested the importance of sensitivity testing of the larynx during an endoscopic swallowing evaluation. What these early studies described was touching or tapping the laryngopharyngeal tissues with the tip of the endoscope and assessing the patient's reaction to such stimulation.[4] Touching or tapping tissues with an endoscope tip is an extremely subjective way to assess sensory capacity. Movement of the endoscope itself may cause a reaction prior to tapping the tissues. Furthermore, it is difficult to translate the reaction to a tissue tap from patient to patient or from the same patient one day to the next.

To perform FEEST, an air-pulse generator is used to send a pulse of air from a specially designed machine through a port in a specially designed flexible nasopharyngoscope. Air pulses can be delivered to the supraglottic larynx and pharynx areas. Using a calibrated puff of air, sensory thresholds can then be determined using one of the psychophysical testing methods. The twitch response of the mucosa suggests the sensory awareness of the stimulus. Video 6–1 shows a FEESST exam. In this exam the endoscope is seen delivering a pulse of air

to the aryepiglottic fold prior to delivering food to the patient. The FEESST provides an accurate indication of the sensory function or dysfunction of the aryepiglottic space, which in turn reflects the degree of awareness of bolus in the oropharynx and the need to protect the airway. A complete protocol for conducting the FEESST is currently available,[5] and it has been shown to be safe when performed following training.[5,6]

Airway protection is determined by administering a pressure- and duration-controlled calibrated pulse of air to the hypopharyngeal tissues innervated by the internal branch of the superior laryngeal nerve (SLN) in order to elicit the **laryngeal adductor reflex (LAR)**, a fundamental brainstem-mediated airway protective reflex.[3] Figure 6–3 shows the examination procedure with a trained SLP conducting the examination. Because swallowing is a complex process that involves interplay between two distinct but related phenomena, airway protection and bolus transport, a test that assesses both sensory and motor components of swallowing

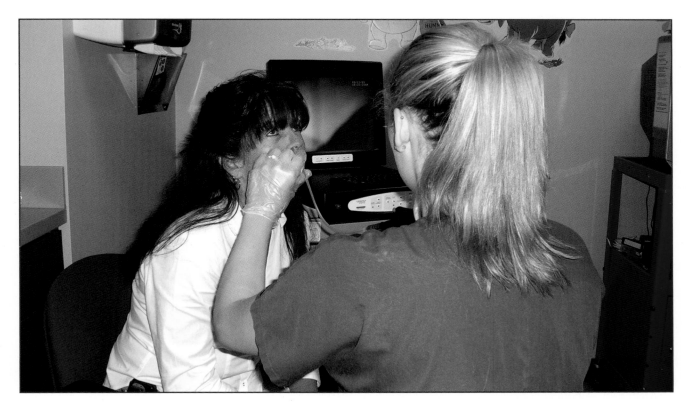

FIGURE 6–3. Trained SLP conducting FEES exam on patient.

is highly advantageous, as opposed to a test that measures the motor component only. Almost all tests of swallowing—**videofluoroscopy** or modified barium swallow (MBS), **manometry**, **esophogram**, flexible endoscopic examination of swallowing (FEES)—specifically look at bolus transport and ignore or infer airway protective capacity. It has been shown that the afferent signal arising from the internal branch of the SLN is necessary for normal deglutition, especially for providing feedback to central neural circuits, which facilitate laryngeal adduction during swallowing.[7] With information obtained from the FEESST regarding the patient's sensory and motor functions, the patient with aspiration is managed quite differently depending on what his or her sensory test results show. The sensory test, along with the food administration portion of the FEESST, provides comprehensive information regarding both sensory and motor functions of the swallowing mechanism. Neither FEES nor MBS alone allow the clinician to safely make decisions to feed the patient or to withhold feeding.[8]

A video camera and recorder coupled to the endoscope provide a permanent record of the examination for later review by the clinician and patient and serve as a baseline to monitor the patient's progress. In selected cases, FEES/FEESST can provide a patient with visual feedback that may aid the rehabilitation process. Figure 6–4 shows the bolus

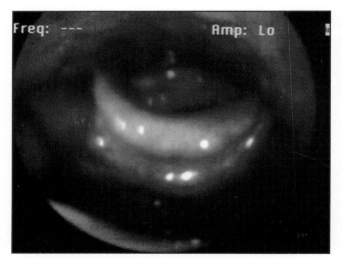

FIGURE 6–4. A portion of the bolus remaining in the hypopharynx after patient swallowed.

penetrating below the epiglottis after the patient attempted to swallow. Video 6–2 shows a FEES video of an individual who had penetration on both liquid and solid materials but produced a cough to clear the penetrated boluses.

MODIFIED BARIUM SWALLOW (MBS)

The modified barium swallow (MBS) is also called a videofluoroscopic swallowing study (VFSS). The MBS is a multidisciplinary evaluation of the swallowing mechanism involving collaboration between a radiologist and an SLP, and was first described by Logemann.[9]

The MBS offers a dynamic assessment of the oral, pharyngeal, and esophageal phases of swallowing by means of videofluoroscopy.

The MBS provides a comprehensive instrumental assessment of swallowing. The decision to recommend an MBS test is often based on the findings of the clinical swallow examination. The test requires a fluoroscopic unit, video recorder, a chair suitable for stabilizing the patient, and various food and liquids that will be coated or mixed with barium.

Under fluoroscopic observation, controlled by the radiologist, the patient ingests barium-coated boluses or liquid barium of varying consistencies, offered at the discretion of the SLP. The MBS usually starts with a liquid barium preparation unless there is evidence of choking on liquids. Thickened barium liquid, pudding, and solids (usually pieces of cookie or a marshmallow coated with barium) are also commonly used in this test. These consistencies are chosen to approximate the consistencies of food that a patient is likely to encounter in his or her daily diet. Clinicians may also ask the patients to bring back their usual foods, such as foods that are specific to their culture and religion, to test the patient's ability to handle different consistencies of food.

Frontal and lateral dynamic x-rays are obtained with the fluoroscope in a fixed position during the MBS with the patient standing or sitting. Video 6–3 is a sample of MBS taken at the lateral position of an individual who had delayed swallow reflex. The MBS is purely dynamic; the complete study is often digitally recorded. Concerns were raised with the number of frames by seconds that are digitized. ASHA recommends that the MBS should be digitized at a rate of 30 frames per second. The MBS can be used with various consistencies, different patient postures in swallowing, or different techniques to manage the bolus. With this recorded information, goals can be set, and treatment can be defined.

MBS Test Observations

The MBS concentrates on the **oral**, **oropharyngeal**, and **hypopharyngeal** phases of deglutition, including the opening of the upper esophageal sphincter; it is also useful to perform a brief evaluation of the esophagus. This dynamic study evaluates formation of the bolus in the mouth, tongue motion, coordination, timing and completeness of swallowing, movement of the epiglottis, elevation of the larynx, and cricopharyngeal contraction. Video 6–4 shows the MBS of a 74-year-old man who was 6 years post stroke and had pharyngeal residue after swallow. Video 6–5 shows the MBS of a 66-year-old man who was 2 years post stroke and had reduced laryngeal elevation and aspiration of thin liquid. Because of the potential danger of excessive exposure to radiation, the clinician must select consistencies wisely in order to limit the patient's radiation exposure.

The MBS is an excellent test for evaluating the oral and pharyngeal phases of swallowing. Pathology that may explain the presence of dysphagia, such as abnormal movements of the tongue in forming the bolus and initiating deglutition, residual barium that pools in the valleculae or piriform sinuses, and aspiration of barium into the airway can be identified. Nasopharyngeal reflux of barium should also be documented during the MBS. Because the entire fluoroscopic study is recorded on videotape or digitally archived, the study can provide a highly detailed analysis of the coordination and timing of swallowing. The MBS may also include testing with compensatory and swallowing maneuvers, such as the chin-tuck, supraglottic swallow, or Mendelsohn maneuver, to name a few. These postures and maneuvers are discussed in Chapter 7.

Radiation Safety During MBS

Studies have shown that the radiation dose level of typical MBS sessions is very low and safe.[10] One study estimated that a patient may receive up to 15 to 40 MBSs annually before exceeding the National Institutes of Health recommended annual radiation dose limit.[11] Often, the patient with a severe problem or a patient undergoing treatment for dysphagia will be given more than 1 MBS within a year but usually no more than 5 MBSs a year. On the other hand, clinicians can easily conduct more than 40 VFSSs per year. Therefore, it is very important for clinicians to protect themselves against radiation exposure during MBS. It is necessary for clinicians to wear protective shields (including a thyroid shield, lead apron, protective glasses, and protective gloves) and a dosimetry badge during MBS. The clinician should also try to keep a distance from the patient and x-ray tube as much as possible. ASHA has issued guidelines on performing VFSS, including a section on radiation safety.

Guidelines for SLPs Performing Videofluoroscopic Swallowing Studies:

Measurement Scales for MBS

Although the MBS is an instrumental measurement of swallowing functions, the interpretation of the MBS is subjective. The reliability and validity of the interpretation may vary depending on the definitions of the analysis parameters, the knowledge, skills, and experience of the clinicians and the quality of the recorded images. Three more commonly used analysis protocols are described below.

Penetration-Aspiration Scale (PAS)

Entry of barium into the airway may be one of the most important observations that the team performing the MBS can make. The clearest and most clinically useful solution to the problem of terminology is to state the location of the barium that extends lowest into the airway. This may be as subtle as a coating of the laryngeal surface of the epiglottis (ie, penetration), or as obvious as gross aspiration of barium into the trachea, as shown in Figure 6–5. Video 6–6 shows the MBS of a 68-year-old man who was 4 years post stroke and had silent aspiration. The location and extent of aspiration should be stated clearly in the MBS report.

Rosenbek and his colleagues[12] proposed an 8-step scale to evaluate the degree of penetration and aspiration seen in the MBS. That scale may be quite useful to monitor changes in a patient's ability to control aspiration and advance to another eating level.

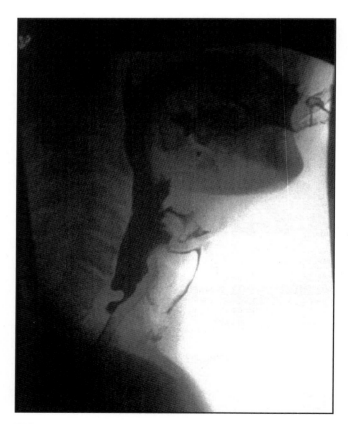

FIGURE 6–5. A lateral radiograph during the modified barium swallow showing significant aspiration.

The 8 steps of the Penetration-Aspiration Scale (PAS) are as follows:

1. Material does not enter airway.
2. Remains above folds/ejected from airway.
3. Remains above folds/not ejected from airway.
4. Contacts fold/ejected from airway.
5. Contacts fold/not ejected from airway.
6. Passes below folds/ejected into larynx or out of airway
7. Passes below folds/not ejected despite effort
8. Passes below folds/no spontaneous effort to eject

Although these steps may not be exact intervals, they do describe decreasing swallow safety, from no penetration to aspiration.

The PAS has been shown to have good reliability and validity and was used to track swallowing changes in individuals with different diseases and disorders.[13–15] Recent study has shown the Penetration-Aspiration Scale may also be applied to the analysis of FEES.[16,17]

Modified Barium Swallow Impairment Profile (MBSImP)

Martin-Harris et al[18] reviewed the findings of the MBS and found that with the number of studies reported in the past 30 years, the degree of validity, reliability, and interpretation of these measures in various patient populations was highly variable. From this review, she and her colleagues developed the Modified Barium Swallow Impairment Profile (MBSImP). The MBSImp is a qualitative measurement tool based on previously validated instruments (such as the PAS, nutritional health status, etc). The MBSImp contains 17 measures, and the scores are based on physiological observations and bolus flow measures. The MBSImp scores were found to correlate significantly with intake recommendations made by SLPs, the Penetration-Aspiration Scale, and measures of quality of life. The authors suggest that the MBSImp demonstrates the importance of obtaining a validated measure of swallowing using a standardized set of terms, a standardized protocol for interpreting the MBS, and a standardized reporting system that can be transferred from institution to institution. Clinicians are required to complete and pass an online training course (takes around 20 to 25 hours and cost involved) before becoming a certified MBSImp clinician, and the certificate needs to be renewed every 5 years.

MBSImp:

Quantitative Analysis of MBS

With advancement and increased availability of free video and image editing software, it is now easier to quantitatively analyze the MBS. Different protocols are tested and described in the literature.[19–21] Common to these protocols is the use of imaging software to guide the analysis. The following steps are usually involved:

1. Digitize the MBS.
2. Identify certain frames in the video clip that correspond to specific moments of the swallow (eg, start of swallow reflex, the frame with the highest laryngeal elevation, or the frame with the maximum pharyngeal constriction).
3. Identify and delineate anatomical landmarks or bolus size.
4. Use the measures obtained from the steps above to calculate specific swallowing-related outcomes (eg, pharyngeal constriction ratio, oral and pharyngeal transit times, laryngeal displacement distance or residue area).

The advantages of using these quantitative measures for MBS are that these measures are objective, reliable, and sensitive to subtle changes in swallowing functions over time. However, it can be time-consuming to obtain these measures. Clinicians will also need to be trained and familiarized with the procedures involved in obtaining these measures.

MBS, FEES, AND SILENT ASPIRATION

The MBS can often provide information as to the cause of aspiration, but it does not necessarily predict aspiration. Silent aspiration may remain undetected on clinical swallow examination and even after the modified barium swallow because limited swallow trials are included.

Silent aspiration is aspiration of foreign materials into the tracheobronchial tree that fails to elicit a normal cough response to clear the materials.

Abnormal motion of the epiglottis, diminished contractions of the pharyngeal constrictor muscles, and abnormal laryngeal "rise" can all be identified on the modified barium swallow, FEES, or FEESST. The use of sensory testing can further be used to predict the risk of silent aspiration. A lack of laryngeal adductor reflex may indicate abnormal laryngeal sensation and an increased risk of silent aspiration. Silent aspiration offers evidence of an underlying neurological dysfunction related to the loss or diminution of sensation.

Leder and Espinosa[22] examined a cohort of subjects using the FEES technique following clinical examination. They found that the clinical examination underestimated aspiration risk in patients who were at risk for aspiration but overestimated aspiration risk in patients who did not exhibit aspiration risk. A retrospective review of the results from the FEESST and videofluoroscopic examinations of 54 subjects by Tabaee et al[23] revealed complete agreement in 52% of the examinations done within a 5-day period. In the other 48%, the disagreements were related to the amount of pooling, penetration, and aspiration. The FEESST tended to lead observers to identify higher percentages of pooling, penetration, and minor aspiration than the videofluorographic exam.

MANOMETRY AND HIGH RESOLUTION MANOMETRY

Pharyngeal manometry refers to the measure of pharyngeal pressure. Manometry is performed with a catheter, a thin tube about 35-cm long and constructed with multiple pressure sensors, which is passed transnasally, and the patient is instructed to perform a series of wet and dry swallows. **High resolution manometry** has pressure sensors that are placed around 1 to 2 cm apart (compared with 3 to 5 cm in conventional ones) and the pressure measures are better presented and analyzed than conventional ones.[24] Pharyngeal manometry can be performed in conjunction with esophageal motility studies. Manometry is used in the evaluation of **esophageal motility disorders**, including achalasia and diffuse esophageal spasm. It is also important in the identification of motor abnormalities associated with other systemic diseases such as scleroderma, diabetes mellitus, and chronic intestinal pseudo-obstruction.

With conventional manometry, the response of the oropharynx to swallowing has two components. First, compression of the catheter against the pharyngeal wall by the tongue results in a high, sharp-peaked amplitude pressure wave followed by a low-amplitude, long-duration wave that reflects the initiation of pharyngeal peristalsis. Second, there is contraction of the middle and inferior pharyngeal constrictor muscles to provide the midpharyngeal response to swallowing, resulting in a rapid, high-amplitude pressure upstroke ending in a single, sharp peak, followed by a rapid return to baseline. Lower esophageal sphincter (LES) pressure is measured at baseline and in response to a swallow. LES pressure is measured as a step up in pressure from the gastric baseline referenced as atmospheric. Complete LES relaxation with a swallow is demonstrated by a decrease in pressure to gastric baseline for approximately 6 seconds. Basal upper esophageal sphincter (UES) pressures can be identified as a rise in pressure above the esophageal baseline. Due to the asymmetry of the UES, this is normally 50 to 100 mm Hg depending on the direction of the pressure sensor (ie, whether lateral or anterior/posterior). Evaluation of UES relaxation and correlation of sphincter relaxation with pharyngeal contraction is obtained by instructing the patient to perform a series of wet swallows. Figure 6–6 shows the conventional manometry catheter in place.

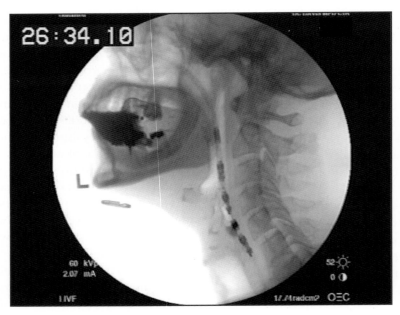

FIGURE 6–6. A radiograph showing the manometry sensing tube in place for study of esophageal motility.

A recent randomized multicenter study comparing the use of conventional and high resolution manometry suggested that high resolution manometry was more consistent than conventional manometry in diagnosing esophageal motility disorders, especially for **achalasia**.[24] The use of manometry to measure the intrabolus pressures during the pharyngeal phase of swallowing may predict which patients will respond to a surgical **myotomy**.

Esophageal manometry with video recording **(videomanometry)** consists of simultaneously recording video radiographic images and solid-state manometry to determine the relationships between intraluminal pressures and movement of the anatomical structures while the bolus passes through the swallowing structures. It provides a qualitative as well as a quantitative assessment of esophageal motility, pressures, and coordination. Videomanometry has been used to document the effects of swallow maneuvers such as the supraglottic swallow, the effortful swallow, and the chin-tuck swallow posture to determine if they are beneficial to patients with oropharyngeal dysphagia.[25] Bülow and colleagues[25] found that none of the three techniques reduced the number of misdirected swallows, but the effortful swallow and the chin-tuck posture did reduce the depth of penetration. Kawahara et al[26] showed that anatomical variations in the esophagus such as the corkscrew esophagus or esophageal atresia are related to abnormal pressure changes that occur in children with esophageal motility disorders. It is apparent that the use of videomanometry has value both for the study of esophageal motility disorders as they are related to dysphagia symptoms and for identifying treatment options once an accurate diagnosis is made.

TONGUE PRESSURE/ STRENGTH MEASUREMENT

The tongue plays an important role during the oral stage of swallowing. The maximal and swallow tongue-palate pressure is a measure of tongue strength. Dysphagic individuals, in general, have been reported to have lower isometric and swallow tongue-palate pressure than healthy individuals.[27,28]

Different tools are available to measure tongue-palate pressure, some allow measuring during swallow (eg, KayPENTAX Swallowing Workstation), and some can only measure during nonswallow tasks (eg, Iowa Oral Performance Instrument, IOPI).

OTHER INSTRUMENTAL TESTS ASSOCIATED WITH SWALLOWING DISORDERS

Table 6–3 summarizes other tests associated with dysphagia and gastroesophageal reflux disease.

Ultrasound

Ultrasound uses high-frequency sounds (>2 MHz) from a transducer held or fixed in contact with skin to obtain a dynamic image of soft tissues. As ultrasound does not penetrate bone, its use is limited to the soft tissues of the oral cavity and parts of the oropharynx.

TABLE 6–3. Diagnostic Tests of Dysphagia and Gastroesophageal Reflux Disease[a]

Test	Indication
Barium esophagram	Structural lesions
Videoradiography	Pharyngeal function
Scintigraphy	Aspiration
Endoscopic ultrasound	Submucosal lesions
Endoscopy	Structural and mucosal lesions
Esophageal manometry	Motility disorders
24-hour pH-metry	Gastroesophageal reflux disease
Sensory testing	Laryngopharyngeal reflux disease
	Cough, throat clearing, excess mucus

[a]Adapted and expanded from Padda and Young.[29(p48)]

Ultrasound is completely noninvasive and does not use ionizing radiation; therefore, repeated studies can be done without risk.

Ultrasound is highly efficient in studying the oral aspects of bolus preparation and bolus transfer. These characteristics render ultrasound as highly useful for children or when multiple studies are required to make a diagnosis. However, if dysphagia due to pharyngeal or laryngeal dysfunction is suspected, ultrasound offers little diagnostic or treatment information.

In ultrasound studies of swallowing, a handheld transducer is placed submentally and is rotated 90°. The swallowing functions of the upper surface of the tongue, the intrinsic tongue muscles, and the soft tissue anatomy of the mouth are within the view of the transducer. Ultrasonography does not require the use of any special bolus or contrast (real food can be used).

Endoscopic Ultrasound

Endoscopic ultrasound is especially important in the evaluation of submucosal lesions, which cannot be adequately assessed with standard endoscopic techniques. Throughout the gastrointestinal (GI) tract, the wall layer echo structure is examined endosonographically (Figure 6–7).

Intraluminal probes are invasive and thus are not tolerated by all patients. The use of ultrasound intraluminal probes requires a high degree of experience and sometimes the probe cannot be passed through a tight stricture. Endoluminal ultrasonography has been used for the study of esophageal and cricopharyngeal diseases, including esophagitis, strictures, and motility disorders.

Electromyography (EMG)

Electromyography (EMG) is the measurement of electrical activity within a muscle. EMG is recommended to ascertain the presence of specific nerve or neuromuscular unit deficits, such as that accompanying vocal fold paralysis or to elucidate or cor-

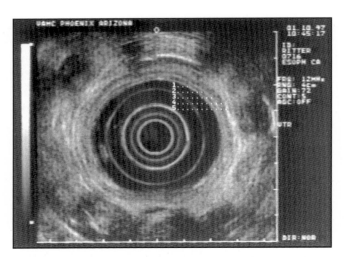

FIGURE 6–7. A photograph of an endoscopic ultrasound image taken in the esophagus. Layer 1 depicts the superficial mucosa, layer 2 is the deep mucosa, layer 3 corresponds to the submucosa, layer 4 corresponds to the muscularis propria, and layer 5 corresponds to surrounding fat in the esophagus, as there is no serosa in the esophagus. Adapted from Padda and Young.[29(p82)]

roborate the presence of a systemic myopathy or degenerative neuromuscular disease. When used for the diagnosis of vocal fold paralysis, laryngeal electromyography (LEMG) may also provide information regarding the prognosis for spontaneous recovery.

The goals of direct LEMG are to detect normal from abnormal activity and localize, and assess the severity of a focal lesion by determining whether there is neuropraxia (physiological nerve block or focal injury, with intact nerve fibers) or **axonotmesis** (damage to nerve fibers leading to complete peripheral degeneration).

Needle LEMG can also evaluate prognosis, providing valuable information to either proceed to definitive surgical correction for a permanent or long-term deficit, or implement temporary measures if spontaneous recovery is likely.

The thyroarytenoid muscle is approached by insertion of a monopolar or concentric electrode through the cricothyroid ligament midline 0.5 to 1 cm, then angled superiorly 45° and laterally 20° for a total depth of 2 cm. The cricothyroid muscle is reached by inserting the electrode 0.5 cm off the midline, then angling superiorly and laterally 20° toward the inferior border of the thyroid cartilage. Figure 6–8 shows a normal recruitment pattern. Reduced motor unit recruitment is observed with focal demyelinating (neuropraxic) lesions such as found after intubation injuries (Figure 6–9). Patients with axon loss lesions, such as partial nerve transection after surgical procedures, will also exhibit decreased motor unit recruit-

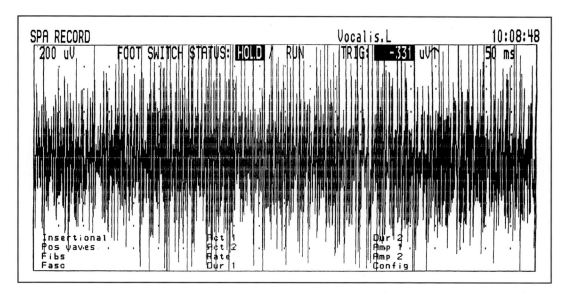

FIGURE 6–8. Normal voluntary motor unit recruitment of the vocalis muscle using the Valsalva maneuver. Note the full interference pattern that obliterates individual motor unit analysis when the sweep speed is set at 50 ms per division. *Source:* Adapted from Munin and Rainer.[30(p88)]

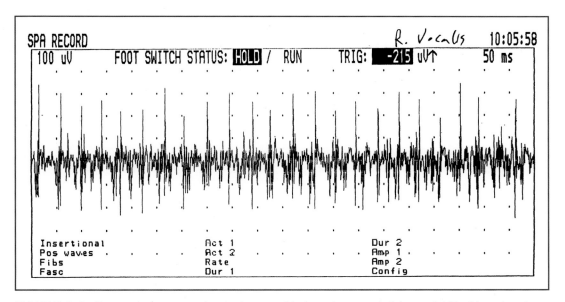

FIGURE 6–9. Decreased motor unit recruitment with the primary unit firing at 24 Hz. Note that there is a decreased interference pattern with the Valsalva maneuver. The sweep speed is 50 ms/division. Adapted from Munin and Rainer.[30(p89)]

ment with normal configuration within the first 6 weeks after injury. However, axonal injuries will exhibit positive waves and fibrillation potentials at rest, which begin 3 to 4 weeks postinjury. Laryngeal nerve regeneration following axon loss lesions can be observed between 6 weeks and 12 months post injury and is characterized by polyphasic motor unit potentials with wide duration.

LEMG is useful in differentiating neurological vocal fold paralysis from laryngeal joint injury. LEMG may also confirm the diagnosis of joint dislocation when a normal recruitment pattern is seen with vocal fold immobility.

The 3 areas of interest for electrodiagnostic evaluation of swallowing are the laryngeal sphincter, the sensory ability of the supraglottic larynx and pharynx (indirectly evaluated through cricothyroid muscle function), and the cricopharyngeal sphincter.

EMG, however, has several pitfalls: the precise site of the lesion cannot be determined, only whether it involves the vagus nerve or brainstem, the superior laryngeal nerve, or the recurrent laryngeal nerve. The posterior cricoarytenoid, which is the main abductor muscle, can be technically difficult to localize. Systemic neuromuscular diseases cannot be differentiated from focal lesions without full neurological evaluation in conjunction with EMG studies of other muscles and nerves.

Magnetic Resonance Imaging (MRI)

High-speed **magnetic resonance imaging (MRI)**, such as fast low angle shot (FAST) or echoplanar imaging, has permitted a dynamic analysis of the pharyngeal phase of swallowing that was impossible using conventional MRI. However, temporal and spatial resolution of MRI is inferior to videofluoroscopy, producing images with poor resolution. MRI is costly, and swallowing in the supine position may not reflect the true physiological mechanism of swallowing.

Functional Magnetic Resonance Imaging (fMRI)

Functional magnetic resonance imaging (fMRI) allows investigators to examine the neural mecha-

nisms of motion-induced tasks such as speaking and swallowing. A number of studies have used fMRI to examine the neural bases of swallowing in healthy individuals and study the cortical changes in dysphagic patients.[31-34] In doing so, functional neural mapping of the events such as swallowing provide information about the neural control under normal conditions and how control may be reestablished after injury to the primary cortical control center.[35] Figure 6–10 shows the activation areas during vocal fold movement in an fMRI.[36]

Positron Emission Tomography (PET)

Positron emission tomography (PET), like fMRI, provides a method of examining neural activity associated with specific motions. Although it is noninvasive, it has the disadvantage of exposure to radiation. Using PET, Smithard[37] demonstrated that swallowing has numerous representations in the brain for both normal healthy volunteers and post-stroke patients. Moreover, he demonstrated that recovery of swallowing following stroke may be spontaneous or may be enhanced by medications. Smithard suggested that recovery of cortical

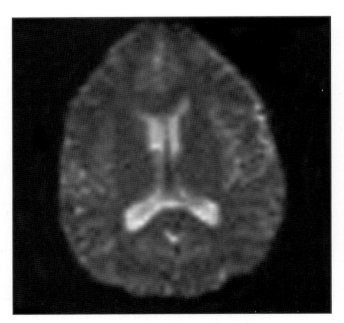

FIGURE 6–10. An fMRI showing the activation areas in white during vocal fold movement.

function does not necessarily follow the same path despite nearly the same location of stroke.

Esophogram (Barium Swallow)/Upper Gastrointestinal Series (UGIS)

The traditional barium swallow evaluates the upper aerodigestive tract between the oral cavity or oropharynx and the gastric fundus or cardia. It is not intended to identify swallow dysfunction, nor dictate treatment, as in the modified barium swallow (MBS).

The barium swallow can identify intrinsic and extrinsic pathology. Intrinsic abnormalities include tumors, cricopharyngeal dysfunction, and aspiration of barium into the airway or reflux into the nasopharynx, diverticula, webs, and esophageal dysmotility. Extrinsic masses such as cervical osteophytes, as seen in Figure 6–11, and an enlarged thy-

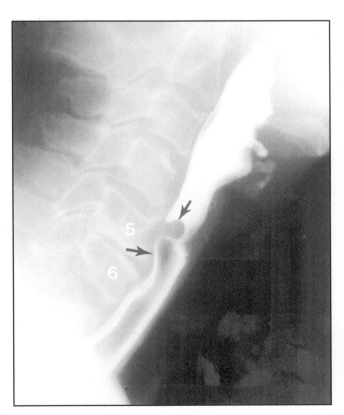

FIGURE 6–11. Lateral view of a barium swallow shows the impression of a prominent cricopharyngeus muscle (*arrow*) on the barium column. An osteophyte at C5-6 causes a smaller impression. *Source:* Adapted from Weissman.[38(p67)]

roid gland may be visualized directly or suspected by their effect on the barium column.

Computed Tomography (CT)

Computed tomography (CT) and MRI are used to delineate the anatomy of a particular region of the head, neck, or other components of the upper aerodigestive tract. The most common use is to identify the site of a lesion, as in the case of a cerebrovascular accident within the central nervous system, or to delineate the extent of a lesion in the intra- or extraluminal space. In general, CT offers direct axial and coronal images that better define the bony anatomy, as opposed to MRI, which better delineates the soft tissue (ie, brain, other neural structures, muscle) in sagittal, coronal, and axial planes, but takes longer to complete the images and thus is more prone to motion artifact.

Esophagoscopy

Endoscopy of the upper aerodigestive tract is recommended to rule out or biopsy a neoplasm that may be suspected as the cause of dysphagia or odynophagia. Occasionally, the endoscopy may be part of the treatment, as in those patients requiring injection of a paralyzed vocal fold, injection of **botulinum toxin**, or dilation of the esophagus for the treatment of cricopharyngeal achalasia or strictures. This procedure is usually conducted by a gastrointestinal specialist.

Dysphagia and odynophagia are common indications for upper GI endoscopy, technically known as an **esophagogastroduodenoscopy (EGD)**, which may be performed as the initial test in the evaluation of these disorders. The esophagus is intubated with a handheld scope of 60 mm under direct visualization of the posterior hypopharynx. The endoscope is usually advanced through the UES, which appears as a slit-like opening in the cricopharyngeus muscle at about 20 cm from the incisor teeth. The entire length of the esophagus is in direct view of the endoscope until its termination at the gastroesophageal junction, which lies at the diaphragmatic hiatus. The esophagus is usually closed at the gastroesophageal junction, but this is easily distended with air insufflation or swallowing. This allows the endoscope to easily advance through the LES into the stomach.

The EGD is the most specific test for identifying esophageal complications of gastroesophageal reflux disease (GERD), esophageal ulcers, infectious disorders, and benign and malignant neoplasms. It is, however, more useful in defining the cause of disease in those patients with solid food dysphagia (transit dysphagia). Contraindications for endoscopy include suspected perforation of the GI tract,

lack of adequately trained personnel, and lack of informed consent. Figure 6–12 shows a summary of pictures from a typical EGD exam.

Recently, a modification of the traditional EGD has been proposed. Transnasal esophagoscopy (TNE)[39] examines the esophagus by passing a small flexible scope through the nose, similar to laryngeal endoscopy. However, the scope is long enough to examine the entire length of the esophagus and the stomach. This test is done with the patient awake; thus, no general anesthesia is needed. Postma and colleagues[40]

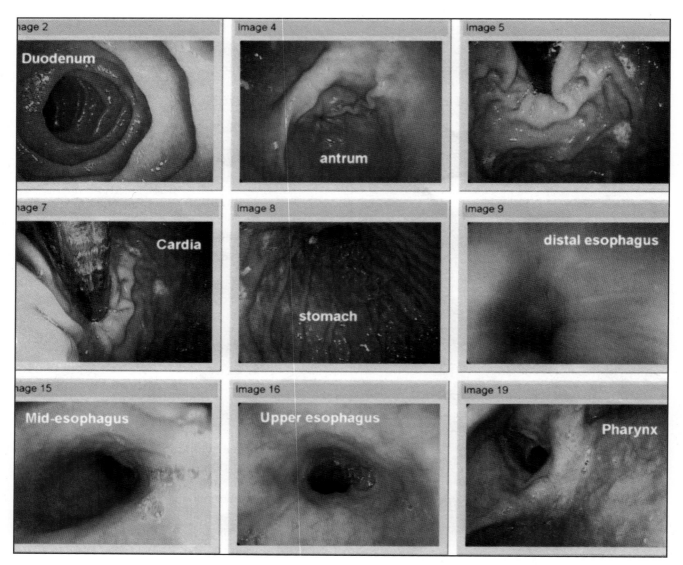

FIGURE 6–12. During the EGD, numerous pictures are taken at various locations along the esophagus and into the stomach. Images can be seen from the hypopharynx (where there is excessive mucous down through the esophagus and into the stomach).

have shown the value of this test when nonspecific symptoms of difficulty swallowing, hoarseness, intermittent heartburn, and cough are present.

Scintigraphy

Scintigraphy is a procedure used to track movement of the bolus and quantify the residual bolus in the oropharynx, pharynx, larynx, and trachea. The patient swallows a small amount of a radionuclide material such as Technetium 99m combined with liquid or food. A special camera (**gamma camera**) records images of the organs of interest over time to obtain a quantitative image of the transit and metabolic aspects.

Scintigraphy can be used to identify trace aspiration and quantify the aspiration over short or long periods of time. Scintigraphy can also be used to calculate the transit time and residual "pooling" of a bolus, before and after treatment, in patients suffering degenerative neuromuscular diseases.

Scintigraphy is typically performed in a specially treated testing suite by trained personnel. Acquisition of data from the oral cavity to the thoracic and even upper abdominal cavities may be dynamic during the swallow and then followed by static images over longer time periods ranging from several minutes to several hours.

The precise amount of aspiration or residual bolus may be identified through computer analysis of the scans made at various time intervals. With the use of scintigraphy, the amount of aspiration in each region may be quantified. Scintigraphy may be more sensitive than barium swallow or MBS studies for long-term assessment of bolus location, and it has the added advantage of permitting the use of common food as the bolus.

Scintigraphy requires cooperation from the patient. Patients with known movement disorders, severe cognitive disorders, and the inability to remain standing or sitting in front of the gamma camera may not be candidates for this test.

Esophageal pH Monitoring

Prolonged (24-hour) esophageal pH monitoring is a test for diagnosing GERD. In addition, ambulatory monitoring devices permit evaluation of the temporal relationship between reflux episodes and atypical symptoms. The monitoring of pH is especially important in the diagnostic evaluation of patients with atypical presentations of GERD. Figure 6–13 shows a reading from part of a dual-probe 24-hour pH metry study. The test is relatively expensive, not available at all institutions, and may not be tolerated by some patients.

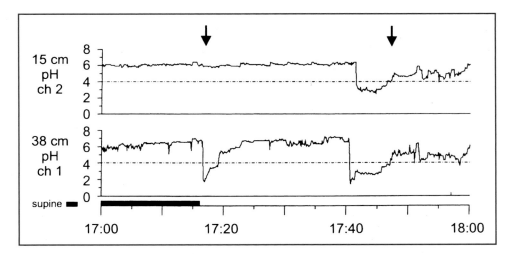

FIGURE 6–13. One hour of a 24-hour ambulatory pH recording from the distal and proximal esophagus, which shows 2 episodes of reflux. Each reflux episode is labeled with an arrow. In the second reflux episode, acid reflux in the distal esophagus reaches the proximal esophagus or higher. Adapted from Padda and Young.[41(p85)]

The identification of lesions that may be caused by GERD requires direct examination (ie, laryngoscopy, esophagoscopy), whereas pH monitoring identifies and quantifies the gastroesophageal reflux.

Dual-probe 24-hour pH monitoring (the use of 2 catheters) is now an accepted protocol for identifying esophageal and gastroesophageal reflux. The 24-hour pH monitoring is usually done following an overnight fast. The pH catheter is inserted transnasally into the esophagus. Standard placement of the distal probe is at a position that is approximately 5 cm above the proximal border of the LES. The proximal probe is located in the upper esophagus just below the esophageal inlet. The probes are attached to a recording device. Patients are asked to note in a diary, or in the recording device, the times that they eat, sleep, or perform any other activities. More importantly, patients will be asked to record any type of discomfort that they have, including heartburn, chest pain, wheezing, and coughing, and to record the time that these symptoms occurred. This information will be used to correlate the pH at the time a symptom or activity took place and a symptom index can be calculated. The most valuable discrimination between physiological and pathological reflux is the percentage of total time that the pH is less than 4. Normal values for the proximal probe have not yet been established. Dual-probe 24-hour pH monitoring is considered to be the most sensitive and specific method of making a diagnosis of laryngopharyngeal reflux disorder (LPRD).[42] The difficulty with pH monitoring is the need to maintain a "routine daily schedule" for 24 hours while wearing a nasal probe. Many patients do not tolerate the probe or alter their daily schedule, which renders the data suspect. Alternatives to the 24-hour pH probe test have been developed. These alternatives involve inserting a small pill-like camera into the esophagus that then travels through the digestive system and out after 48 hours while sending information back to a small, battery-operated device that is worn on a belt. These devices are more easily tolerated than wearing the nasal probe.

SUMMARY

A number of instrumental measures are available to assist in making diagnoses, finding the causes of dysphagia, and designing rehabilitation or management of dysphagia. New tests have been developed in the past 25 years to guide the treatment of swallowing disorders. Some tests remain experimental or may be extremely costly to use on a regular basis. Nonetheless, clinicians should be aware of all of the possible tests for identifying the basis of the swallowing disorder and how the test may aid in treating the problem.

DISCUSSION QUESTIONS

1. FEES and the modified barium swallow are both used in many hospitals and clinics. Discuss the main reasons for using one or the other in
   A. A 67-year-old male who has been diagnosed with a brainstem CVA.
   B. A 35-year-old female who is grossly overweight and who is complaining of food "sticking" in her throat when she swallows.
   C. An 85-year-old otherwise healthy female who has been gradually losing weight over the past 3 months. She does not appear to have had a CVA but has mild slurring of her speech and some slowness to respond to questions.
   Assume that both tests are available and there is someone competent to administer both tests.

STUDY QUESTIONS

1. What radiation safety procedures should be taken by the clinician during a MBS?
   A. Wears a dosimetry badge and leave the MBS suite when exposed to a certain radiation dose level
   B. Wears a thyroid shield, lead apron, protective glasses, protective gloves and a dosimetry badge
   C. Just stand away from the x-ray tube and patient
   D. Only wears a lead apron

2. Laryngeal electromyography is useful in assessing swallowing as it
  A. Provides a prediction of penetration and aspiration
  B. Indicates the status of vocal fold closure during swallowing
  C. Provides a measure of activity in the vocal folds
  D. May be used to replace the clinical bedside assessment in patients who are not cooperative

3. The primary difference between FEES and FEESST is that
  A. One cannot assess sensation
  B. One cannot assess oral function
  C. One provides a calibrated measure of sensory function
  D. One can be done by an SLP and the other cannot

REFERENCES

1. American Speech-Language-Hearing Association (ASHA). *Clinical Indicators for Instrumental Assessment of Dysphagia.* Rockville, MD: ASHA; 2000.

2. Langmore SE, Kenneth SM, Olsen N. Fiberoptic endoscopic examination of swallowing safety: a new procedure. *Dysphagia.* 1988;2(4):216–219.

3. Aviv JE. Sensory discrimination in the larynx and hypopharynx. *Otolaryngol Head Neck Surg.* 1997;116(3):331–334.

4. Bastian RW. Videoendoscopic evaluation of patients with dysphagia: an adjunct to the modified barium swallow. *Otolaryngol Head Neck Surg.* 1991;104(3):339–350.

5. Aviv JE, Murry T, Cohen M, Zschommler A, Gartner C. Flexible endoscopic evaluation of swallowing with sensory testing: patient characteristics and analysis of safety in 1,340 consecutive examinations. *Ann Otol Rhinol Laryngol.* 2005;114(3):173–176.

6. Cohen MA, Setzen M, Perlman PW, Ditkoff M, Mattucci KF, Guss J. The safety of flexible endoscopic evaluation of swallowing with sensory testing in an outpatient otolaryngology setting. *Laryngoscope.* 2003;113(1):21–24.

7. Jafari S, Prince RA, Kim DY, Paydarfar D. Sensory regulation of swallowing and airway protection: a role for the internal superior laryngeal nerve in humans. *J Physiol.* 2003;550(1):287–304.

8. Aviv JE, Liu H, Kaplan ST, Parides M, Close LG. Laryngopharyngeal sensory deficits in patients with laryngopharyngeal reflux and dysphagia. *Ann Otol Rhinol Laryngol.* 2000;109(11):1000–1006.

9. Logemann JA. *Evaluation and treatment of swallowing disorders.* Dallas, TX: Pro-Ed;1997.

10. Chau KHT, Kung CMA. Patient dose during videofluoroscopy swallowing studies in a Hong Kong public hospital. *Dysphagia.* 2009;24(4):387–390.

11. Kim HM, Choi KH, Kim TW. Patients' radiation dose during videofluoroscopic swallowing studies according to underlying characteristics. *Dysphagia.* 2013;28(2):153–158.

12. Rosenbek JC, Robbins JA, Roecker EB, Coyle JL, Wood JL. A Penetration-Aspiration Scale. *Dysphagia.* 1996;11(2):93–98.

13. Kelly AM, Drinnan MJ, Leslie P. Assessing penetration and aspiration: how do videofluoroscopy and fiberoptic endoscopic evaluation of swallowing compare? *Laryngoscope.* 2007;117(10):1723–1727.

14. Hind JA, Gensler G, Brandt DK, et al. Comparison of trained clinician ratings with expert ratings of aspiration on videofluoroscopic images from a randomized clinical trial. *Dysphagia.* 2009;24(2):211–217.

15. Troche MS, Huebner I, Rosenbek JC, Okun MS, Sapienza CM. Respiratory-swallowing coordination and swallowing safety in patients with Parkinson's disease. *Dysphagia.* 2011;26(3):218–224.

16. Colodny N. Interjudge and intrajudge reliabilities in fiberoptic endoscopic evaluation of swallowing (FEES®) using the Penetration–Aspiration Scale: a replication study. *Dysphagia.* 2002;17(4):308–315.

17. Hey C, Pluschinski P, Pajunk R, et al. Penetration-aspiration: is their detection in FEES® reliable without video recording? *Dysphagia.* 2015;30(4):418–422.

18. Martin-Harris B, Brodsky MB, Michel Y, et al. MBS measurement tool for swallow impairment—MBSImp: establishing a standard. *Dysphagia.* 2008;23(4):392–405.

19. Leonard R, Belafsky PC, Rees CJ. Relationship between fluoroscopic and manometric measures of pharyngeal constriction: the pharyngeal constriction ratio. *Ann Otol Rhinol Laryngol.* 2006;115(12):897–901.

20. Molfenter SM, Steele CM. The relationship between residue and aspiration on the subsequent swallow: an application of the normalized residue ratio scale. *Dysphagia.* 2013;28(4):494–500.

21. Thompson TZ, Obeidin F, Davidoff AA, et al. Coordinate mapping of hyolaryngeal mechanics in swallowing. *J Vis Exp.* 2014;(87):e51476.

22. Leder SB, Espinosa JF. Aspiration risk after acute stroke: comparison of clinical examination and fiberoptic endoscopic evaluation of swallowing. *Dysphagia.* 2002;17(3):214–218.

23. Tabaee A, Johnson PE, Gartner CJ, Kalwerisky K, Desloge RB, Stewart MG. Patient-controlled comparison of flexible endoscopic evaluation of swallowing with sensory testing (FEESST) and videofluoroscopy. *Laryngoscope.* 2006;116(5):821–825.

24. Roman S, Huot L, Zerbib F, et al. High-resolution manometry improves the diagnosis of esophageal motility disorders in patients with dysphagia: a randomized multicenter study. *Am J Gastroenterol.* 2016;111(3):372–380.

25. Bülow M, Olsson R, Ekberg O. Videomanometric analysis of supraglottic swallow, effortful swallow, and chin tuck in patients with pharyngeal dysfunction. *Dysphagia.* 2001;16(3):190–195.

26. Kawahara H, Kubota A, Okuyama H, Oue T, Tazuke Y, Okada A. The usefulness of videomanometry for studying pediatric esophageal motor disease. *J Pediatr Surg.* 2004;39(12):1754–1757.

27. Butler SG, Stuart A, Leng X, et al. The relationship of aspiration status with tongue and handgrip strength in healthy older adults. *J Gerontol A Biol Sci Med Sci.* 2011;66:452–458.

28. Stierwalt JAG, Youmans SR. Tongue measures in individuals with normal and impaired swallowing. *Am J Speech Lang Pathol.* 2007;16(2):148–156.

29. Padda S, Young MS. In: Carrau RL, Murry T, eds. *Comprehensive Management of Swallowing Disorders.* San Diego, CA: Singular Publishing; 1999:48, Table 7–1.

30. Munin MC, Rainer M. In: Carrau RL, Murry T, eds. *Comprehensive Management of Swallowing Disorders.* San Diego, CA: Singular Publishing Group; 1999;57–58.

31. Fishman A, Berne R, Morgan H. *American Journal of Physiology. Gastrointestinal and Liver Physiology by the Numbers.* Bethesda, MD: American Physiological Society; 1981.

32. Martin RE, MacIntosh BJ, Smith RC, et al. Cerebral areas processing swallowing and tongue movement are overlapping but distinct: a functional magnetic resonance imaging study. *J Neurophysiol.* 2004;92(4):2428–2493.

33. Li S, Luo C, Yu B, et al. Functional magnetic resonance imaging study on dysphagia after unilateral hemispheric stroke: a preliminary study. *J Neurol Neurosurg Psychiatry.* 2009;80(12):1320–1329.

34. Gracco VL, Tremblay P, Pike B. Imaging speech production using fMRI. *Neuroimage.* 2005;26(1):294–301.

35. Birn RM, Bandettini PA, Cox RW, Shaker R. Event-related fMRI of tasks involving brief motion. *Hum Brain Mapp.* 1999;7(2):106–114.

36. Galgano J, Froud K. Evidence of the voice-related cortical potential: an electroencephalographic study. *Neuroimage.* 2008;41(4):1313–1323.

37. Smithard DG. Swallowing and stroke. *Cerebrovasc Dis.* 2002;14(1):1–8.

38. Weissman JL. In: Carrau RL, Murry T, eds. *Comprehensive Management of Swallowing Disorders.* San Diego, CA: Singular Publishing;1999;65–74.

39. Belafsky PC, Postma GN, Daniel E, Koufman JA. Transnasal esophagoscopy. *Otolaryngol Head Neck Surg.* 2001; 125(6):588–589.

40. Postma GN, Cohen JT, Belafsky PC, et al. Transnasal esophagoscopy: revisited (over 700 consecutive cases). *Laryngoscope.* 2005;115(2):321–323.

41. Padda S, Young MA. In: Carrau RL, Murry T, eds. *Comprehensive Management of Swallowing Disorders.* San Diego, CA: Singular Publishing; 1999:85, Figure 13–3.

42. Richter JE. Diagnostic tests for gastroesophageal reflux disease. *Am J Med Sci.* 2003;326(5):300–308.

Treatment of Swallowing Disorders

A Look at the Chapter

Once the evaluation of the swallowing disorder is completed, a treatment plan is developed and carried out by multiple members of the dysphagia team. This chapter will classify the treatment methods under 2 main types: compensatory and rehabilitative swallowing therapy. Preventive swallowing therapy for head and neck cancer survivors and other emerging swallowing therapies are discussed at the end of the chapter. The treatment methods will be introduced with supporting evidence in the literature and demonstration videos (when appropriate). Changes in diet consistencies and nonoral diets may also be considered as a type of compensatory swallowing therapy and are discussed separately in Chapter 8. Surgical and prosthodontic management for dysphagia are covered in Chapter 11.

INTRODUCTION

As in the diagnostic process, the treatment process involves multiple health professionals and initially focuses on swallow safety. The prevention of aspiration and maintaining good swallowing-related quality of life are the main objectives of most treatment methods. By maintaining the focus on safety, clinicians will find it necessary to rely on multiple approaches, beginning with oral care and hygiene. The major treatment modalities for swallowing disorders include compensatory swallowing therapy and rehabilitative swallowing therapy.

As treatment implies change, clinicians must maintain a high degree of vigilance and monitor changes, both positive and negative. To do so requires accurate understanding of the disorder, acute observational skills, and knowledge of when to use instrumental assessments as part of the decision-making process during treatment. The instrumental assessments described in Chapter 6 form the basis for a treatment plan, which is developed by the treatment team and then presented to the patient and family members. The principles of **Evidence-Based Prac-**

tice should be used to guide clinicians in making clinical decisions.

Changes in patients' swallowing resulting from treatment or simply with the passage of time may be observed through weight changes, speed of eating, types of foods being consumed, or by special scales to assess changes in quality of life brought about through improved swallowing. Such changes can occur throughout the swallowing rehabilitation period.[1] In this chapter, traditional and evolving nonsurgical treatments to enhance swallowing and maintain safety, preventive and alternative treatment for swallowing disorders are described.

EVIDENCE-BASED PRACTICE

ASHA has published a position statement in 2005 that recommends speech-language pathologists to incorporate principles of **Evidence-Based Practice** when making clinical decisions.[2]

Evidence-Based Practice (EBP) promotes the use of best available research evidence, clinical expertise, and client's/caregiver's values and perspectives in making clinical decisions.

There are 4 general steps in EBP. The first step is to generate a clinical question based on the client in need (eg, what are the functional outcomes for poststroke individuals who received muscle strengthening exercises when compared with those who did not receive any exercise?). Then, clinicians should search for available scientific evidence that is relevant to the clinical question raised. A number of organizations have created online platforms for clinicians to find SLP-related evidence. Table 7–1 lists some examples of such online platforms. The third step is to review and evaluate the evidence. The highest level of evidence usually refers to well-designed randomized controlled trial (RCT) and well-designed meta-analysis of more than one RCT. Finally, the last step is to integrate the clinical expertise, client's perspective, and the reviewed scientific evidence together to make the necessary client-specific

TABLE 7–1. Examples of Online Platforms for Gathering Speech-Language Pathology-Related Scientific Evidence

Organization	Name of Platform	Website
American Speech-Language-Hearing Association (United States)	Evidence Maps	http://www.asha.org/Evidence-Maps/
Speech Pathology Database for Best Interventions and Treatment Efficacy (SpeechBITE) (Australia)	SpeechBITE	http://www.speechbite.com
National Institute for Health and Care Excellence (NICE) (United Kingdom)	Evidence search	http://www.evidence.nhs.uk
Taylor & Francis Online	Evidence-Based Communication Assessment and Intervention (journal)	http://www.tandfonline.com/toc/tebc20/current.com

clinical decisions. It is beyond the scope of this chapter to go through the detailed steps of EBP; readers are encouraged to refer to other resources to learn how to implement EBP into their clinical practice.

A number of evidence-based review papers evaluating the impact of swallowing therapy on specific populations (such as individuals with dementia, poststroke or postcancer treatment individuals, elderly) are available.[3–7] In general, it should be pointed out that most of the evidence available was obtained from small groups. There are some difficulties in conducting large-scale or randomized controlled studies in swallowing, such as

- Controlled studies involving the withholding or limiting of treatment or the use of sham treatments may have ethical issues.
- Finding a large sample of patients with identical physical or anatomical deficiencies is not easy.
- Severely dysphagic patients sometimes have concurrent cognitive impairments that prevent them from following the instructions of the swallowing exercises.
- Patients with stroke tend to have some natural recovery of swallow function from the acute phases of the event. Improvement in some cases may simply be related to time since onset of the stroke that brought on the swallowing disorder.

Yet, recent literature reviews suggest that there are increasing numbers of well-designed randomized controlled studies on swallowing therapy in recent years.

Given that many swallowing therapy approaches still need stronger scientific evidence to support their use with patients, the efficacious clinical approach would be to try the methods after a baseline set of reliable objective or subjective tests/assessments were obtained. Clinicians should then make every attempt to document changes that are brought about by the therapeutic process. In that way, they will no longer rely only on clinical impressions that may be misleading but begin to gather evidence related to the exercises.

MULTIDISCIPLINARY APPROACH TO SWALLOWING THERAPY

The primary member of the swallowing team in the nonsurgical management of swallowing disorders is the speech-language pathologist (SLP). Other team members involved include the occupational therapist, physiotherapist, dietitian, nurse, and attending physician. Still others such as the radiologist, otolaryngologist, gerontologist, gastroenterologist, pulmonologist, psychologist, oncologist, practical nurse, and family members may also be involved. Table 7–2 describes the roles of some of the professionals who may be involved in the swallowing team.

> *Treatment is a team process to ensure swallow safety, improve nutrition, and contribute to the overall rehabilitative effort.*

Each person who participates in the patient's treatment either directly or indirectly, whether a professional or a family member, must be acutely aware of the need for swallow safety and prevention of aspiration and aspiration pneumonia.

ORAL HYGIENE

A study has shown that elderly individuals with oropharyngeal dysphagia have poorer oral hygiene than those without dysphagia.[8] Poor oral hygiene and dysphagia are both risk factors for aspiration pneumonia.[9] It is highly recommended that a comprehensive oral hygiene program be implemented to help reduce the risk of developing aspiration pneumonia.[10] A comprehensive oral hygiene program should include self or assisted tooth brushing after each meal, daily denture cleaning, and regular professional dental care. Chlorhexidine-containing mouth rinse is also suggested, but further evidence is needed to confirm its role in preventing aspiration pneumonia.

COMPENSATORY SWALLOWING THERAPY

Compensatory swallowing therapy refers to strategies that aim to ensure safe swallows without directly improving the physiology of swallowing. These strategies should be proven to be effective for the client under instrumental evaluation before rec-

TABLE 7–2. Roles of Professionals Involved in Swallowing Therapy

Professional/Member	Roles
Speech-language pathologist	• Serves as leader in the team • Drives decisions on swallowing management • Implements compensatory or rehabilitation swallowing therapy • Makes referral to other disciplines when necessary
Occupational therapist	• Designs adaptive tools and environment to improve mealtime experience • Implements strategies and tools to improve body posture and arm use for feeding and swallowing
Physiotherapist	• Implements strategies and tools to improve head and body support and positioning during mealtimes • Improves breathing and mobilization to reduce risk of aspiration • Provides physiotherapy management in postaspiration pneumonia rehabilitation
Dietitian	• Performs nutritional assessment • Designs diets to achieve or maintain the client's nutritional and hydration needs • Monitors patient's weight
Dentist	• Assesses and manages oral care • Facilitates oral hygiene
Nurse	• Makes referral to swallowing team when necessary • Ensures clients are following the swallowing team's suggestions on feeding and swallowing (such as diet and posture modifications) • (For client's enteral feeding) Assists in placing and monitoring the enteral feeding tube

ommending them. There are usually no long-term physiological changes associated with these strategies; they are used more as an immediate measure to ensure swallow safety.

Who is suitable for compensatory swallowing therapy?

Compensatory swallowing therapy is suitable for individuals who have

■ Adequate memory and attention to perform the strategies consistently
■ Caregivers who can assist the dysphagic individual to implement the strategies

Who is *not* suitable for compensatory swallowing therapy?

Compensatory swallowing therapy is *not* suitable for individuals who

■ Have severe cognitive impairments
■ Cannot or refuse to follow treatment recommendations

Swallowing Maneuvers

The major aim of implementing the swallowing maneuvers is to better protect the airway immediately before, during, and after swallows. Some of the instructions involved for the maneuvers may be too complex for the elderly, individuals with cognitive impairments, or individuals who have difficulties in muscles control. Clinicians should carefully assess the client's accuracy and consistency in carrying out these maneuvers.

The major maneuvers for placing various aspects of the pharyngeal swallow under the patient's control and for retaining control of the bolus during the pharyngeal swallow are as follows:

1. Supraglottic swallow
2. Super-supraglottic swallow
3. Effortful swallow
4. Mendelsohn maneuver
5. Tongue hold maneuver

The **supraglottic swallow** is a 4-step maneuver: (1) Inhale and hold breath, (2) place bolus in swallow position, (3) swallow while holding breath, and (4) cough after swallow before inhaling.

The effects of the supraglottic swallow maneuver are to close the vocal folds (breath hold) during the swallow and then clear any residue that may have entered the laryngeal vestibule (cough) before breathing again.

This technique is often used with patients who have weak vocal folds, vocal fold paralysis, or laryngeal sensory deficits. This maneuver is considered a voluntary airway closure technique and, when done properly, closes the vocal folds prior to the swallow and keeps them closed during the swallow, thus preventing aspiration.

The **super-supraglottic swallow** is similar to the supraglottic swallow, with the addition of the instruction to bear down once the breath is being held. The effect of bearing down is to increase false vocal fold closure and assist in closing the posterior glottis. For both the supraglottic swallow and the super-supraglottic swallow, the patient is asked to "inhale and hold your breath very tightly." The super-supraglottic exercise adds "bearing down,"

"maintain the hold," "swallow," and then "cough." Although the airway may not be entirely closed, this maneuver offers a degree of protection by having the arytenoid cartilages tilt and possibly come into contact with the epiglottis or tongue base.[11]

The **effortful swallow** is simply a squeeze. The patient is told or shown to "squeeze hard with all of your muscles."

The physiological goal is to increase retraction of the base of the tongue and pharyngeal pressure in order to improve bolus clearance from the valleculae.

This maneuver may be the easiest for patients who have trouble with multiple-stage commands, for children, or for those patients with significant sensory loss. The squeeze may help in propelling the bolus into the oropharynx due to weakness in the tongue. Lazarus reported that this maneuver produces high pharyngeal pressure and results in reduction or elimination of pharyngeal residue.[12] The effortful swallow maneuver should be used with caution if instrumental examination reveals oropharyngeal weakness or lack of vocal fold closure.

The following 2 maneuvers are used as strengthening exercises rather than compensatory swallowing therapy. **Mendelsohn maneuver** is a technique to open the UES by extending the duration of laryngeal elevation. In this maneuver, the patient initiates several dry swallows while trying to feel the thyroid prominence lift.[13] Then, the instruction is to "hold the thyroid up for several seconds."

By keeping the larynx tilted and elevated, it is hypothesized that the UES relaxes to allow food to pass, leaving less residual material in the area.

The Mendelsohn maneuver is useful for treating patients who, for reasons of neurological injury or surgical treatment, cannot obtain adequate laryngeal excursion or elevation or who cannot coordinate the elevation motion with bolus passage. This maneuver is usually used as a strengthening exercise, with or without biofeedback (with surface electromyography, sEMG).

The **tongue hold maneuver** (also referred to as the **Masako maneuver**) is used in an attempt to increase the pressures and time of contact of the tongue base to the pharyngeal wall. As pointed out by Lazarus and colleagues,[12] this technique is efficacious for patients with lingual weakness following surgery for oral cancer. Instructions to the patient are to "hold the tongue between your front teeth and swallow."

Evidence suggests that this maneuver may not actually benefit patients with increased pressures of the tongue base to the pharyngeal wall. Doeltgen et al[14] suggest that the tongue hold maneuver may potentially be contraindicated for individuals with generally decreased anterior hyoid movement. However, a beneficial effect, characterized by increased pharyngeal constrictor strength and ultimately increased pharyngeal pressure gen-

eration, may arise after regular training. Doeltgen et al[14] suggest that the tongue hold maneuver may be useful when accompanied by the **Shaker exercise**.[15]

Pauloski[16] points out that as the maneuver may also result in increased pharyngeal residue, it may be best to do this exercise without food due to the risk of aspirating because of residue remaining as the result of delayed triggering of the pharyngeal swallow. Clearly, further investigation of this maneuver in various patient populations is required.

Table 7–3 summarizes the common swallow maneuvers, the problems for which they were designed, and the rationale. These maneuvers should be slowly explained to the patients, tried first without foods or liquids, and then, ideally, examined during instrumental studies of swallow function before continuous therapy. They may be tried during the CSE on a limited basis as a method for determining the patient's ability to perform the tasks during instrumental examinations.

TABLE 7–3. Swallow Maneuvers and the Problems for Which They Were Designed[a]

Swallow Maneuvers	Problem for Which Maneuver Was Designed	Rationale
Supraglottic swallow	Reduced or late vocal fold closure Delayed pharyngeal swallow	Voluntary breath hold usually closes vocal folds before and during swallow. Closes vocal folds before and during delayed swallow.
Super-supraglottic swallow	Reduced closure of airway entrance	Effortful breath hold tilts arytenoids forward, closing airway entrance before and during swallow.
Effortful swallow	Reduced posterior movement of the tongue base	Effort increases posterior tongue base movement.
Mendelsohn maneuver	Reduced laryngeal movement Discoordinated swallow	Laryngeal movement opens the UES; prolonging laryngeal elevation prolongs UES opening. Normalizes timing of pharyngeal swallow events.
Tongue hold	Lack of posterior pharyngeal wall contact with tongue	Improve contact between tongue base and posterior pharyngeal wall.

[a]Reproduced from Logemann.[19(p451)]

Swallowing Postures

A number of studies have demonstrated that by turning the head to one side, by tucking the chin down toward the chest, or by tilting the head back, swallowing can be facilitated or aspiration can be reduced or prevented.

> *Postures used in swallow exercises can reduce aspiration, improve transit times (oral and pharyngeal), and decrease the amount of residue after the swallow compared to the amount of residue without a postural adjustment.*

The most common swallow postures consist of

1. Head back
2. Chin down
3. Head rotation
4. Head tilt

The **head back posture** relies on gravity to move the bolus out of the oral cavity. Patients with tongue paralysis or partial or total removal of the tongue due to oral cancer may benefit from this posture. Clinicians must ensure that this posture will not increase the patient's risk of aspiration before recommending this posture.

The **chin down posture** (also called the chin tuck or neck flexion posture) improves airway protection by moving the tongue base and epiglottis posterior toward the posterior pharyngeal wall. This, in turn, makes the airway entrance narrower and thus increases airway protection. The chin tuck posture is achieved by tilting the chin down toward the chest, holding that position until the bolus is swallowed. The chin tuck posture was found to be effective in patients with neurological and neuromuscular diseases[17] and in patients following pharyngectomy surgery for cancer.[18] In this flexible endoscopic evaluation of swallowing (FEES) Video 7–1, the patient swallows a liquid bolus and also a cracker. On both, he penetrates and aspirates a small amount of each but coughs it back up. After that he is then given instructions to swallow liquid and a cracker in the chin tuck posture and there is

no aspiration. There was no need to cough after the chin tuck swallow.

The **head rotation posture** is used to promote the flow of the bolus to the more normal side of the pharynx or larynx. Thus, the instruction to the patient is to rotate the head toward the weak or damaged side to attempt to close off that side. This posture is used in patients with unilateral pharyngeal or vocal fold weakness or impairment.

The **head tilt posture** (also called the lateral head tilt) is useful for patients who have unilateral oral or pharyngeal weakness. The instructions to the patient are to tilt the head to the stronger side so that gravity carries the bolus in that direction.

Table 7–4, adapted from Logemann,[19] reports the effects of postures during fluoroscopy and the rationale for using the postures. Especially notable is the chin tuck, which has been shown to significantly increase bolus propulsion through the UES in patients with excessive cricopharyngeal constriction. In addition to the maneuvers reported in Table 7–3, Bulow and colleagues[20] found that the chin tuck did not reduce the number of misdirected swallows in patients with moderate to severe dysphagia but did reduce the depth of bolus penetration. However, Lewin et al[18] did find that the chin tuck eliminated 81% of aspiration when used with esophagectomy patients.

Additional information regarding the chin tuck was reported by Logemann and colleagues.[17] They found that although elderly patients preferred the chin tuck as a method of swallowing, bolus modification was actually more beneficial in preventing aspiration or penetration of the bolus.

> *The importance of teaching the postures prior to the instrumental swallow evaluation is underscored here, as they may be tried during instrumental examinations.*

The data demonstrating the efficacy of these postures have been primarily derived from small groups of patients with various neurological, neuromuscular, and head and neck cancer diagnoses. Each individual patient's ability to improve the speed of swallowing, reduce pooling, and control aspiration

TABLE 7–4. Postural Techniques to Reduce or Eliminate Aspiration or Residue[a]

Disorder Observed on Fluoroscopy	Posture Applied	Rationale
Inefficient oral transit (reduced posterior propulsion of bolus by tongue)	Head back	Uses gravity to clear oral cavity
Delay in triggering the pharyngeal swallow (bolus past ramus of mandible but pharyngeal swallow is not triggered)	Chin down	Widens valleculae to prevent bolus entering airway; narrows airway entrance, reducing risk of aspiration
Reduced posterior motion of tongue base (residue in valleculae)	Chin down	Pushes tongue base backward toward pharyngeal wall
Unilateral vocal fold paralysis or surgical removal (aspiration during the swallow)	Head rotated to damaged side	Places extrinsic pressure on thyroid cartilage, improving vocal fold approximation, and directs bolus down stronger side
Reduced closure of laryngeal entrance and vocal folds (aspiration during the swallow)	Chin down; head rotated to damaged side	Puts epiglottis in more protective position; narrows laryngeal entrance; improves vocal fold closure by applying extrinsic pressure
Reduced pharyngeal contraction (residue spread throughout pharynx)	Lying down on one side	Eliminates gravitational effect on pharyngeal residue
Unilateral pharyngeal paresis (residue on one side of pharynx)	Head rotated to damaged side	Eliminates damaged side of pharynx from bolus path
Unilateral oral and pharyngeal weakness on same side (residue in mouth and pharynx on same side)	Head tilt to stronger side	Directs bolus down stronger side via gravity
Cricopharyngeal dysfunction (residue in piriform sinuses)	Head rotated	Pulls cricoid cartilage away from posterior pharyngeal wall, reducing resting pressure in cricopharyngeal sphincter

[a]Reproduced from Logemann.[19(p451)]

will dictate further treatment. Thus, although all of these techniques show variable results depending on the cause of the swallowing problem, the clinician must consider the information derived from the clinical swallow evaluation, the other team members, and the instrumental assessments to determine when to use the techniques when treating a patient with a swallowing disorder. Factors such as fatigue, attention to the task, and environmental distractions must also be taken into account to determine the length of sessions and the number of swallow trials.

Thermal Tactile Oral Stimulation (TTOS)

Thermal tactile oral stimulation (TTOS) is defined as the stroking or rubbing of one or more of the organs of swallowing with a cold probe. The treatment is generally directed at the anterior faucial pillars. TTOS is often recommended for patients with dysphagia, especially if the dysphagia is caused by sensory deficits. Evidence suggests that TTOS may only lead to immediate changes in swallowing functions and such changes are not long-lasting, therefore, it is classified as a compensatory swallowing therapy. It has been hypothesized by Rosenbek and others that touch and cold stimulation provide heightened oral awareness and an alerting stimulus to the brainstem and brain, causing the pharyngeal swallow to trigger faster than it would without the stimulation.[21-23] Although these authors found slight improvements in the duration of stage transition and the total swallow duration, the amount of time needed varied and was generally extensive.

In Sweden, Bove, Mansson, and Eliasson[24] found no significant differences in healthy individuals in swallowing durational measures following stimulation with a cold laryngeal mirror, but they did find that swallow times were shorter when swallowing cold water compared to swallowing body temperature water. Similar results of the effects of cold stimulation were reported by Sciortino et al.[23] They noted that whatever improvement in latency that was measured following stimulation was short-lived and generally limited to one swallow. To date, there is little research to support the extensive use of cold stimulation to the oral-pharyngeal mucosa to improve swallow function.

A study of tactile stimulation with a sour bolus by Logemann et al[25] found that there was an earlier onset of lingual activity to propel a bolus into the pharynx, triggering the pharyngeal motor response, and a shorter pharyngeal component of the swallow in patients following stroke or a mixed neurological disorder. Other studies of temperature, reported by Bisch et al,[26] and carbonation, reported by Bulow et al,[27] have been equivocal in showing changes in swallow function. However, it remains to be seen if there are cortical effects of these stimuli to alter swallow behavior.

REHABILITATIVE SWALLOWING THERAPY

Rehabilitative swallowing therapy refers to exercises and techniques that aim to achieve long-term improvement in the neuromuscular control of swallowing. These exercises and techniques often follow the general principles of neuromuscular rehabilitation,[28] which are

- Use it or lose it
- Use it and improve it
- Specificity
- Transference

Applying these principles to swallowing therapy means that rehabilitation should encourage patients to swallow as much as possible, even for those who are on a nonoral diet (*use it or lose it; use it and improve it*), and the target exercises should involve swallowing (*specificity*) and training on swallowing-related muscles (*transference*). The frequency and number of repetitions needed to induce changes are also important principles in neuromuscular rehabilitation. Unfortunately, little evidence is available for swallowing therapy in these areas.

Who is suitable for rehabilitative swallowing therapy?

Rehabilitative swallowing therapy is suitable for individuals who have

- Adequate cognitive skills to follow instructions
- Motivation to improve
- Willingness to practice independently or with encouragement from caregivers
- A need to increase muscle strength and range of motion

Who is *not* suitable for rehabilitative swallowing therapy?

Rehabilitative swallowing therapy is *not* suitable for individuals with the following conditions:

- Severe cognitive impairments
- Susceptible to fatigue (eg, patients with myasthenia gravis)

Oral Motor Exercises

Oral motor exercises (OME) have long been suggested as a way to increase control over the swallowing event by increasing strength and volitional control over the movements of lips, tongue, and larynx. Many of these exercises have been derived from the speech and voice literature based on the treatment of **dysarthria**. Because dysarthric speech and voice generally improve when the patient controls the movements of the articulators, the rationale for use of oral motor exercises to treat swallowing disorders is to control the passage of the bolus, increase awareness of the bolus, and maximize the driving force of the bolus in transit to the oropharynx.

Table 7–5 lists the most common exercises for improving lip strength and awareness of the location of the bolus in the oral cavity. These exercises are derived from various articulation treatment protocols and may be applied in treatment plans

TABLE 7–5. Labial Exercises to Improve Strength and Awareness of Control of the Swallowing Mechanism[a]

1. Rapid labial opening and closing using the consonants /p, b/.

2. Extended lip squeeze followed by lip retraction.

3. Repeating the vowels /u, i/ with increased lip movement. Vocalization provides additional stimulation and awareness.

4. Thermal stimulation of the lips with ice. Movement of the ice may be medial-lateral or more focal if drooling on one side is prevalent.

5. Holding different objects between the lips such as straw, tongue blade, plastic spoon, etc, to improve sensory awareness. Objects may be of different sizes, shapes, and weights.

6. Apply various foods to lips, such as yogurt and peanut butter, and encourage the patient to massage the lips together.

7. Use the index finger to apply a sudden or quick stretch to the edges of the upper and lower lips.

8. Practice humming. Cue patient to start and stop humming. When humming stops, the patient should open the lips, then close again.

9. Have patient close the lips. Ask him or her to keep them closed while you try to gently break the lip seal.

10. Practice a "facial squeeze" by squeezing lips together. While keeping lips closed, alternate bringing teeth together and separating them. This mimics chewing activity.

11. Practice inhaling and exhaling through the nose rather than the mouth. The patient may want to watch this activity with a mirror.

12. Prior to swallowing, the patient should hold a glass or cup to the lips. Practice the timing of opening the lips once the cup is laced on the lower lip.

13. Hold small objects such as button (connected to a string) and place it between the lips and teeth. The clinician can put a gentle pull on the string to improve lips strength.

14. Intraoral stimulation of cheeks with a brush, cold objects, or fingers.

15. Resistive exercises. For example, have the patient push the upper lip down while the clinician resists the movement with a tongue blade. Have the patient push the tongue against the cheek while the clinician resists against the outside of the cheek.

[a]Adapted from Murry.[29(p244)]

for patients with swallowing disorders. It can be expected that patients with labial dysfunctions will have difficulty in the preparation of the bolus for transfer. It remains to be seen how these dysfunctions affect the entire coordination of the swallow.

Tongue control provides transmission of the bolus to the hypopharynx. In healthy adults, vocal fold closure is already happening, as the bolus is being propelled through the oral cavity. Lingual strength exercises may constitute a fundamental aspect of swallowing treatment because of the crucial role that the tongue plays in the oral prepara-

tory, oral, and pharyngeal phases of swallowing. Lingual weakness may result from damage to cranial nerves VII, IX, or XII. Tongue strength exercises also aim to improve tongue elevation and lateralization. One of the earliest studies to show the value of tongue strengthening exercises was reported by Lazarus and colleagues, using young healthy adults.[30] The participants were asked to press a rubber bulb or their tongue blade against their hard palate. After a month, both groups showed improved tongue strength compared to a group that received no treatment. Robbins et al[31] found similar results with 8 healthy elderly volunteers and, more recently, Robbins and her group found lingual exercises to improve lingual strength and swallowing outcomes in 6 patients following CVA.[32]

Clark et al[33] reported that although oral motor exercises have long been used to improve articulation in patients with tongue weakness as well as rigidity, arguments have been made that these exercises offer few long-term benefits. They studied normal healthy individuals trained to increase lingual strength, protrusion, and lateralization over 9 weeks. They found improvement in the measures following training but suggested that the gains may diminish when training is stopped. Based on their study and the results of a previous study by Clark[34] and data from Robbins et al,[32] tongue strength exercises appear to be efficacious in the functional improvement of swallowing but must be maintained to retain the improvement.

The oral motor exercises shown in Table 7–6 target tongue strength, tongue lateralization, tongue protrusion, and tongue contact with other struc-

TABLE 7–6. Exercises for Tongue and Mandible Strength and Movement[a]

1. Tongue tip elevation. Place tongue tip on alveolar ridge. Hold it for 2 seconds.

2. Tongue tip sweep. After holding the tongue on the alveolar ridge, sweep posteriorly against the palate.

3. Use the phonemes /t, d/ for rapid contact and release of the tongue tip to the alveolar ridge.

4. Use the "ch" sound to improve tongue contact to the middle of the soft palate. Similarly, the sounds "s" and "sh" help with lateral contact of tongue to palate as well as help to groove the tongue.

5. The /k, g/ phonemes are used to increase posterior tongue to soft palate contact. Combining syllables into quick movements such as "ta-ka" or "cha-ka" is helpful to improve the sweeping motion of the tongue.

6. Range-of-motion exercises can be done by chewing on gauze initially, then adding small amounts of food when it is safe.

7. To improve sensory awareness, use pressure and temperature stimulation:
   a. A cold spoon may be placed on the tip, blade, or back of tongue. Light pressure is applied and the patient is asked to lift the spoon.
   b. The palate is touched with tongue blade or cotton and the patient is asked to touch the area with the tongue.
   c. Cold or sour materials are given to the patient. They may be frozen on a stick if the patient is not yet cleared to swallow.
   d. Various sizes and textures or bolus may be given to identify the size and texture most easily transported by the tongue.

8. Mandible movement. Patients with reduced mandible movement may want to use a device such as TheraBite to increase mouth opening.

9. Resistive exercises to the mandible such as lowering or closing the mandible against the pressure applied by the therapist on the chin.

10. Sucking exercises increase tongue palate contact and help the patient to manage saliva. Sucking may be done with the tongue tip against the alveolar ridge and lips and teeth slightly apart or with teeth closed using a "slurping" or "suctioning" pull of the tongue to the midpalate area. The patient should try to do this with as much sound as possible to increase sensory feedback.

[a]Adapted from Murry.[29(p245)]

tures.[35] Data by Martin-Harris et al[36] suggest that the tongue may even play a role in the laryngeal phase of swallowing.

Martin-Harris and colleagues[36] found that the oropharyngeal swallow consists of a synergistic mechanism in which there are overlapping events that reflect interdependence with each other in order to properly propel the bolus through the swallow channels into the esophagus in a safe manner.

Exercises to increase mouth opening using a device such as the TheraBite allow the clinician and the patient to set goals and track progress. For those patients who can increase mouth opening, the placement of food may significantly increase successful swallowing, especially if surgery or radiation has caused an altering or removal of all or part of some organs.

Airway protection becomes a significant factor in preventing aspiration. When the vocal folds fail to close, the risk of aspiration increases. Table 7–7 lists some of the common procedures to increase vocal fold closure. These exercises have been advanced

TABLE 7–7. Vocal Fold Closure and Laryngeal Elevation Techniques[a]

1. Practice coughing.

2. Increase the loudness of the voice.

3. Initiate voice with a hard glottal onset.

4. Produce sustained phonation. Try to increase the duration while maintaining consistent voice quality.

5. Sustain phonation at various pitches. This helps with anterior vocal fold closure as well as laryngeal elevation.

6. An excellent program of laryngeal exercise has been developed by Ramig and her colleagues. This program is called Lee Silverman Voice Treatment (LSVT).[9] Although this program is designed primarily to increase vocal effectiveness, it also offers promise to those who require increased vocal fold closure to reduce the risk of aspiration.

[a]Adapted from Murry.[29(p246)]

primarily for patients with vocal fold paralysis. Clinicians have tried numerous ways to increase vocal fold closure, including turning the head to the weaker side. Of specific note is item 6 in Table 7–7. The **Lee Silverman Voice Treatment (LSVT)** was developed for treating speech intelligibility in patients with Parkinson's disease. Studies by Ramig and her colleagues have validated the efficacy of these exercises.[37] The focus of this treatment is on increasing the valving ability of the vocal folds.

Sharkawi et al[38] demonstrated that oral and pharyngeal transit times were reduced significantly following the use of LSVT with patients having oropharyngeal dysphagia.

Sharkawi's group[38] found a reduction of 51% in temporal measures of swallowing (oral transit time and pharyngeal transit time) in patients with Parkinson's disease 1 month after completing the LSVT program. They also found a reduction in oral residue following treatment and an increase in vocal intensity for sustained vowel production and oral reading. A review of the LSVT procedure and outcomes can be found in Fox et al.[39]

Specific impairments may benefit from repetition of specific tasks. Table 7–8 lists 13 common impairments or defects found after tissue loss or neurological damage along with goals and tasks to reach each goal.[40] The clinician should use the information derived from the FEES or MBS to focus on 1 or 2 goals at a time. Documentation is important for tracking progress and maintaining patient motivation to continue treatment. Accurate tracking of progress becomes essential not only for continued patient motivation but also for determining when to conduct additional tests of swallowing in order to assess changes that might signal changes in swallowing therapy or the onset of oral eating.

Tongue strengthening exercises such as those in Table 7–6 are useful for improving oral phase swallowing functions such as bolus manipulation, mastication, and bolus clearance in the oral cavity. From a review of the current literature, it appears that only limited empirical data are available to validate neuromotor or oral motor exercises for use in treating

TABLE 7–8. Exercises for Specific Impairments[a]

Impairment	Goal	Tasks May Include
Limited control, agility, or neck rotation, extension, and flexion	Range, control, agility adequate for needed task	Obtain consult from physical therapy, depending on need. Tasks may focus on development of agility of movement as well as control and range of motion (ROM).
Trismus—Inability of the jaw to open due to injury to the trigeminal nerve or muscular deficiency	Adequate opening for feeding route (spoon, fork, cup, or biting), for denture of palatal prosthesis placement, and for oral hygiene	Maintain mandible-maxilla alignment while increasing passive and active range of mandible opening. Movements should be made slowly. Maximum stretch should be maintained ≥15 seconds. The TheraBite is a more sophisticated device, especially useful for marked trismus or when alignment of mandible and maxilla is difficult to maintain.
Weakness or absence of mandibular support/control	Symmetric mandible-maxilla approximation supportive of potentials for posture, oral nutrition/hydration, and speech	Establish optimal alignment passively or actively and present exercises graded for endurance. Increase strength and control using graded for endurance. Increase strength and control using graded resistance and biting. Munching tasks to strengthen muscles of mandibular closure and opening.
Weakness or absence of buccal tone	Increased buccal tone	Isometric tightening of the buccal area or squeezing of soft objects between check and teeth/gums or from buccal sulcus to the molar surface.
Diminished labial opening.	Adequate labial opening size for eating, adequate shaping for speech	Passive stretching and exercises to increase range and strength of lateral commissure movement. Maintain mandible alignment throughout.
Unilateral partial or complete lingual weakness or missing lateral lingual tissue	Posterior bolus retention-release control for airway protection, bolus and airflow control (minimize lateral "leaks")	Maximize lingual symmetry at rest and in a variety of nonspeech and speech gestures. Squeezing and lingual manipulation tasks may be appropriate. Palatal prosthesis may facilitate therapy.
Bilateral lingual weakness	Oral transit with minimum oral loss, maximum coordination with initiation of swallow gestures	Address sectionally, as above.
Absent tongue	Development of compensatory mandibular, labial, and head/neck movement strategies	Develop ROM and agility of movements needed for compensations that take advantage of gravity. Consider mandibular or maxillary shaping prosthesis.
Unilateral or complete weakness or missing tissue of the palate	Adequate velopharyngeal closure if tissue is adequate, effective obturation if tissue is inadequate	Sustained blowing against resistance may strengthen closure. Endoscopic feedback may be helpful even with objurgation. Objurgation may actually recruit improved compensatory participation in closure from the lateral and posterior pharyngeal walls.
Incomplete supraglottic closure	Improved supraglottic closure	Habituate early and effortful laryngeal closure and elevation for swallow. The Mendelsohn maneuver may be used.
Inadequate PES opening for swallow	Maximum PES opening	Maximizing extent and timing of hyoid/laryngeal elevation and the effects of pharyngeal compression of the bolus.

[a]Adapted from Leonard and Kendall.[40]

swallowing disorders.[28] Factors such as the need to increase strength of lip seal, tongue pump, tongue range of motion, and endurance of lip/tongue/jaw coordination remain to be determined.[35] Nonetheless, once the clinician understands the underlying anatomy, physiology, and neural control of these muscle groups, he or she will have a better understanding of whether and when to use a specific exercise.

For patients following head and neck cancer or neurological disorders, it appears that noninvasive exercises that do not require the patient to swallow may have value despite lack of extensive clinical trials. Studies by Logemann,[19] Lazarus et al,[12] Pauloski et al,[41] and Sonies[42] have shown that active participation in a series of neuromuscular swallowing exercises by patients following head and neck surgery improves swallow function.

The use of exercises such as those listed in Tables 7–5 and 7–6 should be based on anatomical and physiological findings from instrumental and clinical assessments. These exercises may be coupled with prosthetic management and other compensatory and rehabilitative swallowing therapy. However, clinicians must guard against blindly treating patients with oral motor exercises unless they can specify a rationale for treatment and document changes related to treatment, swallow safety, quality of life, and/or weight gain. Whenever possible, oral motor exercises should be combined with other treatment approaches.

Shaker Exercise

An important aspect of swallowing is the ability to open the upper esophageal sphincter (UES) to allow the passage of the bolus. Studies by Shaker and others have shown that the UES opening is reduced in the elderly compared to healthy young individuals.[15,43,44] Shaker and his colleagues developed a head lift exercise (HLE) to increase the opening of the UES and therefore decrease the hypopharyngeal intrabolus pressure. In 1997, they studied healthy elderly subjects using manometry and videofluoroscopy to measure intrabolus pressure prior to and following a program of HLEs.[15] The HLE consists of lying in a supine position and doing a series of head lifts while the shoulders remain on the floor or bed. The HLE, or Shaker exercise, was developed to treat UES dysfunction by strengthening the suprahyoid muscles. This would be expected to lead to an increase in the anteroposterior deglutitive opening diameter and cross-sectional area of the upper esophageal sphincter. The goals of the Shaker exercise are to

1. Strengthen the muscles that contribute to the opening of the UES, specifically, the geniohyoid, thyrohyoid, and digastric muscles.
2. Significantly decrease the hypopharyngeal bolus pressure as it enters the UES, thus permitting bolus passage with less resistance.

The Shaker exercise increases UES opening and thus may contribute to the elimination of aspiration in individuals with residue in the pharynx after a swallow due to poor UES opening.[45] Strengthening the suprahyoid muscles through the Shaker exercise should result in a more efficient UES opening.

The original Shaker exercise involves isometric and isokinetic neck exercises while the individual lies in a supine position.[46] The individual alternates between 3 isometric repetitions of sustained 1-minute head raisings and 1-minute rest periods. The individual must raise his or her head high enough to see his or her toes without lifting the shoulders off the ground. The second part of the exercise consists of 30 consecutive head lifts without holding. The shoulders must also be kept on the ground during this portion.[47] The instructions for the patient are shown in Table 7–9. If the patient cannot sustain the head lift for 1 minute, an alternate baseline time can be used at the start of the exercises. Figure 7–1 shows the extended posture for the Shaker exercise once the head is lifted off the ground. Video 7–2 is a demonstration of the exercise.

Not only does the Shaker exercise strengthen the suprahyoid muscles, it also enhances shortening of the thyrohyoid muscle. According to Mepani et al,[48] the thyrohyoid muscle works in conjunction with the suprahyoid muscles to augment UES opening. In their recent study, they compared the effects of traditional dysphagia therapy (focusing on laryngeal and tongue range of motion exercises and swallowing maneuvers) and the Shaker exercise on

TABLE 7–9. Shaker Exercise Protocol

Please perform this exercise 3 times per day for the next _____ weeks.

1. Lay flat on your back on the floor or bed.
2. Hold your head off of the floor looking at your feet for 1 minute. Relax with your head back down for 1 minute and repeat the sequence 2 more times.[a]
3. Raise your head 30 more times and look at your toes. Do not sustain these head lifts.[a]

[a]Do not lift your shoulders while performing this exercise.

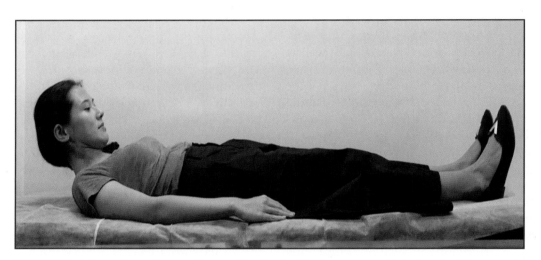

FIGURE 7–1. Depiction of the starting position for the Shaker exercise. Note the shoulders remain in contact with the floor surface.

thyrohyoid shortening across a course of 6 weeks. Thyrohyoid muscle shortening was measured before and after the 6-week period using videofluoroscopy to quantify any gains made in either group. Results from this study showed that the Shaker exercise proved significantly more effective in increasing thyrohyoid shortening compared to the traditional therapy. This would suggest that the Shaker exercise has a positive outcome on deglutition by enhancing UES opening.[48] Although Mepani et al[48] were unable to quantify the statistical significance of changes in thyrohyoid shortening compared to changes in deglutitive UES opening and clinical improvement due to small subject size, they noted a relationship between thyrohyoid muscle shortening and suprahyoid muscle contraction upon UES opening.

Several drawbacks exist with the Shaker exercise. In the Easterling et al[47] study, subjects needed repeated instruction, cueing, and encouragement to accurately perform the exercise. Subjects also reported neck muscle soreness and dizziness during the early weeks of the exercise program.[47] Fatigue may also be a factor for discontinuing the Shaker exercise. A study by White et al[45] found both positives and negatives for the Shaker exercise when looking at the relationship between the exercise and fatigue. Subjects performed the Shaker exercise with surface EMG electrodes positioned to evaluate the progression of fatigue in the suprahyoid muscles, infrahyoid muscles, and the sternocleidomastoid. After a 6-week training program, they found that the Shaker exercise fatigues the sternocleidomastoid, which may preclude the continuation of the exercise in some situations, especially with elderly subjects. This suggests that the Shaker exercise may not be appropriate for individuals prone to fatigue (ie, those with amyotrophic lateral sclerosis or other neuromuscular diseases).

It is important to note that the Shaker exercise cannot be used with individuals who have cervical spine deficits, reduced neck movement ability, and/or cognitive issues that may affect compliance. Unfortunately, these contraindications may eliminate a large group of individuals who would otherwise benefit from the Shaker exercise.

According to Burkhead, Sapienza, and Rosenbek,[49] the principles of exercise found to be effective in other areas such as physical rehabilitation and sports training also extend to exercise treatment of dysphagia. These principles include identifying the optimal volume and duration of the regimen, both of which are involved in the Shaker exercise. It has been shown that the Shaker exercise has been effective in treatment of swallowing dysfunction; however, the optimal volume and duration for the exercise need further investigation. As reported by Burkhead et al,[49] exercises must place a load on the system, involve enough practice, and last for some duration to allow adaptation to the new behavior.

Further research is needed to refine the Shaker exercise, as well as other swallowing exercises to make it as effective as possible and to increase the likelihood of its continuation by patients. Although there are drawbacks in terms of patient populations and need for lengthy use, the Shaker exercise offers the patient whose problems are focused at the cricopharyngeal level an opportunity to improve swallow function.

Expiratory Muscle Strength Training (EMST)

In 2005, Kim and Sapienza[50] reported on a series of studies that demonstrated that expiratory muscle strength training (EMST) improves both ventilatory and nonventilatory functions such as with speech production, cough, and swallow in normal healthy individuals, hypotonic children, and patients with multiple sclerosis. Since then, studies focusing spe-

cifically on swallow function have also shown that EMST may be a valuable adjunctive rehabilitative technique to use with patients who show muscular weakness resulting from neurological or neuromuscular diseases.

> *EMST is a technique of respiratory muscle strengthening through exhaling in a controlled manner into a specific device with a one-way valve that is used to block the expiratory air flow until a sufficient expiratory pressure is produced.*

Strength training of limb muscles has been shown effective for increasing muscle hypertrophy, suggesting that strength training of respiratory muscles may induce the same effect.[51,52] A number of well-designed studies have examined the impact of EMST on swallowing in different populations. Wheeler-Hegland et al[53] studied hyoid movement using surface EMG under three conditions: the Mendelsohn maneuver, effortful swallow, and EMST. They found that EMST achieved higher maximum and average submental surface EMG activity versus normal swallowing. They suggested that the EMST training has the potential to induce strength gains to increase the activation speed in the submental musculature. Other studies have shown that there is evidence of improved swallowing following training with an EMST device such as the one shown in Figure 7–2 for patients with Parkinson's disease, multiple sclerosis, and sedentary elderly.

Swallowing Therapy and Aspiration

It is to be expected that patients recovering from swallowing disorders will experience occasional aspiration. Using the swallowing therapy reviewed in this chapter can be efficacious in reducing aspiration events and preventing aspiration pneumonia. This may be a patient-by-patient experience, given that patients rarely present with a uniform case history and medical status. A summary of the nonsurgical methods to reduce or eliminate aspiration is shown in Table 7–10. Caution should be used by the clinician when applying these approaches.

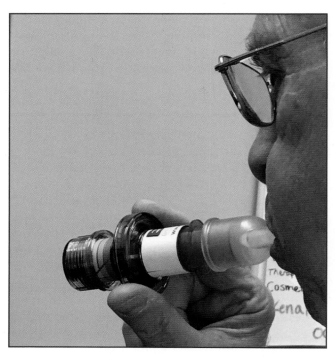

FIGURE 7–2. Shows patient with EMST in place and blowing into it.

A more comprehensive list summarizing the nonsurgical swallowing interventions for head and neck cancer survivors is shown in Table 7–11. These data, taken from a public access manuscript by Pauloski,[55] offer range-of-motion, compensatory, and rehabilitative techniques for the management of various swallow-related disorders.

TABLE 7–10. Nonsurgical Methods for Controlling Aspiration[a]

1. Oral motor exercises:
Lip seal
Tongue retraction and elevation
Tongue strengthening
2. Head position maneuvers:
Chin tuck
Head lift
Rotating head to side of lesion in pharyngeal or vocal fold paresis
3. Postural compensation techniques:
Sitting upright
Lying on side
4. Swallowing retraining:
Supraglottic swallow
Super-supraglottic swallow
Mendelsohn maneuver
Multiple swallows
Frequent throat clearing
5. Diet modification:
Change in bolus size
Change in food consistencies
Changes in temperature and taste
6. Nonoral diet (NPO)

[a]Adapted and revised from Pou and Carrau.[54]

> Groher[55] reported that the variables that separate those who develop aspiration pneumonia from those who do not remain speculative.

To be sure, many more people, with or without swallowing problems, aspirate compared to those who develop aspiration pneumonia. Factors such as prior history of aspiration, mobility, age, state of consciousness, respiration status, upper airway reflexes, instrumental results of swallow evaluation, and the integrity of the lower airway protective mechanism all contribute to prevention of aspiration pneumonia. Clinical judgment suggests that given a decreased medical condition and signs of aspiration, one may ultimately expect aspiration pneumonia and therefore should do everything possible to maintain swallow safety.

PREVENTIVE SWALLOWING THERAPY FOR HEAD AND NECK CANCER SURVIVORS

It is well documented that trismus and long-term dysphagia may occur in post head and neck cancer treatment survivors. Studies have suggested that carrying out swallowing exercises before and during nonsurgical cancer treatment may help to reduce

TABLE 7–11. Swallowing Disorders Most Often Reported for Treated Head and Neck Cancer Patients Are Listed With Associated Postures, Maneuvers, Exercises, and Other Interventions That May Be Effective in Alleviating the Disorder or Reducing Its Negative Impact on Swallowing[a]

Swallow-Related Disorder	Possible Interventions	
Reduced mouth opening	Jaw ROM exercises	
Reduced tongue control/shaping	Chin down posture Super-supraglottic (SSG) swallow Tongue ROM exercises	Bolus manipulation exercises Tongue strengthening exercises
Reduced vertical tongue movement	Tongue ROM exercises Maxillary reshaping prosthesis	
Reduced anterior-posterior tongue movement	Head back posture Multiple swallows Alternate liquids and solids	Tongue ROM exercises Bolus manipulation exercises Maxillary reshaping prosthesis
Reduced tongue strength	Effortful swallow Tongue strengthening exercises	
Delayed pharyngeal swallow	Chin down posture SSG swallow Thermal/tactile stimulation	
Reduced tongue base retraction	Chin down posture Effortful swallow SSG swallow Tongue hold maneuver	Mendelsohn maneuver Tongue ROM exercises Gargle/yawn for tongue base retraction
Reduced laryngeal vestibule closure	Chin down posture SSG swallow Effortful swallow	Mendelsohn maneuver Gargle/yawn for tongue base retraction
Reduced laryngeal elevation	Mendelsohn maneuver Chin down posture SSG swallow	Effortful swallow Laryngeal ROM exercises Shaker exercise
Reduced glottis closure	Head rotation to weaker side SSG swallow Thickened liquids Vocal fold adduction exercises	
Reduced pharyngeal constriction/clearance	Head rotation to weaker side Effortful swallow Mendelsohn maneuver Multiple swallows	Alternate liquids and solids Gargle/yawn for tongue base retraction Tongue hold maneuver
Reduced/impaired cricopharyngeal opening	Head rotation to weaker side Mendelsohn maneuver Shaker exercise Effortful swallow	

[a]From Pauloski.[16]

133

the short- and long-term effect of (chemo)radiotherapy on mouth opening and swallowing functions.[56] A range of exercises have been proposed, such as Shaker, Mendelsohn maneuver, effortful swallow, supraglottic swallow, Masako, and jaw stretching exercises. The selection of exercises is often based on a precancer treatment swallowing evaluation and the type of head-and-neck cancer. There is still no clear evidence as to which exercise clinician should prescribe and when and for how long the patients should practice.[57] Studies have shown that only around 50% of the patients practiced the swallowing exercises during cancer treatment.[58,59] Barriers to adherence to the exercises included pain and fatigue during cancer treatment, not appreciating the importance of the swallowing exercises, lack of support and encouragement to continue with the exercises, and simply forgetting that they had to do the exercises.

OTHER SWALLOWING TREATMENT METHODS

The following swallowing treatment methods have been proposed and tested scientifically. However, there are no strong indications supporting or refuting these methods as yet because of limitations in the studies. Clinicians are recommended to refer to updated evidence before implementing these methods clinically. These methods are often recommended to be used in conjunction with swallowing therapy described above, rather than as a standalone treatment method.

Electrical Stimulation

Different ways are proposed in using electrical stimulation to enhance swallowing. **Neuromuscular electrical stimulation (NMES)** is a technique that has been proposed to stimulate swallow function by applying electrical stimulation to the neck area as a means of stimulating laryngeal elevation. By stimulating the muscles in the neck via surface electrodes, it has been hypothesized that the swallowing musculature will be strengthened or that

the sensory pathways important for swallowing will have heightened awareness. This procedure, also known as transcutaneous electrical stimulation (TES), is noninvasive. Contradictory findings have been reported in the past. A review by Clark et al[60] in 2009 concluded that there were few promising findings related to NMES for swallowing therapy and that there is a need for examining specific issues such as dosage, timing, surface versus intramuscular recording, and applications to specific populations. A recent study has investigated pairing NMES with effortful swallow and swallowing therapy[61] in poststroke individuals. Sixty-one poststroke individuals were recruited, all received NMES, effortful swallow, and "conventional" swallowing therapy. The participants were randomized into 2 treatment methods, one with NMES at motor stimulation intensity and one at sensory stimulation intensity. Results showed that those stimulated at motor stimulation intensity had better anterior and superior hyoid movement and Penetration Aspiration Score than the sensory stimulation group after 6 weeks of treatment. Further studies are necessary to confirm the beneficial effects of NMES in swallowing rehabilitation.

Pharyngeal electrical stimulation (PES) is a technique that uses a transoral or transnasal catheter to place electrodes to the pharyngeal area. Electrical current at an individualized tolerable level is then passed through the electrodes to stimulate the pharyngeal area. Studies have shown that this is a safe and tolerable treatment method.[62] A recent large-scale international,[63] multicenter, randomized, sham-controlled study with 162 subacute stroke patients did not find significant improvement in swallowing functions after 3 daily sessions of PES. This is in contrast with a recent individual patient data meta-analysis study, which concluded that PES was associated with better swallowing outcomes and shorter hospital stay for subacute poststroke survivors.[64]

In contrast to surface stimulation, **intramuscular (IM) stimulation** via hooked-wire electrodes are inserted into specific muscles or electrodes are more permanently implanted into the muscle to direct current locally to increase muscle activity and thus improve swallow functions. Ludlow[65] reviewed the evidence related to electrical stimulation. Her report, including data from up to 2009, suggests that electrical stimulation is most effective when the electrical stimulus is applied directly to the muscle (IM). Intramuscular stimulation using electrodes inserted into these muscles has been shown to produce laryngeal elevation similar to that which occurs during normal swallowing.[66]

Cortical Neuromodulating Treatments

There are 2 types of noninvasive cortical neuromodulating methods proposed for improving swallowing functions, namely, **repetitive transcranial magnetic stimulation (rTMS)** and **transcranial direct current stimulation (tDCS)**. The objectives of these methods are to modulate neuronal activities at targeted cortical regions in order to promote neural changes that may facilitate neuromuscular rehabilitation.

rTMS modulates neuronal activities by discharging electricity to a coil of wire to produce brief, strong magnetic pulses. The coil is usually placed on a targeted area on the head so that the magnetic field will pass through the skull to induce an electrical field. The electrical field will then modulate cortical neural networks. Figure 7–3 shows an example of equipment used for rTMS. Two general types of rTMS have been proposed: low-frequency or inhibitory rTMS (≤1 Hz) and high-frequency or

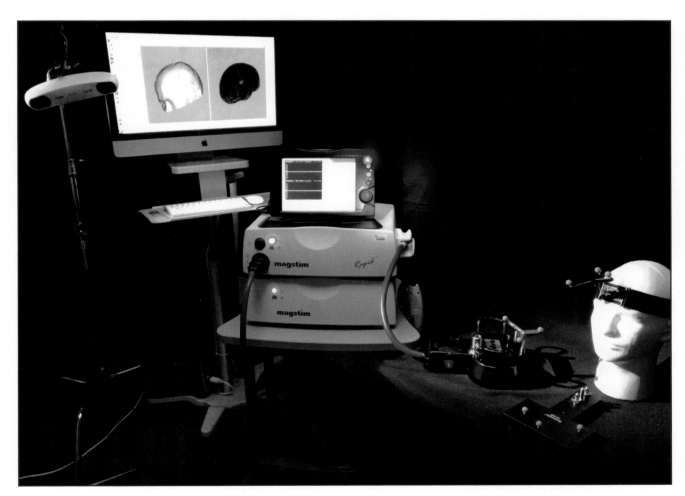

FIGURE 7–3. Equipment used for conducting repetitive transcranial magnetic stimulation. From the left, camera for detecting head and coil location trackers; neuronavigation system for real-time detection and recording of site of stimulation; electric pulse generator and control panel for transcranial magnetic stimulation; head coil; coil trackers calibration block; headband with location trackers.

excitatory rTMS (≥5 Hz). Published studies in the use of rTMS for dysphagia have mainly focused on poststroke individuals. In general, current evidence suggests that rTMS has potential to improve swallowing functions in poststroke individuals.[67] However, different stimulation sites, frequency, and durations of stimulation were studied. Further investigations are needed before rTMS can be used as a clinical tool.

tDCS modulates the excitability threshold of targeted neurons by passing a low-intensity electrical current between two electrodes that are carefully placed at a predefined area of the head. Preliminary findings from the small number of published studies on poststroke population suggest that using tDCS to stimulate the unaffected hemisphere may improve swallowing functions in poststroke individuals.[68] Similar to the rTMS literature, the studies differed in a number of methodological designs, it is not possible to conclude which tDCS protocol would be effective and safe for use as a clinical treatment method. A larger number of well-designed, large-scale randomized-controlled studies are needed before rTMS and tDCS may be recommended as a clinical treatment method for dysphagia.

SUMMARY

Swallowing therapy is now commonly provided for acute and chronic swallowing disorders resulting from postcancer treatment in head and neck cancer, neuromuscular disorders, neurological disorders, and debilitation associated with a cohort of aging conditions that affect the nerves and muscles involved in swallowing. Compensatory and rehabilitative therapies continue to evolve and be tested in both healthy participants and in patients with dysphagia. Procedures such as LSVT and EMST, treatments that were developed for nonswallowing disorders, are now being explored in patients with swallowing disorders. The application of neuromuscular rehabilitation principles such as "use it or lose it," transference, repetition, and intensity in the treatment process offer an improved rationale for the nonsurgical treatment of swallowing. Such

rationale may provide a basis for developing additional evidence for continued exploration of methods to improve swallow safety and quality of life in patients with dysphagia.

DISCUSSION QUESTIONS

1. Most swallowing exercises target a specific organ or posture. Martin-Harris[36] suggests that swallowing is a parallel process, with glottic closure beginning when the bolus has not yet reached the anterior facial arch. Write a rationale for studying one of the exercises in Tables 7–5, 7–6, or 7–7. Discuss the exercise within the framework of parallel processing and suggest how that exercise can improve swallowing and how it will interact and improve the other phases of swallowing.
2. Discuss how the principles of neuromuscular rehabilitation may be applied to rehabilitative swallowing exercises, such as those listed in Tables 7–5 through 7–8.
3. Discuss the roles of different professionals in managing the following clients:
   A. Postcancer treatment patient who is in your SLP clinic for swallowing management but has not gone back to the oncologist for review/follow-up.
   B. A patient who is 6 months post stroke who has swallowing disorders, adequate cognitive functions, limited mobility, and lives in a nursing home.
   C. Individual with Parkinson's disease who is experiencing swallowing difficulties.

STUDY QUESTIONS

1. Exercises for patients with upper motor neuron injury might include
   A. Lip strength
   B. Tongue strength
   C. Mendelsohn maneuver
   D. All of the above

2. The use of the chin tuck during swallowing
   A. Prevents aspiration and penetration
   B. Increases speed of bolus to the oropharynx
   C. Reduces the speed of bolus transit in the oral cavity
   D. Reduces the distance between the thyroid cartilage and hyoid bone

3. The primary outcome from studies using the Shaker exercise is
   A. Significant increase in the anterior excursion of the larynx
   B. Reduced opening of the upper esophageal sphincter
   C. Increase in the speed of a bolus transport to the upper esophageal sphincter
   D. No improvement in the types of liquid patients with UES difficulty could swallow

REFERENCES

1. McHorney CA, Robbins J, Lomax K, et al. The SWAL-QOL and SWAL-CARE outcomes tool for oropharyngeal dysphagia in adults: III. documentation of reliability and validity. *Dysphagia*. 2002;17(2):914.

2. American Speech-Language-Hearing Association (ASHA). *Evidence-Based Practice in Communication Disorders*. Rockville, MD: ASHA; 2005.

3. Frymark T, Mullen R, Musson N, Schooling T. Evidence-based systematic review: oropharyngeal dysphagia behavioral treatments. Part IV—Impact of dysphagia treatment on individuals' postcancer treatments. *J Rehabil Res Dev*. 2009;46(2):205–214.

4. Ashford J, McCabe D, Wheeler-Hegland K, Frymark T, Mullen R, Musson N, Schooling T. Evidence-based systematic review: Oropharyngeal dysphagia behavioral treatments. Part III—Impact of dysphagia treatments on populations with neurological disorders. *J Rehabil Res Dev*. 2009;46(2):195–204.

5. Wheeler-Hegland K, Ashford J, Frymark T, et al. Evidence-based systematic review: oropharyngeal dysphagia behavioral treatments. Part II—impact of dysphagia treatment on normal swallow function. *J Rehabil Res Dev*. 2009; 46(2):185–194.

6. Di Pede C, Mantovani M, Del Felice A, Masiero S. Dysphagia in the elderly: focus on rehabilitation strategies. *Aging Clin Exp Res*. 2016;28(4):607–617.

7. Carnaby G, Madhavan A. A systematic review of randomized controlled trials in the field of dysphagia rehabilitation. *Curr Physical Med Rehabil Rep*. 2013;1(4):197–215.

8. Ortega O, Parra C, Zarcero S, Nart J, Sakwinska O, Clavé P. Oral health in older patients with oropharyngeal dysphagia. *Age Ageing*. 2014;43(1):132–137.

9. Almirall J, Serra-Prat M, Bolibar I. Risk factors for community-acquired pneumonia in adults: a review. *Clin Pulm Med*. 2016;23(3):99–104.

10. van der Maarel-Wierink CD, Vanobbergen JN, Bronkhorst EM, Schols JM, de Baat C. Oral health care and aspiration pneumonia in frail older people: a systematic literature review. *Gerodontology*. 2013;30(1):3–9.

11. Ogura JH, Kawasaki M, Takenouchi S. LXXXVIII neurophysiologic observations on the adaptive mechanism of deglutition. *Ann Otol Rhinol Laryngol*. 1964;73(4): 1062–1081.

12. Lazarus C, Logemann JA, Song CW, Rademaker AW, Kahrilas PJ. Effects of voluntary maneuvers on tongue base function for swallowing. *Folia Phoniatr Logop*. 2002; 54(4):171–176.

13. Ding R, Larson CR, Logemann JA, Rademaker AW. Surface electromyographic and electroglottographic studies in normal subjects under two swallow conditions: normal and during the Mendelsohn manuever. *Dysphagia*. 2002;17(1):1–12.

14. Doeltgen SH, Witte U, Gumbley F, Huckabee M-L. Evaluation of manometric measures during tongue-hold swallows. *Am J Speech Lang Pathol*. 2009;18(1):65–73.

15. Shaker R, Kern M, Bardan E, et al. Augmentation of deglutitive upper esophageal sphincter opening in the elderly by exercise. *Am J Physiol*. 1997;272(6):G1518–G1522.

16. Pauloski BR. Rehabilitation of dysphagia following head and neck cancer. *Phys Med Rehabil Clin North Am*. 2008; 19(4):889–928.

17. Logemann JA, Gensler G, Robbins J, et al. A randomized study of three interventions for aspiration of thin liquids in patients with dementia or Parkinson's disease. *J Speech Lang Hear Res*. 2008;51(1):173–183.

18. Lewin JS, Hebert TM, Putnam JB, DuBrow RA. Experience with the chin tuck maneuver in postesophagectomy aspirators. *Dysphagia*. 2001;16(3):216–219.

19. Logemann JA. Therapy for oropharyngeal swallowing disorders. In: Perlman AL, Schultz-Delrieu K. *Deglutition and Its Disorders: Anatomy, Physiology, Clinical Diagnosis, and Management*. San Diego, CA: Singular Publishing; 1997:449–461.

20. Bulow M, Olsson R, Ekberg O. Videomanometric analysis of supraglottic swallow, effortful swallow, and chin tuck in patients with pharyngeal dysfunction. *Dysphagia*. 2001;16(3):190–195.

21. Rosenbek JC, Robbins J, Willford WO, et al. Comparing treatment intensities of tactile-thermal application. *Dysphagia*. 1998;13(1):1–9.

22. Regan J, Walshe M, Tobin WO. Immediate effects of thermal-tactile stimulation on timing of swallow in idiopathic Parkinson's disease. *Dysphagia*. 2010;25(3):207–215.

23. Sciortino KF, Liss JM, Case JL, Gerritsen KG, Katz RC. Effects of mechanical, cold, gustatory, and combined

stimulation to the human anterior faucial pillars. *Dysphagia.* 2003;18(1):16–26.

24. Bove M, Månsson I, Eliasson I. Thermal oral-pharyngeal stimulation and elicitation of swallowing. *Acta Otolaryngol.* 1998;118(5):728–731.

25. Logemann JA, Pauloski BR, Colangelo L, Lazarus C, Fujiu M, Kahrilas PJ. Effects of a sour bolus on oropharyngeal swallowing measures in patients with neurogenic dysphagia. *J Speech Lang Hear Res.* 1995;38(3):556–563.

26. Bisch EM, Logemann JA, Rademaker AW, Kahrilas PJ, Lazarus CL. Pharyngeal effects of bolus volume, viscosity, and temperature in patients with dysphagia resulting from neurologic impairment and in normal subjects. *J Speech Lang Hear Res.* 1994;37(5):1041–1049.

27. Bülow M, Olsson R, Ekberg O. Videoradiographic analysis of how carbonated thin liquids and thickened liquids affect the physiology of swallowing in subjects with aspiration on thin liquids. *Acta Radiol.* 2003;44(4):366–372.

28. Langmore SE, Pisegna JM. Efficacy of exercises to rehabilitate dysphagia: a critique of the literature. *Int J Speech Lang Pathol.* 2015;17(3):222–229.

29. Murry T. In: Carrau RL, Murry T, eds. *Comprehensive Management of Swallowing Disorders.* San Diego, CA: Plural Publishing; 2006;243.

30. Lazarus C, Logemann JA, Huang C-F, Rademaker AW. Effects of two types of tongue strengthening exercises in young normals. *Folia Phoniatr Logop.* 2003;55(4):199–205.

31. Robbins J, Gangnon RE, Theis SM, Kays SA, Hewitt AL, Hind JA. The effects of lingual exercise on swallowing in older adults. *J Am Geriatr Soc.* 2005;53(9):1483–1489.

32. Robbins J, Kays SA, Gangnon RE, et al. The effects of lingual exercise in stroke patients with dysphagia. *Arch Phys Med Rehabil.* 2007;88(2):150–158.

33. Clark HM, O'Brien K, Calleja A, Corrie SN. Effects of directional exercise on lingual strength. *J Speech Lang Hear Res.* 2009;52(4):1034–1047.

34. Clark H. Clinical decision making and oral motor treatments. *ASHA Leader.* 2005;10(8):8–9.

35. Clark HM. Neuromuscular treatments for speech and swallowing: a tutorial. *Am J Speech Lang Pathol.* 2003;12(4):400–415.

36. Martin-Harris B, Brodsky MB, Michel Y, Lee F-S, Walters B. Delayed initiation of the pharyngeal swallow: normal variability in adult swallows. *J Speech Lang Hear Res.* 2007;50(3):585–594.

37. O'Brien C, Hoehn M, Thompson L. Intensive voice treatment (LSVT) for individuals with Parkinson's disease: A two-year follow-up. *J Neurol Neurosurg Psychiatr.* 2001;71:493–498.

38. El Sharkawi A, Ramig L, Logemann J, et al. Swallowing and voice effects of Lee Silverman Voice Treatment (LSVT®): a pilot study. *J Neurol Neurosurg Psychiatr.* 2002;72(1):31–36.

39. Fox CM, Ramig LO, Ciucci MR, Sapir S, McFarland DH, Farley BG. *The science and practice of LSVT/LOUD: neural plasticity-principled approach to treating individuals with Parkinson disease and other neurological disorders.* Paper presented at: Seminars in Speech and Language; 2006.

40. Leonard R, Kendall K 3rd eds., *Dysphagia Assessment and Treatment Planning: A Team Approach.* San Diego, CA: Plural Publishing; 2013.

41. Pauloski BR, Rademaker AW, Logemann JA, et al. Surgical variables affecting swallowing in patients treated for oral/oropharyngeal cancer. *Head Neck.* 2004;26(7):625–636.

42. Sonies B. Remediation challenges in treating dysphagia post head/neck cancer. A problem-oriented approach. *Clin Commun Disord.* 1992;3(4):21–26.

43. Shaker R, Easterling C, Kern M, et al. Rehabilitation of swallowing by exercise in tube-fed patients with pharyngeal dysphagia secondary to abnormal UES opening. *Gastroenterology.*122(5):1314–1321.

44. Medda BK, Kern M, Ren J, et al. Relative contribution of various airway protective mechanisms to prevention of aspiration during swallowing. *Am J Physiol Gastrointest Liver Physiol.* 2003;284(6):G933-G939.

45. White KT, Easterling C, Roberts N, Wertsch J, Shaker R. Fatigue analysis before and after Shaker exercise: physiologic tool for exercise design. *Dysphagia.* 2008;23(4):385–391.

46. Shaker R, Antonik S. The Shaker exercise. *US Gastroenterol Rev.* 2006;1:19–20.

47. Easterling C, Grande B, Kern M, Sears K, Shaker R. Attaining and maintaining isometric and isokinetic goals of the Shaker exercise. *Dysphagia.* 2005;20(2):133–138.

48. Mepani R, Antonik S, Massey B, et al. Augmentation of deglutitive thyrohyoid muscle shortening by the Shaker exercise. *Dysphagia.* 2009;24(1):26–31.

49. Burkhead LM, Sapienza CM, Rosenbek JC. Strength-training exercise in dysphagia rehabilitation: principles, procedures, and directions for future research. *Dysphagia.* 2007;22(3):251–265.

50. Kim J, Sapienza CM. Implications of expiratory muscle strength training for rehabilitation of the elderly: tutorial. *J Rehabil Res Dev.* Mar-Apr 2005;42(2):211–224.

51. Baker S, Davenport P, Sapienza C. Examination of strength training and detraining effects in expiratory muscles. *J Speech Lang Hear Res.* Dec 2005;48(6):1325–1333.

52. Chiara T, Martin D, Sapienza C. Expiratory muscle strength training: speech production outcomes in patients with multiple sclerosis. *Neurorehabil Neural Repair.* May-Jun 2007;21(3):239–249.

53. Wheeler-Hegland KM, Rosenbek JC, Sapienza CM. Submental sEMG and hyoid movement during Mendelsohn maneuver, effortful swallow, and expiratory muscle strength training. *J Speech Lang Hear Res.* Oct 2008;51(5):1072–1087.

54. Pou AM, Carrau RL. In: Carrau RL, Murry T, eds. *Comprehensive Management of Swallowing Disorders.* San Diego, CA: Singular Publishing; 1999:157, Table 23-1.

55. Groher ME. Determination of the risks and benefits of oral feeding. *Dysphagia.* Fall 1994;9(4):233–235.

56. Kulbersh BD, Rosenthal EL, McGrew BM, et al. Pretreatment, preoperative swallowing exercises may improve dysphagia quality of life. *Laryngoscope.* Jun 2006;116(6): 883–886.

57. Paleri V, Roe JWG, Strojan P, et al. Strategies to reduce long-term postchemoradiation dysphagia in patients with head and neck cancer: an evidence-based review. *Head Neck.* 2014;36(3):431–443.

58. van der Molen L, van Rossum MA, Burkhead LM, Smeele LE, Rasch CR, Hilgers FJ. A randomized preventive rehabilitation trial in advanced head and neck cancer patients treated with chemoradiotherapy: feasibility, compliance, and short-term effects. *Dysphagia.* Jun 2011;26(2): 155–170.

59. Shinn EH, Basen-Engquist K, Baum G, et al. Adherence to preventive exercises and self-reported swallowing outcomes in post-radiation head and neck cancer patients. *Head Neck.* Dec 2013;35(12):1707–1712.

60. Clark H, Lazarus C, Arvedson J, Schooling T, Frymark T. Evidence-based systematic review: effects of neuromuscular electrical stimulation on swallowing and neural activation. *Am J Speech Lang Pathol.* Nov 2009;18(4):361–375.

61. Park JS, Oh DH, Hwang NK, Lee JH. Effects of neuromuscular electrical stimulation combined with effortful swallowing on post-stroke oropharyngeal dysphagia: a randomised controlled trial. *J Oral Rehabil.* 2016;43(6): 426–434.

62. Fraser C, Power M, Hamdy S, et al. Driving plasticity in human adult motor cortex is associated with improved motor function after brain injury. *Neuron.* 2002;34(5): 831–840.

63. Bath PM, Scutt P, Love J, et al. Pharyngeal electrical stimulation for treatment of dysphagia in subacute stroke: a randomized controlled trial. *Stroke.* Jun 2016;47(6):1562–1570.

64. Scutt P, Lee HS, Hamdy S, Bath PM. Pharyngeal electrical stimulation for treatment of poststroke dysphagia: individual patient data meta-analysis of randomised controlled trials. *Stroke Res Treatment.* 2015;2015:8.

65. Ludlow CL. Electrical neuromuscular stimulation in dysphagia: current status. *Curr Opin Otolaryngol Head Neck Surg.* Jun 2010;18(3):159–164.

66. Burnett TA, Mann EA, Cornell SA, Ludlow CL. Laryngeal elevation achieved by neuromuscular stimulation at rest. *J Appl Physiol.* Jan 2003;94(1):128–134.

67. Michou E, Raginis-Zborowska A, Watanabe M, Lodhi T, Hamdy S. Repetitive transcranial magnetic stimulation: a novel approach for treating oropharyngeal dysphagia. *Curr Gastroenterol Rep.* 2016;18(2):1–9.

68. Pisegna JM, Kaneoka A, Pearson WG Jr, Kumar S, Langmore SE. Effects of non-invasive brain stimulation on post-stroke dysphagia: a systematic review and meta-analysis of randomized controlled trials. *Clin Neurophysiol.* Jan 2016;127(1):956–968.

Chapter 8

Nutrition and Diets

A Look at the Chapter

Individuals with dysphagia often need to modify their nutritional intake to ensure safe swallowing. The diet modifications may involve thickening fluids, changing the texture of solid food, or changing to a nonoral diet. In this chapter, the different types of diet modifications are described. Students should be aware that different terminologies or systems are used to describe different levels of liquid and food consistency. This chapter introduces the more common systems used internationally. The ethics involved in managing nutrition in dysphagia are also addressed in this chapter. When a speech-language pathologist or other team member recommends a change in diet, especially to a nonoral diet, the patients and their family may not comply or agree with the recommendations. Ethical dilemmas relating to diet changes are discussed especially in relation to patients with dementia or at end of life.

INTRODUCTION

The importance of proper nutrition cannot be over-estimated in the management of swallowing disorders. Nutritional status can have a significant impact on recovery from disease and swallowing rehabilitation, especially those factors related to self-esteem, psychosocial concomitants of oral eating, and overall quality of life.

The highest priority in the management of the dysphagic patient is swallow safety. The dysphagia team must also ensure that, no matter how the dysphagic patient is managed, he or she must receive adequate nourishment, measured by the amount of calories received, the content of the calories, and the degree of satisfaction when eating or drinking those calories.

Failure to achieve proper nutrition, whether it is via an oral or nonoral pathway, will result in **malnutrition**, a major complication in the recovery process.

In this chapter, the properties of liquids and foods are examined in relationship to the safety and nutrition of the dysphagic patient. Oral diets and nonoral feeding alternatives are reviewed. Malnutrition and its consequences as they relate to dysphagia are considered. Nutrition and its importance in the recovery from sickness, injury, or surgery are extensive topics and have far-reaching implications. Comprehensive reviews of nutrition including enteral feeding requirements and calorie intake calculation are summarized, and references are provided for those who need specific patient requirements.

Proper nutrition can be achieved through oral or nonoral diets or from a combination of the two. In the recovery process from head and neck cancer, nutrition usually begins with a nonoral diet, often a nasogastric tube, and then proceeds to a combined oral and nonoral diet and finally an oral diet in most cases.

Stroke recovery is similar; however, with the stroke patient, the patient's cognitive status, degree of alertness, and understanding of the nutritional process must also be taken into account.

For these reasons, the nutritional status of the stroke patient must be managed carefully.

DIETITIAN AND DYSPHAGIA

A comprehensive dysphagia treatment program involves extensive input from the nutritionist/dietitian (the term **"dietitian"** is used in this chapter in reference to **"registered dietitian"**) in order to prevent malnutrition, maintain or increase strength, and maintain immune status.

The dietitian is a trained professional who selects the proper calorie and nutrition content of the diet and monitors the nutritional status and continuing needs of the patient.

As such, it is important for the speech-language pathologist (SLP) and dietitian to work together, as nutritional needs will change with changing medical status. The dietitian may elect to perform a comprehensive nutrition assessment, as seen in Table 8–1, or may limit the assessment to the specific needs of the patient at treatment modification stages. The dietitian also works closely with other rehabilitation team members to select foods or supplements for oral feeding that provide proper nourishment while at the same time maximize proper oral control, transit, and timing of swallowing. If nutrition is nonoral, the dietitian monitors and determines amounts and timing of enteral feeding to assure proper energy requirements and to ensure that the foods/supplements selected do not interfere with other conditions such as cardiac disease and diabetes. A comprehensive review of the roles of the dietitian may be found in the publications of the Academy of Nutrition and Dietetics.[1,2]

What is an RDN and DTR?:

What an RDN Can Do for You:

TABLE 8–1. Comprehensive Examination in Conjunction With a Nutritional Assessment by a Dietitian[a]

Medical History
Primary diagnosis
Planned medical procedures
Medical comorbidities
Current cognitive status
Gastrointestinal history
History of pneumonia
Neurological status
Review of medications
Review results of previous swallow studies
Physical Assessments
Current weight and recent weight change
Coordination skills
Dentition
Edema
Handedness and recent change in handedness
Feeding skills
Living status
Nutritional History
Diet history
Recent diet changes
Tolerances to foods
Use of nutritional supplements
Medical restrictions to types of foods
Vitamin supplements
History of anorexia
Alcohol intake
Recent Biochemical Data
Albumin, Transferrin, Prealbumin
Glucose
Electrolytes
Hemoglobin/hematocrit
BUN/creatine

[a]Adapted and revised from Molseed.[3(p150)]

PROPERTIES OF LIQUIDS AND FOODS

Rheology is the study of the deformation and flow of matters. The need to use the proper thickeners and food textures in treating patients with dysphagia has influenced the recent development of this science specific to swallowing disorders.

Although their clinical significance is not completely determined, the rheological properties of food may be useful for the study and development of standard dysphagia diets and feeding protocols.

More importantly, by obtaining a set of standards for different food and liquid consistencies, instrumental testing (whether it is the Modified Barium Swallow [MBS], flexible endoscopic evaluation of swallowing [FEES], or other instrumental testing) can also approach standardization.

Recently, the International Dysphagia Diet Standardisation Initiative (IDDSI) has developed a comprehensive framework establishing standards for foods and drinks.[4] Fluids and solid foods are categorized according to their rheological properties. To understand this analysis completely goes beyond the scope of most members of the dysphagia team. However, a basic knowledge of rheology and how it relates to dysphagia is important to the clinician (Table 8–2).

TABLE 8–2. Rheology Terminology

Creep test	A test to determine the deformation of a material exposed to a constant stress. These are like relaxation tests, but a constant stress is applied, rather than a constant strain. The simplest creep test would be to apply a weight on top of a sample and record the change in shape (strain) over time; for example, placing a book on a cake and measuring the deformation over time.
Density	The compactness of a substance; the ratio of its mass to its volume measured in grams per milliliter (g/mL) or kilograms per milliliter (kg/mL).
Homogeneous	Well mixed and compositionally similar regardless of location.
Incompressible	Material that shows no change in density when a constant stress is applied (eg, water).
Isotropic	The material response is not a function of location or direction.
Kinematic viscosity	Viscosity divided by the density of the material.
Laminar flow	Nonturbulent flow.
Linear viscoelasticity	Viscoelasticity within the region where stress and strain are linearly related.
Newtonian fluid	A fluid with a linear relationship between shear stress and shear rate with a yield stress. The fluid viscosity of a newtonian fluid does not vary with shear rate.
Non-newtonian fluid	Any fluid deviating from newtonian behavior (eg, fluids that are suspensions). The attractive force between suspended particles weakens as shear rate increases.
Rheogram	A graph showing rheological relationships.
Rheometer	An instrument used for measuring rheological properties. This device is used in creep tests.
Shear (strain) rate	Change in strain with respect to time.
Strain	Relative deformation.
Viscoelastic	A material having both viscous and elastic properties.
Viscosity	Resistance to flow or alteration of shape by a substance as a result of molecular cohesion. This is perhaps the most important property when planning a diet for someone with a swallowing disorder. **Newton's postulate** reasons that if the shear stress is doubled, the velocity gradient (shear strain rate) within the fluid is doubled. For fluids, strain is measured in terms of shear rate, and the shear stress may be expressed as some function of shear rate and viscosity. For newtonian fluids, the viscosity function is constant and called the coefficient of viscosity or **newtonian viscosity**.
Viscometer	A device used to measure the resistance of a material to flowing.

Applications of Rheology

Viscosity is a prime variable in the study of newtonian fluids. For simplicity, the clinician may view the viscosity of a fluid as being proportional to the force required to move it through. A bolus that is twice as viscous requires roughly twice as much power from the swallow musculature to transport the bolus. Viscosity sheer rate profiles for different types of fluids can be found in the literature.[5–7]

Density also plays a role in the analysis of liquids. Density can be affected by temperature and the thickening agent. As the compactness of a substance changes, its flow will also change. Thus, the density may decrease as the compactness decreases. Moreover, if a product stays in the oral cavity for any length of time, its denseness may change, leading to misinterpretation of the type of fluid a patient can or cannot swallow.

ORAL NUTRITION AND DYSPHAGIA DIETS

Oral nutrition is the goal for most patients with dysphagia due to stroke or for those who have undergone head and neck cancer surgery. Conversely, for patients with progressive neuromuscular diseases, oral nutrition may be the starting level of intervention, with progression to an enteral feeding stage due to the progress of the disease.

Oral nutrition diets are organized on the basis of viscosity of the foods and liquids. Safe swallowing requires temporal management of the neuromuscular behaviors at each stage of the swallow.

All dysphagia diets should adjust food/liquid intake for (1) amount, (2) viscosity, (3) consistency, and (4) timing of the meal to achieve maximal nutrition and maintenance of the desired viscosity over the course of the feeding period.

Diets and Consistencies

The management of oral feeding requires an understanding of liquid viscosities and food textures. The **International Dysphagia Diet Standardisation Initiative (IDDSI)** proposed 7 levels to describe foods and drinks of different viscosity and texture. The use of standardized terminologies across countries will allow ease of comparisons across studies and gather more evidence for the use of diet modifications as a dysphagia treatment option. Figure 8–1 shows the 7 levels of foods and drinks proposed by the IDDSI.

IDDSI—Food Description:

Drinks: According to the IDDSI framework, there are 5 levels of drinks (Table 8–3):

Thin: eg, Clear liquids, milk, coffee and tea, and broth-based soups

Slightly thick: eg, "antiregurgitation" infant formula

Mildly thick: eg, honey, nectar

Moderately thick: eg, smoothie

Extremely thick: eg, puree

Liquid modification may be used to increase or decrease the viscosity of the liquid in order to achieve bolus control. Thin or thick liquids may require thickening agents to modify the consistency. It should be remembered that these thickeners may also alter other aspects of the bolus, such as cohesiveness, taste, appearance, and flow. A number of food thickeners are now available in supermarkets, pharmacies, and health food stores.

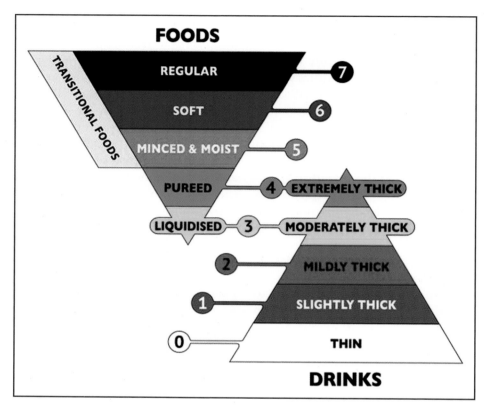

FIGURE 8–1. International Dysphagia Diet Standardization Initiative. From http://www. iddsi.org. The IDDSI Framework and Descriptors are licensed under the CreativeCom mons Attribution Sharealike 4.0 Licence.

TABLE 8–3. Descriptors of the IDDSI Liquid Levels

Liquid Level	Examples	Suggested Target Population	IDDSI Flow Test
0 (Thin)	• Water • Apple juice	• For individuals who can safely swallow all levels of liquids	• Flows through completely in 10 seconds
1 (Slightly thick)	• Antiregurgitation (AR) infant formula • Buttermilk	• Mainly used in the pediatric population as a thickened drink	• Leaves 1–4 mL in the syringe after 10 seconds
2 (Mildly thick)	• Gravy • Yogurt drinks	• Individuals who have slightly reduced tongue control	• Leaves 4–8 mL in the syringe after 10 seconds
3 (Moderately thick)	• Molasses • Yogurt	• More reduced tongue and oral control than Level 2	• Leaves >8 mL in the syringe after 10 seconds
4 (Extremely thick)	• Pureed fruits • Avocado spread	• Poor tongue control • Increased risk of residue	• No flow or drop through after 10 seconds

Table 8–4 lists some common thickening agents that may be used. Because new products are being developed and marketed constantly, it is not the purpose of this chapter to recommend one manufacturer over another. Rather, clinicians will have to keep up with new materials and with the modifications that companies offer. The amounts to be mixed will vary substantially, and the clinician may resort to "trial-and-error" mixture consistency for each individual. The key is to clearly document how to prepare the final consistency that suits each individual.

The current commercially available thickeners or prethickened beverages vary in their thickening ingredients. They may be starch based, xanthun gum based, or a mixture of both. Table 8–5 lists the different types of thickeners that may be used to alter the viscosity of fluids. Although there has been a significant increase in the number of thickeners available, there remains a need to identify the rheological properties as they relate to viscosity, because viscosity plays a major role in the consistency of the fluid swallowed.

There is no clear evidence from the literature that suggests which viscosity levels should be used for different levels of dysphagia severity. In general, studies showed that thicker fluids flowed more

TABLE 8–4. Common Agents for Modifying the Viscosity of Food and Drinks

Noncommercial Agents		
Thinning Agents/Blenderizing Agents	**Thickening Agents**	
Milk	Cornstarch	
Gravy	Baby cereal (or other dehydrated baby food)	
Juice	Mashed potato flakes	
	Instant pudding	
	Unflavored gelatin	
Commercial Thickening Agents		
Company	**Ready-to-Consume Products**	**Product Basis**
Nestle Nutrition http://www.nestlenutritionstore.com	X	Modified cornstarch
Woodbury Products http://www.thickit.com	✓	Starch and gum based
Simply Thick http://www.simplythick.com	X	Xanthan gum
Hormel Health Labs http://www.hormelhealthlabs.com	✓	Starch and gum based
Nutricia Nutilis http://nutilis.com/products	✓	Xanthan gum
Flavour Creations https://www.flavourcreations.com.au	✓	Xanthan gum
Fresenius Kabi http://www.fresenius-kabi.com	X	Modified food starch

TABLE 8–5. A Comparison of Commercially Available Liquid Thickeners

	Starch-Based Thickeners (powders)	Gum-Based Thickeners (with starch powder ingredients)	Gel Thickener	Prethickened Beverages (starch or gum based)	Prethickened Drink Mixes (starch powder based)
Mixed in any beverage	Yes	Yes	Yes	• Ready-to-drink	• Only with water
Appearance when added to clear beverage	• Appear cloudy • Slightly grainy texture	• Remain clear • Smooth slightly slippery texture	• Remain clear • Smooth slightly slippery texture	• Clarity depends on type of thickener used	• Appear cloudy • Slightly grainy texture
Consistency changes over time	Yes	No	No	No	Yes

slowly down the swallowing tract and increased the duration of the swallowing events[8–12] than thin fluids. Thicker fluids and harder foods were reported to require greater tongue, jaw, pharyngeal, and laryngeal efforts to swallow.[10,13–16] When focusing on dysphagic patients, studies showed that thicker fluids reduced the amount of penetration and aspiration, but at the same time increased the amount of post-swallow pharyngeal or vallecular residue.[10–12,17–19]

> The key to recommending thickened fluids as a treatment option is to find a consistency that allows maximal protection from penetration and aspiration, but at the same time minimal level of postswallow residue.

The decision to use which viscosity level is often made after studying the swallow patterns with the modified barium swallow (MBS). Clinicians should note the type and consistency of the barium used during testing. Where regular MBS studies are done, premixed barium consistencies should be available to the clinician so that when a report is generated, the treatment team will know the conditions under which the patient was evaluated. An instrumental assessment of swallowing provides an indication of acceptable viscosities for maximum safe swallowing once it has been shown that the patient has adequate sensation. It is important that the entire team understands the viscosities and uses consistent mixtures during the treatment.

Examples of pre-mixed barium consistencies

When clinicians are using premixed barium products or ready-to-drink thickened fluids, they should be aware that the viscosity of these products might vary from brand to brand even when they are labeled to be representing the same level of fluid thickness. Strowd et al[6] published a summary of various dysphagia diet foods (DDFs) that are available for thickening. They found that the viscosity of honey-thick DDF was consistent with the National Dysphagia Diet (NDD) guidelines, but other products that represented other consistencies were not. In general, they also found that the premixed barium drinks for MBS had higher viscosity than the NDD guidelines. Factors such as temperature, shaking up the substances before use, flavor selection, and stability over time were all capable of changing the viscosity. Payne et al[7] also found that there was a large range of viscosities over a number of commercially available starch products used in thickening liquids in Great Britain. They noted that the physical properties of the materials changed after opening, despite correct storage procedures.

> *For drinks that are thickened using starch-based thickeners, the consistency may change over time and when the drinks are mixed with saliva. When a patient retains foods or drinks in the oral cavity for lengthy periods of time, the viscosity and density are no longer the same as when the foods or drinks was prepared.*

Speech-language pathologists may perform their own flow test on products that they will use in MBS and in treatment to ensure the appropriate fluid thickening level is recorded for communication among the dysphagia team and for future treatment planning. The IDDSI proposed a simple 10-second flow test for fluids using a 10-mL syringe. The results of the flow test for each fluid level in the IDDSI framework are clearly listed in their guidelines.

IDDSI—Drinks Description:

YouTube Video—IDDSI Syringe Test Instructions:

Liquid modifications often involve the preparation of the thickened drinks by the health care team member responsible for the dietary consistency. Ide-ally, a liquid should be thickened to the consistency as recommended by the speech-language pathologists. Most manufacturers list the mixing instructions on their thickening products. Garcia et al[20] found that in a study of 42 health care providers, the range of thickened materials did not compare favorably to the published findings of laboratory viscosity measures or to the ranges of the NDD. Final thickened products were either too thick or too thin in their relationship to the target values. Reasons for this may be as simple as not following the guidelines on the product or perhaps may be related to the actual range in the makeup of the thickener itself.

> *It is important that speech-language pathologists provide clear and simple written guidelines on food and drink preparation to family members or health care providers who are responsible for daily preparation of meals and drinks. Regular training and monitoring on diet modifications should also be conducted.*

An additional issue associated with thickened liquids is the risk of dehydration because of reduction in fluid intake, especially in the older adult populations.[21–23] Limited access to thickened liquids, change in taste and texture, and inability to quench thirst are some of the factors that may be associated with poor intake of thickened liquids. With the aim to improve hydration level, a rehabilitation hospital proposed a **Fraizer Water Protocol** (or also known as **Free Water Protocol**).[24] The protocol proposes that free water access is given to patients who are on thickened liquids and nonoral diets. The protocol clearly specified when and how thin water may be given and cases where this protocol would not be recommended. Recent studies have found that patients who were mobile and had good cognitive functions benefited from this water protocol in terms of increased level of hydration and improved quality of life without increasing the risks of aspiration pneumonia.[25–27] If the free water protocol is recommended, it is crucial that the SLP and other members of the dysphagia team review the protocol guidelines thoroughly to avoid misuse of the protocol.

Foods

Texture refers to the composition of foods. The goal of normal swallowing is oral intake of all foods, liquids, as well as solids. The intake of solid foods is related to the severity of impairment, adequate dentition for chewing, and muscular strength and coordination for bolus transit and control. According to Bourne,[28] there are 5 characteristics for defining food texture. These characteristics and examples of the textures related to these characteristics are shown in Table 8–6.

Texture modifications: According to the IDDSI's framework, there are 5 levels of foods:

Liquidized: Food that is blended with added liquid as needed to form a smooth, moderately thick fluid.

Pureed: Food that is blended with added liquid as needed to form a smooth, extremely thick fluid.

Minced and moist: eg, finely mashed or minced tender meat that is served with a thick smooth sauce that is mixed with the foods.

Soft: eg, naturally soft foods that require minimal amount of chewing, minced cooked tender meats with no bones or small pieces of vegetables that are steamed or boiled.

Regular: Daily foods of different textures

TABLE 8–6. Characteristics of Food Textures as Outlined by Bourne[28] and the 8 Most Common Textures That Have a Significant Role in Dysphagia Diets, According to the American Dietetic Association[a]

Characteristics of Food Texture

1. It is a group of physical properties that derive from the structure of the food.
2. It consists of a group of properties, not a single property.
3. It is sensed by touch, usually in the mouth but hands may also be used.
4. It is not related to chemical senses of taste or odor.
5. It can be measured objectively by means of mass, distance, and time.

8 Textures Most Significant in Dysphagia Diets and Treatments

1. Adhesiveness—The work required to overcome the attractive forces between the surface of a food and another surface to which it has contact (eg, amount of work required to remove peanut butter from the palate)
2. Cohesiveness—The degree to which the food deforms (eg, when a moist bolus of cracker is compressed between tongue and palate)
3. Firmness—The force required to compress a semisolid food (eg, compressing pudding between the tongue and palate)
4. Fracturability ("Biteability")—The force that causes a solid food to break (eg, biting peanut brittle with the incisors)
5. Hardness—The force required to compress a solid food to attain a certain deformation (eg, chewing a hot dog just prior to when it begins to shear)
6. Springiness—The degree or rate that a sample returns to its original shape after being compressed (eg, marshmallows)
7. Viscosity—The rate of flow per unit force (eg, the rate at which a milkshake or nectar is drawn through a straw)
8. Yield Stress—The minimum amount of shear stress that must be applied to food before it begins to flow (eg, force required to get ketchup to flow from a bottle)

[a]Adapted from National Dysphagia Diet Task Force.[29]

Little evidence is available in the literature in relation to the effect of texture modifications to improve swallow safety. Studies have shown that it takes longer and larger force to chew and swallow harder solid foods.[30-33] Given the lack of evidence-based guidelines on texture modifica- tions, clinicians should carefully assess each individual's responses to different types of texture modifications and clearly explain to the patient and his or her caregivers the rationale for the diet modifications and the preparation methods (Table 8–7).

TABLE 8–7. Description of Different Levels of Foods Level Preparation According to IDDSI

Food Level	Examples	Characteristics	IDDSI Fork Pressure Test
3 (Moderately thick liquidized)	• Thick pumpkin soup • Thick gravy and sauces	• Increased time for oral control • Alleviates pain on swallowing	IDDSI flow test: • leaving >8 mL in the syringe after 10 seconds
4 (Pureed extremely thick)	• Mashed potato • Greek yogurt • Clotted cream	• Suitable for those with significantly reduced tongue control and those with no teeth/denture issues as no biting or chewing is required • Alleviates pain on chewing or swallowing • Beware of residue	• A clear pattern on the surface • The food retains the indentation from the fork • No lumps
5 (Minced & Moist)	• Finely chopped or minced meat served in extremely thick, smooth, non-pouring gravy • Mashed fruits with excess juices drained • Thick and smooth cereal with 2-4mm lumps, with excess milk or fluid drained	• Requires some tongue force • Suitable for those with missing teeth or denture issues as biting is not required • Requires minimal chewing • Tongue force required to move the bolus • Alleviates / prevents pain or fatigue from chewing	• The particles should easily be separated between and come through the prongs of a fork • Can be easily mashed with little pressure from a fork
6 (Soft)	• Cooked, tender meat served in sizes of 1.5 cm x 1.5 cm • Casseroles, stews, and curries containing small solid pieces that are soft and tender, no hard lumps • Steamed or boiled vegetables in final cooked size of 1.5 cm x 1.5 cm	• Requires adequate tongue force for oral and oral-pharyngeal stage processing • Suitable for those with missing teeth or poorly fitted dentures as no biting is required • Requires chewing • Prevents pain or fatigue on chewing	• Pressure from a fork held on its side can be used to "cut" or break this texture into smaller pieces • When a sample is pressed with the base of a fork, the sample squashes and changes shape, and does not return to its original shape when the fork is removed
7 (Regular)	• Normal, everyday foods of various textures • Any method may be used to eat these foods	• Requires good chewing and tongue control • Suitable for those with adequate swallow safety	N/A

Foods and drinks may behave differently in persons with different tongue force, range of movement, and amount of saliva. Clinicians should carefully explore a range of food and drinks with different levels of modifications that are specific to the individual's preference, needs, and culture.

Table 8–8 presents 3 categories of foods that are not well tolerated by individuals with swallowing problems.

Dysphagia Diet Guidelines

Different organizations around the world have issued descriptions of different types or levels of dysphagia diet as clinical guidelines. Table 8–9 highlights some of these. These guidelines are often used regionally to allow communication across organizations and dysphagia team members. There is still a need to develop empirical evidence to support the use of these specified diet levels for any particular group of patients or dysphagia severity.

National Dysphagia Diet—United States

Dysphagia diets vary considerably from facility to facility. Although many hospitals, clinics, and nursing homes are beginning to adopt many of the recommendations and features of the National Dysphagia Diet,[34] considerable variation for specific patients remains. The NDD requires both the specification of food consistency and its viscosity. Traditional oral dysphagia diets are typically a stepwise progression to the normal diet in 4 levels and liquids are described as 4 levels of viscosity/consistency boluses.

Dysphagia Diet Food Texture Descriptors—United Kingdom

The Descriptors[35] were developed by the National Patient Safety Agency (NPSA) Dysphagia Expert Reference Group in 2011. The descriptors only cover

TABLE 8–8. Three Categories of Foods That Are Not Well Tolerated by Individuals With Swallowing Problems

Crumbly and Noncohesive Foods	
Plain ground meat, chicken, or fish	Cornbread
Scrambled eggs	Cottage cheese
Jello	Coconut
Crackers	Nuts and seeds
Peas, corn, or legumes	
Mixed Consistency Foods	
Vegetable soup	Salad with dressing
Soup with large pieces or chunks of food	Canned fruit
Cold cereal with milk	Gelatin with fruit
Citrus fruit	Yogurt with fruit
Sticky Foods	
Dry mashed potatoes	
Peanut butter	
Fresh white or refined wheat bread	
Fudge or butterscotch sauce/caramel	
Bagels or soft rolls	

TABLE 8–9. International Guidelines on Dysphagia Diet[a]

Name	Country	Levels of Diet	Levels of Liquid
The National Dysphagia Diet (NDD)	United States	• Dysphagia Pureed (NDD 1) • Dysphagia Mechanically Altered (NDD 2) • Dysphagia advanced (NDD 3)	• Spoon-thick • Honey-like • Nectar-like • Thin: includes all beverages
Dysphagia Diet Food Texture Descriptors	United Kingdom	• Thin Puree Dysphagia Diet (B) • Thick Puree Dysphagia Diet (C) • Pre-mashed Dysphagia Diet (D) • Fork Mashable Dysphagia Diet (E)	• Extremely thick (pudding/Stage 3) • Moderately thick (honey/Stage 2) • Mildly thick (nectar/Stage 1)
The Australian Clinical Food Texture Grading Scale; The Australian Clinical Fluid Texture Grading Scale	Australia	• Texture A (Soft): soft foods, moist or served with a sauce • Texture B (Minced and Moist): soft and moist, easily forms into a ball • Texture C (Smooth Pureed): smooth and lump free	• Level 150 (Mildly Thick) • Level 400 (Moderately Thick) • Level 900 (Extremely Thick)
Irish Consistency Descriptors for Modified Fluids and Food (Based on the Australian Scales)	Ireland	• Texture A (Soft): soft foods, moist or served with a sauce • Texture B (Minced and Moist): soft and moist, easily forms into a ball • Texture C (Smooth Pureed): smooth and lump free • Texture D (Liquidized): smooth, pouring, uniform consistency, lump free	• Grade 1 (Very mildly thick) • Grade 2 (Mildly thick) • Grade 3 (Moderately thick) • Grade 4 (Extremely thick)

[a]Adapted from McCullough, Pelletier, and Steele[34]; National Patient Safety Agency[35]; Atherton et al.[36]; and IASLT.[37]

food texture but not for fluids. There are 4 levels of texture modifications. The guidelines provided detailed descriptions on how to prepare different types of food for each level of modification.

Australian Standardised Definitions and Terminology for Texture-Modified Foods and Fluids

The Australian foods and fluids[36] scales were consensus standards adopted by Speech Pathology Australia and the Dietitians Association of Australia. The scale includes a regular food texture, 3 levels of modified food textures, a level of regular fluid consistency, and 3 levels of thickened fluids. Descriptions of each level were provided, together with food and drink examples.

NONORAL DIETS

Introduction

A large number of patients are unable to take adequate nutrition orally. This may be temporary in patients who have had surgery for oral, pharyngeal, or laryngeal disease or patients who are acutely recovering from a stroke or those patients with a neuromuscular degenerative disorder who no longer can manage oral nutrition.

Enteral feeding is a type of feeding that occurs by way of the intestine. In patients who are unable to take adequate nutrition by mouth but otherwise have a functioning gastrointestinal (GI) tract, this type of feeding can be used. The enteral approach may reach the stomach, duodenum, or jejunum via a feeding tube placed through the nose or directly to the GI tract. **Parenteral feeding** (intravenous nutrition) is a type of feeding that bypasses the gastro-intestinal tract and directly injects the nutrition into the body through the veins. A special liquid mixture that contains proteins, carbohydrates, fats, vitamins, and minerals is given intravenously. It may be a temporary or long-term feeding method. Table 8–10

TABLE 8–10. Characteristics and Possible Complications of Different Types of Tube Feeding

Type of Nutrition Delivery	Characteristics	Possible Complications
Simple IV/peripheral parenteral nutrition (PPN); central total parenteral nutrition (CTPN)	• Intravenous • May need surgical placement to CTPN • Simple IV solution or complete solution for nutrition	• PPN: infection, bleeding, weakened and collapsed veins • CTPN: air embolism, pneumothorax, blood clot, infection, sepsis
Nasogastric (NG tube)	• Temporary alterative to oral intake • Minimally invasive • Easy placement and removal • Transitional to bolus feeding • Stomach must be uninvolved with primary disease	• Misplacement into the airway • Discomfort • Risk of sinusitis and nasal ulceration • Cosmesis: feeding tube is visible • May impact swallow function and increased risks of reflux and aspiration • Lack of intact gag reflex may contribute to aspiration and reflux
Nasoduodenal/Nasojejunal	• Minimally invasive • Easy placement • Suitable for short-term use • Useful in conditions of gastroparesis or impaired stomach emptying • Useful if esophageal reflux present • Requires radiographic confirmation of placement • (Nasojejunal) placement of tip further down GI tract minimizes dislocation to stomach	• Cosmesis: feeding tube is visible • More prone to plugging if not properly maintained
Gastrostomy (G-tube)/ Percutaneous Endoscopic Gastrostomy (PEG)	• Suitable for long-term feeding • Concurrent oral intake is possible in certain cases • Cosmesis: feeding tube can be hidden under clothing • Easy tube replacement • Insertion site care needed • Lowers risk of tube migration and aspiration	• Insertion may require surgery • Risk of infection, excoriation, and skin irritation at gastrostomy site • Potential fistula at insertion site after tube removal • Potential risk of pulmonary aspiration and reflux • Risk of nausea, vomiting, diarrhea, constipation
Jejunostomy (J-tube)	• Same advantages as gastrostomy, except oral feeding is not recommended • Good alternative feeding route if stomach is impaired • Requires special nutrition formula	• Insertion requires surgery • Loss of controlled emptying of the stomach • Misplacement • Risk of diarrhea and dehydration

summarizes the common types of nonoral feeding, with their characteristics and possible complications. The decision to opt for nonoral feeding is often a critical one for the patient and family.

> *Instrumental testing provides the basis for the decision to opt for nonoral feeding, but the decision is not based solely on radiographic, manometric, or endoscopic assessment.*

Other factors used to decide in favor of nonoral feeding include (1) time required to swallow, (2) energy level of patient, (3) need for alternative route for medications, (4) repeated episodes of dehydration, (5) history of pneumonia, and (6) unexplained weight loss or signs of malnutrition. All of the issues, those related to diagnostic finding as well as the clinical observations, must be discussed with the patient and family when the option for nonoral feeding is part of the treatment plan. Clinicians should remember that regular reviews and concurrent rehabilitative treatment (if appropriate) should still be provided. Studies have reported that nonoral feedings are associated with poor quality of life.[38–39] Where possible, clinicians should assist non-oral-fed patients to return to oral feeding as early as possible.

It is equally important to present to the patient a strong rationale to elect nonoral feeding when there is a progressive neuromuscular disease such as amyotrophic lateral sclerosis (ALS). Logemann[40] has pointed out that the time to complete one swallow has diagnostic significance. This factor, along with those noted above, should be considered when a feeding tube is planned.

> *The patient with ALS and other patients with neuromuscular degeneration will benefit from a feeding tube when they still have the energy and desire to maintain their nutrition.*

Waiting until the patient is at or near the end of life denies him or her the quality of life that might otherwise remain if nutrition was maintained.

Nasogastric, Nasoduodenal, and Nasojejunal Tubes

Nasogastric (Ryles) tubes (NG tubes) are the most commonly placed tubes. The nasogastric tube is inserted through the nose and terminates in the stomach. Their use is typically short term (up to around 4 weeks), and they are placed with the expectation that swallow rehabilitation will be aggressive and fast paced. There are places and reasons (eg, recent history of pneumonia) where the NG tube is kept for a longer period of time. In some cases, the NG tube must be replaced by a more permanent nonoral feeding tube, but these cases are usually the result of additional morbidity that was not expected at the time of NG placement. Figure 8–2 shows a typical NG feeding tube that may be used for both short-term or long-term nutritional support. The tube is usually first placed by the physician and replaced or re-inserted by nurses or physician assistants at a later time, and usually an x-ray is taken to validate the final location of the tube. A pH test of tube aspirate is recommended to be carried out before each feeding to ensure the tube has not shifted to the airways.

Nasoduodenal tubes are also used for short-term dysphagia. They are useful when there is a strong suspicion of **esophageal reflux** or **gastroparesis** (inability to empty the stomach due either to bilateral vagotomy or neural damage to the vagus nerve).

Nasojejunal tubes terminate in the jejunum, which is the midsection of the small intestine. In the jejunum are small fingerlike outgrowths that allow for digested food or liquid to be absorbed, thus providing the needed nutrition even when the stomach cannot tolerate foods or liquids.

Gastrostomy Tubes

A gastrostomy tube is surgically placed directly into the stomach. Feedings via gastrostomy tube can be administered by continuous feeding or by bolus feeding.

When long-term enteral feeding is required, gastrostomy tubes are preferred because they usually

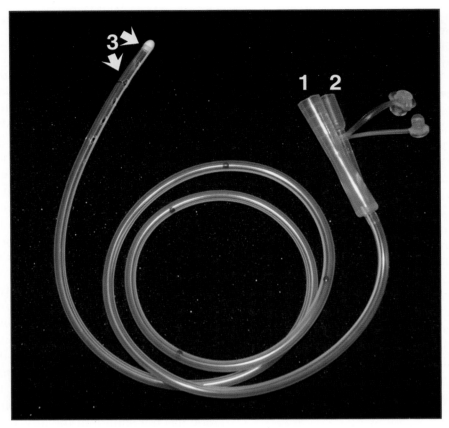

FIGURE 8–2. Kendall Argyle silicone Salem Sump tube, 16-Fr., 48″ length (Tyco/Healthcare). Dual lumen. Y-connector with (1) suction drainage lumen/feeding port, (2) suction vent lumen, and (3) closed-end tip with multiple exit ports. From Leonard and Kendall.[41(p151)]

last longer, require less replacement, and are less likely to become clogged or dislodged than nasal tubes. The replacement of gastrostomy tube is easier and creates less discomfort for patients than nasal tubes. Gastrostomy is also cosmetically more acceptable and will not create nasal ulceration. A gastrostomy can be created by endoscopic method, surgically or by radiological guided method (Figure 8–3).

Endoscopic method, **percutaneous endoscopic gastrostomy (PEG)**, has become the procedure of choice in current practice because it can be performed quickly in endoscopy room under local anesthesia. It is relatively low risk with a high success rate.[42]

Surgical gastrostomy requires mini-**laparotomy**. It is a surgical procedure that has to be performed in a surgical suite and is relatively more complicated than PEG. It is performed for patients who cannot open the mouth wide enough for PEG (eg,

head and neck cancer patients after radiotherapy) or there is significant obstruction in the esophagus (eg, patients with esophageal cancer).

Radiological guided gastrostomy, **percutaneous radiologic gastrostomy (PRG)**, can be used for patients who are not suitable for PEG and surgical gastrostomy.[43] It is the first choice of gastrostomy for some centers where endoscopy service is not readily available. It is performed under fluoroscopic guidance; therefore, both the operators and patients are exposed to radiation.

Only a few postoperational complications are related to gastrostomy.[44] PEG and PRG may have a very small chance of perforating other abdominal organs, especially the large bowel. Exit site infection is rare with the routine use of prophylactic pre-operation antibiotic.[42] Long-term complications are also uncommon.[44] Most reported long-term prob-

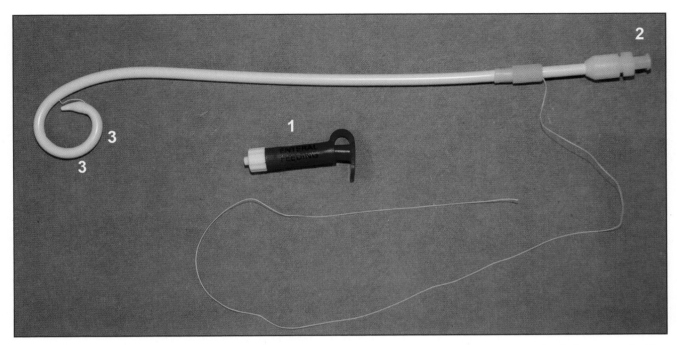

FIGURE 8–3. Deutsch gastrostomy catheter with AQ hydrophilic coating, 16-Fr., 25-cm long with Cook-Cope-type locking loop. (1) Enteral feeding adapter with male Luer lock fitting, (2) Luer lock tube opening, and (3) exits ports. From Leonard and Kendall.[43(p153)]

lems include skin irritation around exit site due to leakage of gastric content, granuloma causing bleeding, and discharge known as **buried bumper syndrome,** which can be fatal but is very uncommon. With simple good gastrostomy care, these problems can be easily prevented and solved.

Gastrostomy is not permanent. When the patient's swallowing functions improve, the gastrostomy tube can be removed and the gastrostomy site will close down after several days with appropriate nursing care. On the other hand, the gastrostomy site will not close down immediately after the gastrostomy tube is dislodged.

MALNUTRITION AND DEHYDRATION

Patients with swallowing disorders should be monitored for signs of **malnutrition** and **dehydration**. The dietitian regularly reviews body weight, caloric intake, liquid intake, feeding schedules (oral and nonoral), medication/nutrition interactions, and biochemical data. However, it is up to the entire dys-phagia team to be alert for those factors that lead to dehydration and malnutrition.

Stroke

Stroke patients may be the largest group of individuals with dysphagia to be at risk for malnutrition and dehydration. Cognitive defects, hemiparesis, spatial neglect, and motor disabilities all contribute to the risk of malnutrition in stroke patients. Malnutrition in stroke patients may be as high as 62% during the acute or chronic phase.[45–47]

Malnutrition occurs as a result of poor or inadequate oral or nonoral intake. **Protein-calorie malnutrition (PCM)** is one of the most common types of malnutrition.

> *PCM has the power to fatigue muscles, alter the neuromuscular function of the swallow muscles, and contribute to increasing the severity of dysphagia.*

Other factors such as increased stress reaction, higher incidence of respiratory and urinary infections, and bedsores come into play once malnutrition is present. Given these comorbidity factors, one might expect longer hospital stays, poorer outcome, and greater risk of further illness with the presence of malnutrition.

In a systematic review of nutritional status during the acute and rehabilitation periods, Foley et al[47] found malnutrition ranging from a low of 8% to a high of 52.6%. Interestingly, the findings of malnutrition were increased during the rehabilitation period compared to the acute stroke period (0 to 7 days postonset). Others have found that malnutrition in the stroke patient is also related to the severity of the stroke[48] and to the lack of swallowing therapy during the poststroke period.[49]

Head and Neck Cancer

The problems with nutrition following head and neck cancer relate primarily to the loss of organs for swallowing during surgery or cancer treatment.

Patients with cancers in the head and neck often have significant swallowing problems prior to surgery.

They may already be suffering from malnutrition due to their inability to tolerate foods and liquids either due to the pain, the inability to move foods through the mouth, or the blockage of food by tumors in the pharynx or esophagus. Following surgery, the pathway to swallowing may be significantly altered. If radiation therapy is prescribed, further difficulties occur with mucositis, pain, or simply fatigue. A greater incidence of tracheostomy dependence and increased incidence of aspiration are noted when structures that have previously contributed to valving have been removed (eg, supraglottic laryngectomy, partial laryngectomy).[50]

Long-term effects of head and neck cancer also contribute to malnutrition due to the changing and fibrosing structures associated with radiation. PEG dependency rates increase due to the inability of the postradiation patient to manage bolus transfer due to tissue fibrosis and achalasia.[51]

When there is a concern about malnutrition, weight, or weight history, serum albumin and prealbumin are capable of identifying the majority of patients requiring nutritional attention. In the acute and rehabilitation settings, weight should be checked every 2 days. For home health care, weight should be checked at every visit.

For patients undergoing longer treatments such as radiation therapy or chemotherapy, weight should be checked weekly and nutritional reviews should be done if a weight change is noted from one period to the next.

Patients should understand that a feeding tube need not be a permanent nutritional route but rather a part of the rehabilitation from the underlying condition, whether it be a stroke or treatment for head and neck cancer. Whenever signs of malnutrition and dehydration are observed, a dietitian should be consulted.

Dementia

Dementia is an increasingly prevalent condition globally, especially in the aging population.[52] Malnutrition and dehydration are common concerns for individuals with different stages of dementia. The causes may range from an inability to recognize food, loss of appetite, difficulties in coordinating head, hands and arms movement, and in cases of advanced dementia, difficulty with swallowing. Individuals with dementia are often on a modified diet and/or require feeding assistance to ensure swallowing safety. Studies have found that the nutrition and moisture level of modified texture food varied greatly with different methods of preparation, and this may have significant impact on the nutrition and hydration level of the patients.[53–54]

The speech-language pathologists should work closely with dietitians and caregivers to ensure patients with dementia have adequate nutrition and hydration. This includes calorie counts and proper mix of protein, fats, and carbohydrates.

Studies have found that providing training to carers who are responsible for providing feeding assistance to dysphagic patients may help to improve the patients' amount of food intake and reduce feeding difficulties.[55-57] There is moderate evidence in support of using nutritional supplements to improve the nutritional status of patients with dementia.[58,59]

A Cochrane systematic review on the use of tube feeding in older adults with advanced dementia concluded that there is not enough strong evidence to support (or oppose) the use of tube feeding in this population.[60] Only 7 observational controlled studies were identified in the literature, and they found that tube feeding neither prolonged life nor improved nutritional status, when compared with assisted feeding. However, a recent study in Japan showed that individuals who were on PEG or home parenteral nutrition had significantly longer survival than those who were on self-feeding oral intake.[61] Given that the current evidence is not clear on the use of tube feeding in older adults with advanced dementia, studies have suggested providing "comfort feeding" and informed decision making on feeding options[62-64] using decision aids for this population.

> SLPs need to carefully balance the benefits and risks of diet modifications and enteral feeding and fully involve the patients and surrogate decision maker into the decision-making process.

NUTRITION IN THE AGING POPULATION

Presbyphagia is used to describe the continuous and degenerative changes in swallowing functions in healthy aging. When swallowing functions deteriorated to a level that is not tolerated or compensated for by the elderly, dysphagia would then occur. Up to 84% of elderly may develop changes in swallowing functions that would be considered as "abnormal" in younger healthy adults.[65] Swallowing problems with advancing age are a major health problem in the elderly but otherwise well individuals, as well as in hospitalized individuals and nursing home residents.

> Studies estimated that 30% to 68% of nursing home residents have signs of swallowing disorders.[66-69]

In this group and elderly patients in general, nutrition and eating play an important part of life, whether to maintain health or to aid in recovery from disease or sickness.[70] Because of the importance of eating, no diet should be recommended simply on the basis of a diagnosis or on the basis of an instrumental test. There are many factors that go into the nutritional needs of patients with dysphagia, as we have reviewed above. This is especially true in elderly patients, including those restricted to nursing home care or those otherwise healthy elderly individuals with other comorbidities. In both groups, the diet should be as liberal as swallowing safety allows. The elderly dysphagic population may face many problems affecting nutrition, such as poor eyesight, eating alone, and limited hand mobility. All of these problems have a bearing not only on what the patient may or may not eat but also on the patient's quality of life. The importance of qualified dietitians to oversee the content of meals for the elderly should not be overlooked in the rehabilitation process. However, the dietitian should not undertake the management of nutrition in the elderly as his or her responsibility solely.

> Especially in elderly patients, the dietitian must work with the SLP, the physical therapist, and the attending physician to make sure that the nutrition needs are met within the framework of the medical conditions present, the physical abilities and limitations of the patient, and the quality of life that apply to each particular patient.

In some patients, this may mean a more liberalized diet to enhance quality of life; in others, it may mean restrictions in certain food groups or viscosities.[71]

Table 8–11 summarizes the major considerations that must be considered when preparing diets for elderly individuals. The SLP and dietitian must take all of these into consideration, along with the nutrition requirements of each individual.

TABLE 8–11. Considerations When Planning a Nutritional Rehabilitation Program for the Elderly Patient

Body structures and functions
Swallow safety
Dentition
Physical disabilities and limitations
Cognitive functions
Motivation and appetite
Communication ability
Emotional functions
Nutritional needs—weight maintenance, weight gain, weight reduction
Activities and Participation
Social interactions at mealtime
Religious preferences
Ethnic food preferences
Environmental factors
Living situation
Family or friends support
Available community diet services
Meal delivery systems

These considerations are important because it is not always possible to do the proper tests or complete tests in elderly individuals. Thus, the choice of food consistencies and the viscosities and combinations of viscosities may be more subjective than objective. There is a need to talk to the families if available, other caregivers such as nurses and attendants, and roommates or neighbors to get a feel for what the elderly patient's needs are when the patient himself or herself cannot or does not express those needs. In all elderly patients, no diet should be so restrictive that it discourages oral intake. The Academy of Nutrition and Dietetics advocates a liberalized policy when considering diets for the elderly.[72]

The Academy encourages health care professionals to carefully balance the benefits and risks associated with "therapeutic diets" (including modified diets). The elderly clients should be involved in the decision making as far as possible to increase the desire to eat and quality of life.

ETHICAL CONSIDERATIONS

Ethical dilemmas may occur when considering whether to recommend nonoral feeding or highly restrictive modified diets. SLPs may have identified high aspiration risks or inadequate nutritional and hydration intakes, warranting a medical need to modify the oral diet and/or the use of enteral feeding. However, the situation may become more complicated and ethically challenging when the patient has an **Advanced Directives** or Living Will, or when the patient or the **surrogate decision maker** does not agree with the recommendations. The following case is a hypothetical situation that may be seen in rehabilitation hospitals:

Mrs. P is a 69-year-old lady who had a severe stroke a month ago, resulting in severe global aphasia and dysphagia. She had a PEG tube placed a week ago. Mrs. P's swallowing functions are slightly and slowly improving over the last week. Mrs. P's daughter produced Mrs. P's advanced directives (AD) to the physicians and demanded Mrs. P's feeding tube to be removed as Mrs. P indicated in her AD that she does not want to live on tube feeding. Mrs. P's daughter made repeated comments to the treatment team that she feels stressed and lost, wondering if this is how her mother wishes her life to end.

There is no straightforward recommendation that can be applied to all similar cases as the one above. A number of clinical settings have published decision-making algorithm or guidelines to aid health care providers to make decisions on diet modifications or tube feeding.[73–76]

A number of common themes to these guidelines are as follows:

1. Accurately identify the current progress and prognosis of the patient.
2. Educate the patient and family members of the risks and benefits of the dysphagia management recommendations.
3. Involve the patient and family in the decision making.

4. Encourage regular follow-up after a decision has been made.

These guidelines can help to ease the burden on health care providers and the patient's family.

SUMMARY

This chapter discussed the importance of integrating the work of the dietitian with that of the SLP to avoid such problems as dehydration and malnutrition that can occur with patients following stroke, head and neck cancer, or other diseases leading to dysphagia. The SLP who treats swallowing disorders must not only use behavioral techniques to improve oral nutrition, but must also maintain knowledge of the properties of the foods and liquids that are being swallowed.

> *Bolus size, consistency, viscosity, and food texture all affect the ultimate success of the patient's ability to achieve oral nutrition that results in adequate protein-calorie intake.*

Proper viscosity allows the patient to control the speed of fluid transit and ultimately reduce the probability of penetration and/or aspiration. Diets for patients with dysphagia are organized on the basis of rheological properties and protein-calorie balance. Safe swallowing requires a combination of the proper consistency and viscosity along with the management of neuromuscular behaviors at each stage of the swallow. Viscosity modifications, either by changing the foods themselves or by modifying liquids and foods with thickening or thinning agents, provide the clinician with a range of options that can be used with various postures and techniques to achieve a safe swallow and advance the patient closer to a regular diet.

If oral nutrition is not possible, other means of nutrition must be invoked. The SLP who understands the basis of nonoral feeding, whether through a PEG or other means, can monitor the progress of the patient, along with the nutritionist.

DISCUSSION QUESTION

Diabetic patients are a special group when it comes to nutrition requirements and limitations. Review additional literature to discuss the nutritional requirements and limitations for adult diabetes (usually type 2 diabetes) as well as for childhood diabetes (usually type 1 diabetes). How will oral (including the use of thickeners) and nonoral nutritional needs have to be adjusted for these groups?

STUDY QUESTIONS

1. The prime variable for studying the properties of liquids is
   A. Density
   B. Flow
   C. Viscosity
   D. Shear rate

2. Viscosity represents a characteristic of a liquid that can be described more simply as
   A. Thickness
   B. Resistance to flow
   C. Degree of elasticity
   D. Type of texture

3. Chewing provides an opportunity for a food texture to be
   A. Equally dense
   B. Equally homogeneous
   C. Equally cohesive
   D. All of the above

REFERENCES

1. Nutrition management in dysphagia. *Manual of Clinical Dietetics.* 5th ed. Chicago, IL: American Dietetic Association; 1996.
2. Lewis MM, Kidder JA. *Nutrition Practice Guidelines for Dysphagia.* Chicago, IL: American Dietetic Association; 1996.
3. Molseed L. Clinical evaluation of swallowing: The nutritionist's perspective. *Comprehensive Management of*

Swallowing Disorders. San Diego, CA: Plural Publishing; 2006.

4. Cichero J, Steele C, Duivestein J, et al. The need for international terminology and definitions for texture-modified foods and thickened liquids used in dysphagia management: foundations of a global initiative. *Curr Phys Med Rehabil Rep.* 2013;1(4):280–291.

5. Cichero JA, Hay G, Murdoch, BE, Halley M. Videofluoroscopic fluids versus mealtime fluids: Differences in viscosity and density made clear. *J Med Speech Lang Path.* 1997;5:210.

6. Strowd L, Kyzima J, Pillsbury D, Valley T, Rubin BR. Dysphagia dietary guidelines and the rheology of nutritional feeds and barium test feeds. *Chest Journal.* 2008;133;6:1397–1401.

7. Payne C, Methven L, Fairfield C, Bell A. Consistently inconsistent: commercially available starch-based dysphagia products. *Dysphagia.* 2011;1;26;1:27-33.

8. Goldfield EC, Smith V, Buonomo C, Perez J, Larson K. Preterm infant swallowing of thin and nectar-thick liquids: changes in lingual–palatal coordination and relation to bolus transit. *Dysphagia.* 2013;28(2):234–244.

9. Bisch EM, Logemann JA, Rademaker AW, Kahrilas PJ, Lazarus CL. Pharyngeal effects of bolus volume, viscosity, and temperature in patients with dysphagia resulting from neurologic impairment and in normal subjects. *J Speech Lang Hear Res.* 1994;37(5):1041–1049.

10. Bingjie L, Tong Z, Xinting S, Jianmin X, Guijun J. Quantitative videofluoroscopic analysis of penetration-aspiration in post-stroke patients. *Neurol India.* 2010;58(1):42.

11. Lin P-H, Hsiao T-Y, Chang Y-C, et al. Effects of functional electrical stimulation on dysphagia caused by radiation therapy in patients with nasopharyngeal carcinoma. *Support Care Cancer.* 2011;19(1):91–99.

12. Troche MS, Sapienza CM, Rosenbek JC. Effects of bolus consistency on timing and safety of swallow in patients with Parkinson's disease. *Dysphagia.* 2008;23(1):26–32.

13. Lee J, Sejdic E, Steele CM, Chau T. Effects of liquid stimuli on dual-axis swallowing accelerometry signals in a healthy population. *Biomed Eng Online.* 2010;9(7).

14. Anderson K, Throckmorton G, Buschang P, Hayasaki H. The effects of bolus hardness on masticatory kinematics. *J Oral Rehabil.* 2002;29(7):689–696.

15. Youmans SR, Youmans GL, Stierwalt JA. Differences in tongue strength across age and gender: is there a diminished strength reserve? *Dysphagia.* 2009;24(1):57–65.

16. Karkazis H, Kossioni A. Surface EMG activity of the masseter muscle in denture wearers during chewing of hard and soft food. *J Oral Rehabil.* 1998;25:8–14.

17. Chen MY, Peele VN, Donati D, Ott DJ, Donofrio PD, Gelfand DW. Clinical and videofluoroscopic evaluation of swallowing in 41 patients with neurologic disease. *Gastrointest Radiol.* 1992;17(1):95–98.

18. Lee KL, Kim WH, Kim EJ, Lee JK. Is swallowing of all mixed consistencies dangerous for penetration-aspiration? *Am J Phys Med Rehabil.* 2012;91(3):187–192.

19. Barata LF, de Carvalho GB, Carrara-de Angelis E, de Faria JCM, Kowalski LP. Swallowing, speech and quality of life in patients undergoing resection of soft palate. *Eur Arch Oto-Rhino-Laryngol.* 2013;270(1):305–312.

20. Garcia JM, Chambers I, Clark M, Helverson J, Matta Z. Quality of care issues for dysphagia: modifications involving oral fluids. *J Clin Nurs.* 2010;19(11–12):1618–1624.

21. Cichero JA. Thickening agents used for dysphagia management: effect on bioavailability of water, medication and feelings of satiety. *Nutr J.* 2013;12(1):1–8.

22. Castellanos VH, Butler E, Gluch L, Burke B. Use of thickened liquids in skilled nursing facilities. *J Am Diet Assoc.* 104(8):1222–1226.

23. Whelan K. Inadequate fluid intakes in dysphagic acute stroke. *Clin Nutr.* 20(5):423–428.

24. Panther K. The Frazier Free Water Protocol. *SIG 13 Perspect Swallowing Swallowing Disord (Dysphagia).* 2005; 14(1):4–9.

25. Frey KL, Ramsberger G. Comparison of outcomes before and after implementation of a water protocol for patients with cerebrovascular accident and dysphagia. *J Neurosci Nurs.* 2011;43(3):165–171.

26. Karagiannis MJ, Chivers L, Karagiannis TC. Effects of oral intake of water in patients with oropharyngeal dysphagia. *BMC Geriatr.* 2011;11(1):1–10.

27. Karagiannis M, Karagiannis TC. Oropharyngeal dysphagia, free water protocol and quality of life: an update from a prospective clinical trial update from a prospective clinical trial. *Hellenic J Nucl Med.* 2014;17:26–29.

28. Bourne M. *Food Texture and Viscosity: Concept and Measurement.* San Diego, CA: Academic Press; 1982.

29. National Dysphagia Diet Task Force (NDDT), American Dietetic Association. *National Dysphagia Diet: Standardization for Optimal Care.* Chicago, IL: American Dietetic Association; 2002.

30. Ruark JL, McCullough GH, Peters RL, Moore CA. Bolus consistency and swallowing in children and adults. *Dysphagia.* 2002;17(1):24–33.

31. Igarashi A, Kawasaki M, Nomura S-i, et al. Sensory and motor responses of normal young adults during swallowing of foods with different properties and volumes. *Dysphagia.* 2010;25(3):198–206.

32. Inagaki D, Miyaoka Y, Ashida I, Yamada Y. Influence of food properties and body position on swallowing-related muscle activity amplitude. *J Oral Rehabil.* 2009;36(3):176–183.

33. Ashida I, Iwamori H, Kawakami SY, Miyaoka Y, Murayama A. Analysis of physiological parameters of masseter muscle activity during chewing of agars in healthy young males. *J Texture Stud.* 2007;38(1):87–99.

34. McCullough G, Pelletier C, Steele C. National dysphagia diet: What to swallow? *ASHA Leader.* 2003;8(20):16–27.

35. Dysphagia Diet Food Texture Descriptors. London, UK: National Patient Safety Agency; 2011.

36. Atherton M, Bellis-Smith N, Cichero J, Suter M. Texture-modified foods and thickened fluids as used for individu-

als with dysphagia: Australian standardised labels and definitions. *Nutr Diet.* 2007;64(2 suppl):s53–s76.

37. IASLT. Irish Consistency Descriptors for Modified Fluids and Food. Dublin, Ireland: Irish Nutrition and Dietetic Institute; November 2009.

38. Roberge C, Tran M, Massoud C, et al. Quality of life and home enteral tube feeding: a French prospective study in patients with head and neck or oesophageal cancer. *Br J Cancer.* 2000;82(2):263–269.

39. Kwok T, Lo RS, Wong E, Tang, WK, Mok V, Wong, KS. Quality of life of stroke survivors: a 1-year follow-up study. *Arch Phys Med Rehabil.* 2006;87(9):1177–1182.

40. Logemann JA. Factors affecting ability to resume oral nutrition in the oropharyngeal dysphagic individual. *Dysphagia.* 1990;4(4):202–208.

41. Leonard R, Kendall K. *Dysphagia Assessment and Treatment Planning: A Team Approach.* 2nd ed. San Diego, CA: Plural Publishing; 2007; 151.

42. Friginal-Ruiz AB, Lucendo AJ. Percutaneous endoscopic gastrostomy: a practical overview on its indications, placement conditions, management, and nursing care. *Gastroenterol Nurs.* 2015;38(5):354–366.

43. Shin JH, Park A-W. Updates on percutaneous radiologic gastrostomy/gastrojejunostomy and jejunostomy. *Gut Liver.* 2010;4(suppl 1):S25.

44. Clarke E, Pitts N, Latchford A, Lewis S. A large prospective audit of morbidity and mortality associated with feeding gastrostomies in the community. *Clin Nutr.* 2016. doi:10.1016/j.clnu.2016.01.008.

45. Axelsson K, Asplund K, Norberg A, Eriksson S. Eating problems and nutritional status during hospital stay of patients with severe stroke. *J Am Diet Assoc.* 1989;89(8): 1092–1096.

46. Bouziana SD, Tziomalos K. Malnutrition in patients with acute stroke. *J Nutr Metab.* 2011;2011. doi: http://dx.doi.org/10.1155/2011/167898.

47. Foley NC, Martin RE, Salter KL, Teasell RW. A review of the relationship between dysphagia and malnutrition following stroke. *J Rehabil Med.* 2009;41(9):707–713.

48. Crary MA, Carnaby-Mann GD, Miller L, Antonios N, Silliman S. Dysphagia and nutritional status at the time of hospital admission for ischemic stroke. *J Stroke Cerebrovasc Dis.* 2006;15(4):164–171.

49. Lin LC, Wang SC, Chen SH, Wang TG, Chen MY, Wu SC. Efficacy of swallowing training for residents following stroke. *J Adv Nurs.* 2003;44(5):469–478.

50. Wein RO, Weber RS. The current role of vertical partial laryngectomy and open supraglottic laryngectomy. *Curr Probl Cancer.* 2005;29(4):201–214.

51. Corry J. Feeding tubes and dysphagia: cause or effect in head and neck cancer patients. *J Med Imaging Radiat Oncol.* 2009;53(5):431–432.

52. Prince M, Bryce R, Albanese E, Wimo A, Ribeiro W, Ferri CP. The global prevalence of dementia: a systematic review and metaanalysis. *Alzheimers Dementia.* 2013; 9(1):63–75.e62.

53. Beck AM, Hansen KS. Meals served in Danish nursing homes and to Meals-on-Wheels clients may not offer nutritionally adequate choices. *J Nutr Elder.* 2010;29(1): 100–109.

54. Durant M. A comparison of energy provision by diet order in a long-term care facility. *Can J Aging.* 2008;27(02): 225–227.

55. Suominen MH, Kivisto SM, Pitkala KH. The effects of nutrition education on professionals' practice and on the nutrition of aged residents in dementia wards. *Eur J Clin Nutr.* 2007;61(10):1226–1232.

56. Wright L, Cotter D, Hickson M. The effectiveness of targeted feeding assistance to improve the nutritional intake of elderly dysphagic patients in hospital. *J Hum Nutr Diet.* 2008;21(6):555–562.

57. Chang CC, Lin LC. Effects of a feeding skills training programme on nursing assistants and dementia patients. *J Clin Nurs.* 2005;14(10):1185–1192.

58. Allen VJ, Methven L, Gosney MA. Use of nutritional complete supplements in older adults with dementia: systematic review and meta-analysis of clinical outcomes. *Clin Nutr.* 2013;32(6):950–957.

59. Liu W, Cheon J, Thomas SA. Interventions on mealtime difficulties in older adults with dementia: a systematic review. *Int J Nurs Stud.* 2014;51(1):14–27.

60. Candy B, Sampson EL, Jones L. Enteral tube feeding in older people with advanced dementia: findings from a Cochrane systematic review. *Int J Palliat Nurs.* 2009;15(8):396.

61. Shintani S. Efficacy and ethics of artificial nutrition in patients with neurologic impairments in home care. *J Clin Neurosci.* 20(2):220–223.

62. Hanson LC, Carey TS, Caprio AJ, et al. Improving decision-making for feeding options in advanced dementia: a randomized, controlled trial. *J Am Geriatr Soc.* 2011; 59(11):2009–2016.

63. Einterz SF, Gilliam R, Chang Lin F, McBride JM, Hanson LC. Development and testing of a decision aid on goals of care for advanced dementia. *J Am Med Dir Assoc.* 15(4):251–255.

64. Palecek EJ, Teno JM, Casarett DJ, Hanson LC, Rhodes RL, Mitchell SL. Comfort feeding only: a proposal to bring clarity to decision-making regarding difficulty with eating for persons with advanced dementia. *J Am Geriatr Soc.* 2010;58(3):580–584.

65. Ekberg O, Feinberg MJ. Altered swallowing function in elderly patients without dysphagia: radiologic findings in 56 cases. *Am J Roentgenol.* 1991;156(6):1181–1184.

66. Maeda K, Akagi J. Sarcopenia is an independent risk factor of dysphagia in hospitalized older people. *Geriatr Gerontol Int.* 2016;16(4):515–521.

67. Nogueira D, Reis E. Swallowing disorders in nursing home residents: how can the problem be explained? *Clin Interv Aging.* 2013;8:221–227.

68. Steele MC, Greenwood C, Ens I, Robertson C, Seidman-Carlson R. Mealtime difficulties in a home for the aged: not just dysphagia. *Dysphagia.* 1997;12(1):43–50.

69. Park Y-H, Han H-R, Oh B-M, et al. Prevalence and associated factors of dysphagia in nursing home residents. *Geriatr Nurs.* 34(3):212–217.

70. Centers for Disease Control and Prevention. *Healthy Aging Improving and Extending Quality of Life Among Older Americans.* Atlanta, GA: National Center for Chronic Disease Prevention and Health Promotion; 2009.

71. Kuczmarski M, Weddle D. Position paper of the American Dietetic Association: nutrition across the spectrum of aging. *J Am Diet Assoc.* 2005;105(4):616–633.

72. Dorner B. Position of the American Dietetic Association: individualized nutrition approaches for older adults in health care communities. *J Am Diet Assoc.* 2010;110(10): 1549–1553.

73. Kaizer F, Spiridigliozzi A-M, Hunt MR. Promoting shared decision-making in rehabilitation: development of a framework for situations when patients with dysphagia refuse diet modification recommended by the treating team. *Dysphagia.* 2011;27(1):81–87.

74. Brady Wagner LC. Withholding and withdrawing tube feeding for persons with dysphagia: exploring complications of advance directives and the obligations of a rehabilitation team. *Top Stroke Rehabil.* 2001;8(1): 56–59.

75. Angus F, Burakoff R. The percutaneous endoscopic gastrostomy tube: medical and ethical issues in placement. *Am J Gastroenterol.* 2003;98(2):272–277.

76. Rabeneck L, McCullough LB, Wray NP. Ethically justified, clinically comprehensive guidelines for percutaneous endoscopic gastrostomy tube placement. *Lancet.* 1997;349(9050):496–498.

Pediatric Dysphagia: Assessment of Disorders of Swallowing and Feeding

A Look at the Chapter

In this chapter, the focus is on a thorough assessment of the infant. The importance of the case history is emphasized, as that may be the only data available in order to begin treatment. The birth records, the parents' history, and input from others who may be involved with the growth and development of the child are reviewed. The anatomy and physiology of the child is discussed with attention to developmental milestones of feeding and eating. The importance of changes in the child's behavior as they relate to eating is considered. This chapter includes a survey of the most common swallowing disorders that occur in children.

INTRODUCTION

Pediatric swallowing and feeding disorders result from multiple medical problems that develop either prior to, during, or following birth. Because of their inability to swallow normally, these children are at a greatly increased risk for difficulties at every stage of development. Specialized care must be provided to minimize the dangerous consequences of events like aspiration, pneumonia, and other conditions that cause failure to thrive. Clinically, the methods used to examine and assess feeding in the newborn, infant, and young child must be specific to those populations. It is critical the clinician not treat pediatric dysphagia as simply an adult condition on a smaller scale.

The scope of pediatric swallowing disorders includes latching, sucking, feeding, and breathing, as well as the sensory and motor components that coordinate these functions. Disruption at any point of this process can cause swallowing dysfunction, which can lead to food and/or liquids entering the airway. Once this occurs, children start to cough, choke, and eventually avoid eating altogether. This, in turn, causes failure to thrive, behavior problems, and delays in normal physical and mental development.

Feeding and swallowing disorders in the pediatric population may result from multiple conditions such as congenital or acquired neurological issues, anatomical and physiological problems, genetic syndromes, behavioral conditions, and systemic illnesses. These may be isolated conditions or seen in combination, especially in the preterm infant. Additionally, the effects of seemingly benign situations in adults are often much worse in the younger patient. For example, an adult usually tolerates a small amount of liquid in the lungs, but it may be fatal for the infant who lacks pulmonary reserve and the ability to cough. To successfully treat infants and children with feeding and swallowing problems, the clinician must work with an expanded team that incorporates medical professionals as well as psychologists and social workers to target all aspects of the child's care.

This chapter reviews the physiology of swallowing, as well as epidemiology, pathogenesis, and the various etiologies, clinical courses, and objective measures of diagnosis and treatment in children with feeding and swallowing disorders. In addition to discussing problems related to neurological, anatomical, and physiological conditions, this chapter addresses feeding issues that can sometimes result from common pediatric conditions.

DEFINITION

Pediatric dysphagia, which for the purposes of this chapter includes any problem with the initiation and/or execution of swallowing or feeding, encompasses a wide variety of causes that preclude a generic definition. As each condition affects swallowing and feeding differently and maybe in multiple ways, a thorough understanding of the disease in question would require a disease-specific discussion. Select conditions are reviewed later; however, there are some general guidelines employed in the clinical setting that are useful to review.

The World Health Organization (WHO) defines health as the "state of complete physical, mental, and social well being and not merely the absence of disease or infirmity."[1] For more than a century, the

WHO has depended on the *International Classification of Diseases* (ICD) to define and characterize individual disorders, but the language is medically focused and lacks a discussion of function. More recently, the International Classification of Functioning, Disability, and Health (ICF),[2] developed by WHO in 2001, has been the framework for defining diseases on a functional level, to include problems with swallowing and feeding. The ICF includes sections discussing disability, contextual factors (eg, environmental), and personal factors (eg, background, past experiences). The ICF is a complement to the ICD and allows for better understanding of how health conditions affect one's ability to interact with the environment and carry out activities of daily life.[3] The ICF's section on swallowing is represented under Body Functions entitled, "Functions of Digestive, Metabolic, and Endocrine Systems." It could be used, for example, to help clarify the ICD code 787.2 for dysphagia, which does not differentiate between children with mild problems

swallowing and those with profound dependence on feeding tubes.[3] ICF and ICD are useful means to help define pediatric dysphagia in both clinical and research settings.

ETIOLOGY

Appropriate swallowing and feeding in the newborn, infant, and young child depend on a complex system of reflexes, neurological and physiological maneuvers, and behavioral components. A disruption at any point along this pathway could ultimately lead to dysfunction. Given the complexity of the actions required, there is a large number of disorders and diseases that cause difficulty with swallowing and/or feeding, and it is beyond the scope of this chapter to discuss them all. The more common etiologies with incidences are presented in Table 9–1.

TABLE 9–1. Common Conditions Associated With Pediatric Dysphagia[a]

Neurological/Neuromuscular	Anatomic/Congenital
Cerebral palsy	Cleft of palate, lip
Bulbar palsy	Laryngomalacia
Myasthenia gravis	Subglottic stenosis
Arnold Chiari formation	Tracheoesophageal fistula
Poliomyelitis	Esophageal stricture
Muscular dystrophy	Foreign body sensation
Tardive dyskinesia	Esophageal tumor
Inflammatory	Pierre Robin syndrome
Laryngopharyngeal reflux	Tachypnea (>60 breaths/min)
Gastroesophageal reflux	Piriform aperture stenosis
Caustic injection	Choanal atresia
Infections	**Behavioral**
Epiglotitis	Depression
Esophagitis	Oral/taste aversion
Adenotonsilitis	Conditioned dysphagia
Pharyngitis	Autism spectrum disorder

Adapted and organized from [a]Arvedson (1994), Newman,[10] Rudolph.[26]

EPIDEMIOLOGY

The available data on the prevalence and incidence of swallowing and feeding problems in the pediatric population are limited. There are various reasons for this including the reporting of diseases rather than symptoms (eg, dysphagia), the lack of standardized protocols for establishing diagnoses in infants and young children, inconsistent use of terminology, and the misinterpretation of findings that may reflect multiple underlying conditions (eg, an infant with low birth weight and gastroesophageal reflux disease [GERD]).[3] Additionally, some children have feeding problems specifically (eg, cleft lip), while others may have swallowing difficulty (eg, esophageal stenosis). These issues often get combined and further confuse the data. This deficiency may change as more standardized test batteries are employed for classification.

Currently, the estimated prevalence of feeding problems ranges from 25% to 45% in the normally developing child, and 33% to 80% in those with developmental delays.[4–6] While the exact incidence of pediatric dysphagia is unknown, it is thought to be increasing as a result of increased survival of premature infants (<37 weeks), those with low birth weight (<2500 g, 5.5 lb), and those with complex medical conditions.[7,8] The percentage of infants delivered prematurely has increased by 20% since 1990, and the proportion of those born with low birth weight is the highest ever recorded in the last 50 years.[7] Over the past 20 years, children with dysphagia-associated diseases like cerebral palsy (CP) and other developmental disabilities (eg, autism spectrum disorders), have also seen a greater life expectancy, contributing to the rising rates of pediatric feeding and swallowing disorders.[9]

Numerous studies have looked at rates of dysphagia in specific pediatric conditions. Of all children examined for feeding and/or swallowing problems, 37% to 40% were born prematurely,[5,9–12] up to 64% to 78% have disorders of development,[5,10–12] and 90% have at least one medical diagnosis. Table 9–2 summarizes the major reasons why children may have difficulty with swallowing or refuse to eat. Children may have more than one reason for refusing liquids or foods, and the clinician must be alert to this when detailing the case history.

One of the most common medical diagnoses associated with feeding and swallowing problems is gastroesophageal disease (GERD).[11] Neurological conditions such as Pompe disease, Prader-Willi syndrome, and Down syndrome all have high rates of GERD with associated dysphagia, as do select cardiovascular disorders.[14,15]

CLINICAL CONSIDERATIONS

Anatomy of Swallowing and Feeding

The anatomy and physiology of swallowing has been described in Chapter 2. In the pediatric population the anatomy is under constant change resulting from the typical growth and development of the child. The act of swallowing normally relies on a highly functional sensorimotor system with coordinated reflexes integrated at the brainstem level. Newborns and infants have the added component of breathing while sucking and swallowing, further complicating an already complex process.

Unlike children and adults, infants acquire nutrition by virtue of a suck-swallow-breathe sequence.

There are several key differences between the anatomy of the adult and that of the infant. These include the size and shape of the oral cavity, the placement of the tongue, and the relative positions of the velum, hyoid bone, epiglottis, and larynx. Figure 9–1 shows the outline of the infant head and neck at birth and at approximately 2 to 3 years of age. The relative size of the oral cavity in the infant is small with respect to overall head size due to the smaller and more posteriorly placed mandible.[16] More of the tongue exists within the oral cavity, and the hard palate is flatter when compared to that of the adult. As a result, the tongue is relatively restricted in movement upward or forward.

TABLE 9–2. Common Pediatric Conditions and Associated Rate of Dysphagia

Medical Condition	Incidence of Dysphagia	Source
Head trauma/traumatic brain injury (TBI)	Average 5.3%, 68% for severe TBI, 15% for moderate TBI, 1% for mild TBI	Morgan, Ward, Murdoch, Kennedy, and Murison, 2010[45]
Hemiplegia and diplegia	25%–30%	Stallings, Charney, Davies, and Cronk, 1993[44]; Dahl, Thommessen, Rasmussen, and Selberg, 1996[42]; Reilly, Skuse, and Poblete, 1996[30]
	11.44%	Rommel, De Meyer, Feenstra, and Veereman-Wauters, 2003[11]
Neurological	44%	Field, Garland, and Williams, 2003[15]
	28% continuous drooling of saliva, 56% choked with food	Sullivan, Lambert, Rose, Ford-Adams, Johnson, and Griffiths, 2000[52]
	56%	Newman, Keckley, Petersen, and Hamner, 2001[43]
Cerebral palsy	32%	Field, Garland, and Williams, 2003[15]
	57% sucking problems	Reilly, Skuse, and Poblete, 1996[30]
	38% swallowing problems	Reilly, Skuse, and Poblete, 1996[30]
	89% needed help with feeding	Reilly, Skuse, and Poblete, 1996[30]
	27%	Waterman, Koltai, Capria Downey, and Cacace, 1991[46]
	Oral and pharyngeal abnormalities present in almost all patients	Arvedson, Roger, Buck, Smart, and Msall, 1994[53]
Spastic quadriplegia or extrapyramidal CP	50%–75%	Stallings, Charney, Davies, and Cronk, 1993[44]; Dahl, Thommessen, Rasmussen, and Selberg, 1996[42]
Gastroesophageal reflux	56%	Field, Garland, and Williams, 2003[15]
Gastrointestinal issues	14%	Field, Garland, and Williams, 2003[15]
Isolated gastrointestinal	42.45%	Rommel, De Meyer, Feenstra, and Veereman-Wauters, 2003[11]
Gastrointestinal-neurologic	6.14%	Rommel, De Meyer, Feenstra, and Veereman-Wauters, 2003[11]
Gastrointestinal-genetic	1.66%	Rommel, De Meyer, Feenstra, and Veereman-Wauters, 2003[11]
Gastrointestinal-ENT-orofacial	2.49%	Rommel, De Meyer, Feenstra, and Veereman-Wauters, 2003[11]

continues

TABLE 9–2. *(continued)*

Medical Condition	Incidence of Dysphagia	Source
Gastrointestinal-nephrologic	1.66%	Rommel, De Meyer, Feenstra, and Veereman-Wauters, 2003[11]
"Other combined medical pathologies"	18.57%	Rommel, De Meyer, Feenstra, and Veereman-Wauters, 2003[11]
Developmental delays	74%	Burklow, Phelps, Schultz, McConnell, and Rudolph, 1998[5]
	33%–80%	Linscheid, 2006[4]; Burklow, Phelps, Schultz, McConnell, and Rudolph, 1998[5]
Autism	24.4%	Field, Garland, and Williams, 2003[15]
Down syndrome	39.9%	Field, Garland, and Williams, 2003[15]
Prematurity	38%	Burklow, Phelps, Schultz, McConnell, and Rudolph, 1998[5]
	37%	Newman, Keckley, Petersen, and Hamner, 2001[10]
	40%	Hawdon, Beauregard, Slattery, and Kennedy, 2000[12]
	Prevalence and incidence estimates of feeding problems in extremely preterm infants are limited	Arvdeson, Clark, Lararus, Schooling, and Frymark, 2010[41]
Structural-neurological-behavioral	30%	Burklow, Phelps, Schultz, McConnell, and Rudolph, 1998[5]
Neurological-behavioral	27%	Burklow, Phelps, Schultz, McConnell, and Rudolph, 1998[5]
Structural-behavioral	9%	Burklow, Phelps, Schultz, McConnell, and Rudolph, 1998[5]
Structural-neurological	8%	Burklow, Phelps, Schultz, McConnell, and Rudolph, 1998[5]
Pneumonia	44%	Taniguchi and Moyer, 1994[47]
	49%	Newman, Keckley, Petersen, and Hamner, 2001[43]
Genetic	3.32%	Rommel, De Meyer, Feenstra, and Veereman-Wauters, 2003[11]
Genetic: Infantile Pompe disease	100%	Jones, Muller, Lin, et al, 2009[49]
Cardiologic	2.82%	Rommel, De Meyer, Feenstra, and Veereman-Wauters, 2003[11]
ENT-orofacial	3.32%	Rommel, De Meyer, Feenstra, and Veereman-Wauters, 2003[11]

TABLE 9–2. *(continued)*

Medical Condition	Incidence of Dysphagia	Source
Metabolic	1.66%	Rommel, De Meyer, Feenstra, and Veereman-Wauters, 2003[11]
Oncologic	2.49%	Rommel, De Meyer, Feenstra, and Veereman-Wauters, 2003[11]
Nephrologic	1.99%	Rommel, De Meyer, Feenstra, and Veereman-Wauters, 2003[11]
Cardiopulmonary	35%	Field, Garland, and Williams, 2003[15]
Anatomical anomalies	13%	Field, Garland, and Williams, 2003[15]
Post open heart surgery	18%	Kohr, Dargan, Hague, et al, 2003[48]
Apnea	23%	Newman, Keckley, Petersen, and Hamner, 2001[43]
Tube fed	21%	Newman, Keckley, Petersen, and Hamner, 2001[43]
Infants with oxygen-dependent chronic lung disease (CLD)	39.66%	Shaw, Ohlesson, Halliday, et al, 2003[51]
CHARGE syndrome	90% on tube feeding at some point in time	Dobbelsteyn, Peacocke, Blake, Crist, and Rashid, 2007[50]

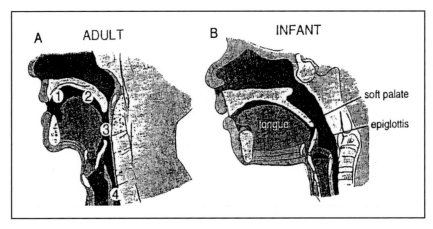

FIGURE 9–1. View showing the changes that take place in the anterior oral cavity (1), palate (2), pharynx (3), and esophagus (4) from infancy to adulthood. Reprinted with permission from Link, Willging, Miller, Cotton, and Rudolph.[21]

To overcome this anatomical condition in mobility, the newborn and infant must employ a **suckling motion** to feed. This motion requires the tongue to move anteriorly to posteriorly. As the child develops, the suckling motion becomes a **sucking motion** that incorporates a superior to inferior and side-to-side tongue motion as well. Eventually the sucking motion declines and the normal child begins to swallow. Age of normal swallow varies due to environmental conditions, parental feeding, and normal development.

A relatively small oral cavity and positions of the buccal fat pads allow the lips, cheeks, and tongue to work in close proximity to aid in suckling and sucking. Table 9–3 reviews the normal coordination of sucking, swallowing, and breathing in the infant. Normal coordination in this activity precedes normal feeding, and children who display difficulty with this movement must be evaluated for an underlying neurological cause.[17]

In the pharynx, the high position of the epiglottis appears attached to the tongue and contact is often made with the soft palate. This may cause the child to cough. The high position of the epiglottis, the lack of space for the tongue, and the overall oral cavity size become an ideal passage for liquids but not food.

There are several other important anatomical differences in the pharyngeal region as well. The epiglottis is relatively high in the infant (often appearing attached to the tongue base) and can often make contact with the soft palate during normal swallowing. On occasion this may trigger a cough reflex. The infantile larynx rests at the level of the C1-C3 vertebrae and, along with the hyoid bone, lies almost directly beneath the tongue base. This anatomical arrangement allows the tongue, soft palate, and epiglottis to approximate and separate respiration from swallowing.[17] By age 2, the larynx descends and this becomes impossible. This

movement highlights the evolutionary importance of feeding in an infant as a pause need not occur even to breathe. Furthermore, should food become blocked or slowed within the pharynx, it does not occlude the airway as it would in a child or adult with a relatively lower larynx.

These relationships are subject to change due to the constant growth of the infant. It is believed that at around 4 to 6 months of age, respiratory instability may occur due to changes in the anatomic relationships of the mandible, tongue, and palate, or due to the neuromuscular developments that increase the activity of the tongue.[18] As the hyoid bone and larynx descend and separate from the base of tongue, the coordination of swallowing becomes increasingly complex. It is generally accepted that by age 2 or 3, the respiratory and swallowing pathways are no longer functionally separate. It is at this point that aspiration becomes more possible, and can happen with poor oral control of a food bolus, poor pharyngeal coordination, or impaired vocal fold closure at the level of the glottis.

Physiology of Swallowing and Feeding

The physiology of swallowing was described in Chapter 2. The pediatric physiology is undergoing constant change along with the anatomy. In healthy children, the changes are gradual and coordinated. In a child with anatomical or neurological pathology, the changes may not occur or they may occur without coordination causing the child to choke or to assume that each swallow will be just the same as the previous one. A coordinated normal swallow is one of the most fundamental and complex pathways known. Table 9–4 summarizes the body systems involved and their associated functions.

In general, normal feeding relies on a series of inherent reflexes controlled largely within the brainstem, and calls for a great deal of physical and mental coordination, to include coordinated breathing. As the newborn becomes an infant, and the infant a child, the neuromuscular system matures with normal development to keep up with the changes to ensure continued feeding success.

Early information on the neurology of infant swallowing was hypothesized from animal studies

TABLE 9–3. Normal Coordination of Sucking, Swallowing, and Breathing in the Infant

1. A well-coordinated feeding pattern creates the maximum sucking pressure when breathing out; swallowing takes place between breaths and just before the onset of the next suck.

2. An efficient sucking pattern is characterized by each suck having a relatively low pressure and long duration.

3. When coordination breaks down, breathing is typically the limiting factor; infants become unable to maintain adequate ventilation while continuing to suck and swallow.

TABLE 9–4. Physiologic and Behavioral Systems Involved in Normal Feeding[a]

Systems	Required for
Oral motor function	Sucking, munching, chewing, and movement of the bolus; also needed for speech
Respiratory system	Maintaining normal oxygen exchange, coordinating suck and swallow, coughing to protect airways
Cardiovascular system	Maintaining normal blood pressure and oxygenation of the tissues
Pharyngeal coordination	Coordinating swallowing and breathing, safely transporting the bolus to the esophagus
Gastrointestinal system	Esophageal transporting of the bolus to the stomach and lower esophageal sphincter to avoid reflux. Gastric emptying to the duodenum and transporting throughout the bowel
Gross motor	Maintaining head in midline and upright position, sitting stability on the chair
Fine motor	Finger feeding, using a spoon, holding a cup
Expressive language	Asking for more or saying no
Nonverbal communication games	Pointing for food, opening mouth to receive food, gesturing, playing
Receptive language	Comprehension of the meaning of words "food, bottle," understanding of commands
Hypothalamus	Controlling hunger and satiety
Cognitive	Recognizing foods by color, appearance, taste, and so on; learning the associations related to feeding (ie, sound of the bottle = food is coming); learning to self-serve food
Social	Giving positive feedback to the caregiver, eye contact
Caregiver (socioeconomic)	Providing appropriate amount and type of food
Caregiver (emotional)	Funneling positive emotional support of a child during the learning process, setting rules and limits

[a]Data merged from Arvedson,[19] Wiedmeier JE, et al,[34] Rudolph and Link,[26] Stevenson and Allaire.[54]

for many years. More recently, careful investigators have looked at both healthy infants and those with neurological or anatomical disorders impairing swallowing.[9,18–23] These studies have focused on the developmental aspects of infant swallowing and further elucidated this process.

Neural control of swallowing primarily involves two areas within the medulla, the *nucleus of tractus solitarius* (NTS) and the *nucleus ambiguus* (NA). The NTS is made up of the visceral afferent fibers of cranial nerves (CN) VI, IX, and X (abducens, glossopharyngeal, and vagus), as well as those of the superior laryngeal nerve (sensory from CN X). The NTS is the first synaptic point for several inputs relaying information on taste and deglutition in addition to cardiovascular and respiratory signals. The NA leads to the brachial efferent motor fibers of CN X as well as to the efferent motor fibers of CN IX. These motor fibers terminate in various laryngeal and pharyngeal muscles, as well as the stylopharyngeus.

Integrated into this neurological pathway is a unique system of reflexes that help to protect the infant or young child from aspiration. This is largely achieved at the level of the larynx and pharynx.

> *The three reflexes responsible for both facilitating swallowing and preventing aspiration are the* laryngeal adductor reflex *(LAR), the* pharyngoglottal closure reflex *(PGCR), and the* esophagoglottal closure reflex *(EGCR).*[25]

Additional barriers to the prevention of aspiration at the laryngeal level are the contractions of the aryepiglottic folds and the posterior and inferior motion of the epiglottis during swallow. Finally, the ability to produce a strong cough is the last defense against material that has penetrated the laryngeal complex.

Aspiration may also occur from material moving in a retrograde direction. In the pediatric population, this is associated with high upper esophageal sphincter pressures that slow passage of food through the pharynx. In addition, regurgitation and vomiting are common occurrences in infants and young children due to the rapid rise of esophageal pressure during feeding and the relatively small stomach, as well as the high prevalence of GERD in these populations. This can result in a high level of acid and bile surrounding the laryngeal inlet. In response to this retrograde motion of food and gastric materials, the EGCR and PGCR have the additional critical roles of preventing aspiration from below. While these reflexes may be present in the premature infant, they seem to respond at slower rates.[26] Recently, Jarcherla et al found a relationship between normal maturation and the ability of the infant to respond to stimuli based on dose of stimuli. Thus normal reflexes adapt to neural maturation.[27]

Coordination of Apnea in Swallowing

For infants and children who have lost the functional separation of breathing and swallowing, the coordination of apnea is another critical component in the normal swallow. If not conducted properly, an ill-timed inhalation could result in a significant aspiration event. This is even more important in the infant who naturally has a faster respiratory rate. Conditions that further increase breathing rate and cause tachypnea (eg, systemic illness) greatly increase the risk of aspiration.

The amount of apnea required during the swallow depends on several factors. The age and respiratory rate of the infant or child are important. Also, swallows that are nutritive (involved with the passage of food) are shorter than those that are non-nutritive, and therefore require shorter periods of apnea. This is likely because the food bolus moves at a higher velocity than just saliva, accounting for the shorter swallowing time.[28]

CLASSIFICATION OF DYSPHAGIA

A dysfunction along any point in the complex feeding mechanisms described above can lead to difficulty with swallowing and/or feeding. Therefore, it is useful to section disorders of feeding and swallowing into several general categories. In basic terms, feeding disorders can be divided into Anatomic/Congenital, Neurological, Inflammatory, and Behavioral. These were presented in Table 9–1. Anatomic/congenital etiologies include those that cause difficulty with breathing (eg, pyriform aperture stenosis, choanal atresia, laryngomalacia), those that impair latching or sucking (eg, cleft lip/palate), and those that cause physical barriers or diversions to swallowed food (eg, esophageal stenosis, tracheoesophageal fistula, laryngeal cleft, tumors). All of these conditions will hinder the normal coordination of sucking, swallowing, and breathing.

Neurologic Causes

Neurologic causes include any condition or disorder that impairs the brain's ability to connect the brainstem with the physical structures of feeding. This includes neuromuscular diseases such as myasthenia gravis, muscular dystrophy, and tardive dyskinesia, all of which can show dysfunction of the swallowing muscles. Infants and children who have problems with the structure or function of the brainstem (eg, Arnold Chiari malformation, traumatic brain injury) may be unable to appropriately relay signals from the nucleus tractus solitarius and/or nucleus ambiguous, and could also have difficulty with swallowing reflexes. Additionally, issues with more global cerebral dysfunction may cause dysphagia as may be seen in children with cerebral palsy and autism spectrum disorders.

Inflammatory Conditions

Inflammatory conditions can affect feeding in several ways. The most common is the development of pain or swelling in the oral cavity or throat that discourages eating. Adenotonsillitis is a frequent illness in the pediatric population and is often associated with decreased oral intake. Another common inflammatory condition is GERD, which can present as vomiting in the infant, throat or chest pain in the older child, or simply insufficient weight gain. Careful consideration for the diagnosis of GERD must be kept in any child exhibiting a failure to thrive.[10] Diet modifications and timing of eating and rest often resolve the problem. In some cases, a mild antireflux medication is prescribed.

Behavioral Conditions

Behavioral conditions can also be associated with swallowing and feeding problems. Psychiatric conditions such as depression or neglect can often lead to poor oral intake. Infants who are recovering from oral or lip surgery (with the associated painful postop exams) occasionally develop an oral aversion and show reluctance to latch to a nipple or bottle. Behavioral conditions entail more of a contextual difficulty with feeding and depend on the child's ability to interact with and cope with the surrounding environment. A study of 103 children with feeding disorders found that the structural-neurological-behavioral paradigm was the most common classification of feeding disorders, underscoring the importance of treating behavioral factors to achieve normal feeding.[5]

Swallowing disorders, more specifically, can also be classified based on the point at which dysfunction occurs during the swallowing maneuver.[26] These categories are based on the phases of swallowing and include the *Pre-oral phase, Oral phase, Pharyngeal phase, Esophageal phase,* and *Gastrointestinal phase.*

> *While a typical swallow is rapid and the phases blend without discrete transition points, it is helpful to think about the process in phases. Especially relevant for the pediatric population are the pre-oral and oral phases, since they differ most drastically from adults.*

The pre-oral stage includes the child's level of alertness, the selection of the appropriate food, and the proper manner of delivering the food to the oral cavity. Children, especially those with behavioral disorders, are sensitive to environmental cues and stimuli that play a role in the pre-oral stage of eating. If not addressed carefully, adverse sensations during this stage of feeding may lead to oral aversion and/or food refusal.[19]

The oral phase consists of sucking or chewing followed by transfer of a food bolus to the oropharynx. While the sucking and chewing portions can be assessed easily, the transfer portion of this phase can only be observed when actual food is being swallowed. Children with poor oral motor function may have difficulty managing the food bolus and delivering it posteriorly, which sets up problems in the subsequent phases.

The pharyngeal phase is involuntary and begins once the bolus reaches the tonsillar pillars (oropharynx). At this point there is a pause in respiration, the larynx rises to meet the epiglottis, the vocal folds close, and the upper esophageal sphincter opens. Once the food bolus enters the esophagus, the larynx descends and the vocal folds open, allowing respiration to resume.

> *A great amount of coordination is required during this phase, and this is the time of highest risk for aspiration.*

During the esophageal phase, there are involuntary esophageal muscle contractions that create a wave-like motion to carry the bolus past the lower esophageal sphincter and into the stomach. Various disorders of the esophagus may disrupt this activity, and the contents of the bolus may be regurgitated if not passed completely into the stomach. Finally, the gastrointestinal phase involves the processing of the bolus in the stomach and delivery into the small intestine for digestion.

DIAGNOSIS

There are various reasons a child might be brought for evaluation of a problem with feeding or swallowing, and parents are usually the first to sense that something is wrong. Table 9–5 presents some common parental concerns that lead to an instrumental evaluation.

Pediatricians and general practitioners are the first line of clinicians to perform these exams and must be skilled to diagnose a wide range of conditions. Occasionally, infants and young children will be referred to a specialist including an otolaryngologist (ENT), swallow therapist, nutritionist, or speech-language pathologist.

TABLE 9–5. Indications, Signs, and Symptoms for Referring a Child for an Instrumental Swallowing Examination

Failure to thrive: remains at or recedes to a low weight
Vomiting, regurgitation
Coughing, gagging, or drooling
Voice quality changes during feeding
Known or suspected structural abnormalities
Refusal to eat
One or more episodes of pneumonia
Lack of coordination in oral structures
Positive chest x-ray (infiltrates)
Lack of or reduced sensation noted in clinical examination
Suspected structural disorders (TE fistula, vocal fold paralysis)

Some of the more common parental concerns that prompt a feeding or swallowing evaluation include one or more of the following: newly observed difficulty swallowing,[15,19] refusal to eat,[15] oral motor delays,[15] and problems with transitioning to developmentally appropriate foods and textures.[12,15,28] In some cases at presentation, the signs may be characteristic of an underlying etiology. For example, oral motor issues are common in children suffering from developmental delays, and occur in up to 80% of children diagnosed with Down syndrome,[15,29] and 90% of those diagnosed with CP.[30] Children with a disorder of the autism spectrum, however, are more likely to show discrimination of specific types and textures of foods rather than oropharyngeal dysphagia.[15,19]

Clinical Examination

The evaluation of swallowing disorders in the pediatric population begins with a thorough history. Questioning should include birth-related information including the birth-mother's general medical condition, the patient's medical history, including previous illnesses, immunizations, medications, eating and nutrition history, and especially incidents or events that occurred around the onset of the swallowing problem. Specific investigation should include the type and timing of milk feeding as well as the use of various supportive devices in case the child's muscle tone is not fully developed.[31,32] The clinician should also inquire about swallowing problems in other children in the family and how those family members were diagnosed and treated.

After a complete history, the child should undergo a clinical examination including a complete oral motor examination. The clinical examination begins by noting the child's overall awareness of the surroundings, as well as his or her social and environmental interactions. The clinician should observe general motor ability including head and trunk support, sitting posture, and the need for assistive devices for support or movement. Neck flexion especially should be identified. The ability to suck (assessed by placing a pacifier on the tongue) and the presence of breathing through the mouth and nose at rest should be noted. Special consideration should also be paid to the child's overall cooperation in the assessment. Table 9–6 is a comprehensive summary of feeding development along with motor and language skills from birth to 3 years of age.

> The goal of the clinical examination is to establish whether the child has appropriate sensory and motor developmental maturity.

Oral-Motor Examination

This specific portion of the examination includes an assessment of the structure, symmetry, tone, coordination, and function of the lips, tongue, palate, and jaw. Assessment of the uvula hanging from the soft palate should be made to rule out deviation or bifidity, which may be present in cases of submucous cleft. The tongue, hard palate, gumline, and teeth (if present) should all be evaluated to ensure they appear normal. Poor dental health is also important to recognize. Assess strength of the lips, tongue, and cheeks as well. Additionally, speaking with the child may allow for the evaluation of his or her voice, which should include assessment of voice quality, loudness, and pitch. Children with impaired vocal cord function may have hoarseness or problems with projection. These children may be at increased risk for aspiration, and therefore, feeding should be discouraged until a formal evaluation by a laryngologist or speech-language pathologist is conducted. If the child is not at risk for aspiration and has been eating previously, it may be appropriate to attempt trial feedings in the office. Special consideration should be given to the use of suitable utensils and eating posture. At this point, management of saliva and food in the mouth can be evaluated, in addition to the behavior of the child while eating.

Assessment of Early Reflexes

An important component of a thorough feeding/swallowing exam includes an evaluation of the child's developing reflexes. These are a series of reflexes that mature during early life and are critical for the establishment of a safe and successful swallow. Oral reflexes develop and adapt most rapidly in the first 12 months of life. These reflexes may be absent or diminished in preterm infants, and although readiness to feed can sometimes "catch up" to the full-term infant, delays in feeding skills are common in children born prematurely.[33,34]

Clinical examination of an infant's feeding reflexes will depend on the age of the child. For children under the age of 4 months, several primitive reflexes are important to identify. The *suck reflex* is assessed by placing a finger softly onto the palate and feeling for the pull created against the finger towards the palate. The *bite reflex* is subtle and usually observed by the up/down motion of the mandible when pressure is applied to the gum line. The suck and bite reflexes usually disappear by 6 months of age. The *rooting reflex* is another early reflex that is thought to help the infant find a food source. It is defined as an orientation toward tactile stimulation in the perioral region or visual stimulation near the face[35] and is assessed by stroking the infant's cheek and observing for head turn in that direction. This reflex is usually gone by 5 months of age. Another basic reflex is the *tongue protrusion reflex*, which is tested by placing a small amount of food or thickened liquid on the tongue. The tongue in the infant will move forward instead of back. If the tongue protrusion reflex lasts beyond 4 months, it usually indicates the child is not ready for solid foods.

The *gag reflex* is different from the reflexes previously mentioned, as it can remain present throughout life. To test for it, a small tongue blade is placed on the back of the tongue. The tongue will generally move upward and backward, and frequently cause the child to cough. On occasions, it is absent but this usually does not hinder swallowing.

The *swallow reflex* is an important indicator of appropriate laryngeal response to swallowing. It remains present throughout life and is assessed by feeling for elevation of the cricoid cartilage when the child is given food to eat. It suggests that the larynx is moving upward appropriately toward the epiglottis to decrease the chance of aspiration during the swallow.

TABLE 9–6. Normal Feeding Development for First 3 Years[a,b]

Mo.	Feeding Skills	Oral Motor Skills	Food Type	Fine Motor Skills	Gross Motor Skills	Cognitive/ Sensory Skills	Language: Expressive/ Receptive Skills	Socio-emotional Development Skills
1	Suck and swallow reflex. Starts interaction with caregivers. Pushes food out when placed on tongue. Initial swallow involves posterior part of the tongue.	Suck and swallow reflex, rooting reflex. Bite reflex.	Liquids (breastfeeding, bottle).	Palmar grasp reflex.	Holds head up.	Visual fixation and tracking.	E = Coos R = Alert to sounds	Regulation of states. Interest in the world. Can be calm. Eye contact and mutual gaze.
2		Suckling pattern. Extension and retraction movements of the tongue.			Holds chest up.		R = smiles when stroked or talked	
3	Anterior part of the tongue starts to be involved in initial swallow, facilitating the ingestion of semisolids.	Corners of mouth become active during sucking. Extends tongue in anticipation.		Unfisted grasp.		Recognition of parents.		Smile. Mother-child interaction.
4	Voluntarily grasps with both hands. Sits with support.	Transfers bolus from anterior tongue to pharynx. Rooting reflex disappears.	Pureed food. Fed by caregiver, taken passively from spoon.	Starts reaching for objects. Objects to midline.	Rolls front to back.	Anticipates feeding.	E = Laughs R = Orients to voice	Shows positive affect to caregivers. Displays negative affect. Responds with pleasure to social interactions.
5	Upright supported position for spoon-feeding. Approximates lips to rims of the cup.	Sucking pattern.		Transfers objects.	Rolls back to front, sits with support.	Stereoscopic vision. Enjoys looking around environment.	E = Razzes, blows bubbles, "Ah-goo" R = Orients to bell/keys	

Mo.	Feeding Skills	Oral Motor Skills	Food Type	Fine Motor Skills	Gross Motor Skills	Cognitive/Sensory Skills	Language: Expressive/Receptive Skills	Socio-emotional Development Skills
6	Initiation of finger feeding. Drinks from the cup.	Chewing pattern emerges. Closes lips around spoon. Biting reflex disappears.	Pureed foods and teething crackers. Cup introduced.	Unilateral reach, raking grasp.	Sits.	Visual interest in small objects. Oral exploration of objects.	E = Babbles	Referential look. Reciprocal vowel play.
7	Able to eat crackers. Starts helping spoon find mouth.	Lips begin to move while chewing.		Radial grasp.			R = Localizes bell indirectly	
8	Begins use of cup.	Lip closure achieved.			Sits/crawls.	Object permanence.	E = Dadda (not specific)	Stranger anxiety.
9	Pincer approach to food. Holds bottle.	Tongue lateralization of food bolus emerges.	Ground and mashed table foods.	3-finger grasp.	Pull to stand/cruises.		R = Understands no/gesture games.	Plays pat-a-cake, peek-a-boo. Interacts in a purposeful manner. Initiates interactions.
10	Finger feeding.						E= Mama/Dada R = Orients to bell directly	
11	Drinks from cup (mother holds it).			Mature pincer.	Walks alone.		E = first word other than mama or dada R = 1-step command with gesture	
12	Reaches for food. Plays with food (throwing food, spoon, etc). Tries to keep spoon for self.	Munching with improved lateralization. Licks food from lower lip.	Soft table foods (easily chewed).	Voluntarily release.		Help dressing. Imitates actions.	E = 2 words other than mama.	

continues

TABLE 9–6. *(continued)*

Mo.	Feeding Skills	Oral Motor Skills	Food Type	Fine Motor Skills	Gross Motor Skills	Cognitive/ Sensory Skills	Language: Expressive/ Receptive Skills	Socio-emotional Development Skills
15	Begins using cup.			Tower 2 blocks.	Runs, creeps up stairs.	Use of tolls.	E = Jargon/4–5 words R = Command no gesture	Comprehends, communicates, elaborates sequences of interactions.
18	Prefers to feed self over longer periods of time. Imitates others during feeding.	Mature chewing and drinking.		Turns pages.	Throws ball from standing.	Imitates parents in tasks.	E = Mature jargon R = Points to body parts	Imitates parents in tasks.
21	Eats with spoon, but spills. Holds glass with both hands.		Soft table foods (easily chewed).	Tower 5 blocks.	Goes up steps.	Asks for food or toilet.	2-word phrases.	
24	Correct use of spoon. Distinguishes between food and inedible materials.			Turns 1 page.	Up/down stairs alone.	Help with undressing.	E = 50 words. R = Follows 2-step commands	Pretend play (representational capacity of ideas).
30	Spear with fork.		Table food. Vegetables, meat.	Unbuttons.	Jumps.		E = Pronouns appropriately R = Concept of 1	
3 years	Straw drinking, can eat by himself or herself, can serve cup.			Copies circle.	Rides tricycle, throws ball.	Undresses completely.	E = Plurals/250 words/3-word phrase R = Concept of 12	

[a]Data merged from Arvedson,[19] Wiedmeier, et al,[34] Rudolph and Link,[26] Stevenson and Allaire.[54]

[b]V9-1 FEES: Infant No 1. Five-month-old. This is a FEES examination of a 5-month-old infant who has been treated twice for pneumonia. She was born prematurely at approximately 32 weeks' gestational age to a mother who had no prenatal care. The examination followed evaluation by a neurologist who diagnosed her with neurological deficits based on her sluggish reflexes. The FEES study shows a rapid respiration rate, penetration of the 5-mL thickened liquid, a cough that does not clear the bolus entirely, and postswallow aspiration.

Early development changes in the oral cavity and neuromuscular network help the infant learn volitional eating. By 12 months of age, the primitive reflexes have faded and the normal developing child begins to self-feed, showing voluntary control of swallowing.

Delays or difficulties with this process may indicate early neurological problems. Additionally, failure to meet the appropriate feeding milestones shown in Table 9–6 suggests further evaluation may be necessary. Performing an instrumental examination generally does this.

Instrumental Examinations

Significant information can be obtained from a thorough history and physical examination. An instrumental examination represents the next step in diagnosis available to the clinician and can aid in cases where either more specific information is required about the anatomy or physiology of a child's swallow, or if the child was not cooperative enough to perform a complete clinical examination. However, the objective measures discussed in this section also require a certain degree of patient cooperation and should not be pursued if the diagnosis can be made based on findings already obtained from the clinical exam. The available options for performing an instrumental exam consist of a radiologic or flexible endoscopic examination. Regardless of which technique is employed, the study must meet 3 important criteria prior to proceeding:

1. The examination will give additional information needed for diagnosis and formation of a treatment plan.
2. The infant or child will behave appropriately during the exam.
3. The examination team is fully competent to provide a safe testing environment for the child, including children with special needs. If all requirements are met then the instrumental examination may be arranged. Above all else, priority is placed on maintaining a safe swallow throughout the testing procedure.

Radiologic Examination

In general, static lateral neck x-rays and computed tomography (CT) scans have a limited role in the evaluation of feeding and swallowing disorders. Occasionally, a CT scan is performed if there is concern for specific anatomical abnormalities or infectious issues that might be impacting swallowing such as a retropharyngeal abscess. Effects on swallowing, however, must then be inferred as a CT scan says nothing about the dynamic nature of the child's swallow. The most specific information about the functional swallow is obtained with a modified barium swallow (MBS) study.

A team consisting of a radiologist, a fluoroscopic technician, and a speech pathologist usually conducts the MBS. It is performed in a specialized x-ray suite that contains age-appropriate equipment to help with positioning in the younger or uncooperative patient. It is often helpful to discuss the upcoming exam and show parents and the child (if applicable) photos of the exam room and machines used prior to bringing the child into the exam room. It is also helpful to withhold food for a short period before the study to encourage the child to swallow during the test. This will minimize the time required to perform the exam, as well as limit the radiation exposure to the child. Depending on the cooperation level of the child and the level of information needed for diagnosis, sufficient data can usually be obtained by fluoroscopically recording 4 or 5 specific swallows.[10] This is done from the lateral neck position and should include the time when food is placed into the mouth until the bolus is passed into the esophagus, leaving time to assess for management of residual food in the hypopharynx. Generally, a 30- to 120-second recording is sufficient. In some cases, different textures or types of foods can be used to obtain more specific information on swallowing ability. If applicable, movement of the child should be minimized as it can limit the information obtained during the test. Once adequate videos are made, a radiologist who specializes in swallow exams to assess for abnormalities reviews the videos.

Flexible Endoscopic Examination

The use of a flexible endoscope to evaluate swallowing function was first described in 1988,[36] and now the flexible endoscopic evaluation of swallowing (FEES) has become a staple in the armamentarium of clinicians who treat dysphagia. Video 9–1 is an example of a child who presented with a behavioral problem related to feeding. Note the movement in the larynx. The child was later referred to a neurologist for further diagnosis and found to have minimal brain damage related to head injury. The FEES test for this child was performed with the patient in the upright-seated position and, with the mother holding the child in her lap. Older children may not need to be held but an upright chair that prevents moving around is often helpful. If required, topical anesthesia can be sprayed into the nasal cavity with care taken to use a minimal amount, so as to avoid anesthetizing the larynx. A pediatric endoscope is then placed into the nasal cavity and guided into the nasopharynx, oropharynx, and hypopharynx under direct visualization. The examiner then visualizes the larynx and vocal folds to determine normal movement and closure. While maintaining this view and keeping the tip off the endoscope above the epiglottis, food is introduced and the swallow is observed, allowing for direct evaluation of both coordination and effectiveness.

The FEES is an ideal instrument in the evaluation of pediatric dysphagia as there is no radiation exposure and it requires only limited patient cooperation. It can also be performed in children as young as 1 month.[21] The use of familiar foods rather than radiopaque material also makes for a smoother testing experience.

In 1993, Aviv and colleagues introduced an added procedure enabling the clinician to assess the sensation of the larynx by delivering a short burst of air through a channel attached to the endoscope.[37] Combining this technique with the FEES gave birth to the flexible endoscopic evaluation of swallowing with sensory testing (FEESST). In a normal patient, when air is directed onto the supraglottic structures supplied by the superior laryngeal nerve, the laryngeal adductor reflex (LAR) is activated and the vocal cords twitch closed. This adjuvant test is useful to evaluate laryngopharyngeal sensory deficits as they relate to aspiration risks in patients who suffered a stroke or other injuries that may affect the superior laryngeal nerve. Although occasionally a child may not tolerate the slightly larger size of the scope with sensory channel, FEESST has been shown to be a safe and useful addition in evaluating pediatric dysphagia.[21]

Ultrasound Imaging

The use of ultrasound imaging has been in existence for many years.[38] This examination is used primarily to assess the oral phase of swallowing as it images the tongue and floor or the mouth. Ultrasound visualizes soft tissue by using high-frequency sound waves that reflect different shades of light depending whether it is focusing on bone, soft tissue, or fluids such as mucous. The pharynx, which is a critical area of assessment in the infant, cannot be studied easily nor simultaneously with ultrasound. If, on examination, the clinician feels that the oral cavity is a significant area of swallowing dysfunction, ultrasound is a useful imaging tool to further examine the child since it does not require x-ray. Geddes et al[39] have shown the value of ultrasound in the study of breastfeeding. They detected movement of the milk bolus through the pharyngeal area of a breastfeeding infant to show the pattern of mild flow. Ultrasound does not require the use of restraints and the duration of the study is not limited by x-ray exposure. Thus, it has a value in the study of infant feeding, especially in the study of the oral cavity and during breastfeeding.

SUMMARY

It is essential that children not be treated as small adults. Everything about their biology is unique. Normal children are constantly undergoing physical, neurological, and behavioral development that factors into every aspect of daily life. Occasionally, problems arise that hinder these processes and affect such functions as swallowing and feeding. These issues can range from congenital causes, to degenerative conditions, to behavioral problems. Depending on the underlying reason for swallowing or feeding dysfunction, children may experience difficulty transitioning through appropriate steps of development.

Beginning in infancy, children with feeding and swallowing problems should be under the care of a multidisciplinary team that focuses on all aspects of the child's health. Unlike adults, treating dysphagia in the infant or young child does not simply mean preventing aspiration. Rather, the objective is to ensure the child receives adequate nutrition for growth and development. Treatment may include a comprehensive program that aims to overcome obstacles such as low birth weight or prematurity, and improve oral-motor skills to promote self-feeding. Several formal programs have been designed to serve this purpose. They use techniques such as food selection, oral-motor exercises, and behavioral modification to improve feeding skills. If children are unable to maintain appropriate oral intake, gastrostomy tube feeding or parenteral nutrition can assist with nutrition. Regardless of the approach used, long-term care is sometimes required, and frustration is common on the part of the caretakers. The ultimate goal in treating children with a feeding or swallowing disorder is to produce safe oral feeding to maximize growth and quality of life.

DISCUSSION TOPICS

1. How would you go about discussing the need for an instrumental swallow study for a 9-month-old child who is underweight, often rejects foods and liquids and cries during feeding time? Is there also any other testing or assessment procedure that you would suggest for this child?
2. Look at Video V-1 again. What information is in this segment of the exam that would guide you to developing a treatment plan?

STUDY QUESTIONS

1. The condition that has been shown to be the primary basis for feeding disorders in newborn infants is
   A. Neurological disorders
   B. Prematurity
   C. Parental feeding skills
   D. Birth weight

2. A child born at full birth weight and at full term is likely to have
   A. Minor swallowing disorders
   B. Normal feeding and swallowing

C. Weak oral motor control for liquids
D. 25% to 30% probability of aspiration at birth

3. The true incidence of feeding and swallowing problems in premature infants
   A. Is about 25%
   B. Can be found at the Centers for Disease Control and Prevention
   C. Remains relatively unknown due to the problems of counting diseases versus symptoms
   D. Is recorded at the National Institutes of Health

4. The infant tongue is rather large compared to the oral cavity space. Therefore,
   A. The tongue motion is limited in newborn infants
   B. The tongue can move only from side to side in the newborn
   C. The proximity of the tongue to the cheeks and lips helps in suckling and sucking
   D. The tongue is less important in the infant than in the older child for swallowing purposes

5. Glottal closure reflexes in the infant are dependent upon
   A. The ability to produce a strong cough
   B. Normal sensory stimulation of a bolus
   C. Normal function of the pulmonary system
   D. All of the above

REFERENCES

1. Constitution of the World Health Organization. *Am J Public Health Nations Health.* Nov 1946;36(11):1315–1323.
2. World Health Organization. *International Classification of Functioning, Disability, and Health.* Geneva, Switzerland: Author; 2001.
3. Lefton-Greif MA, Arvedson JC. Pediatric feeding and swallowing disorders: state of health, population trends, and application of the international classification of functioning, disability, and health. *Semin Speech Lang.* Aug 2007;28(3):161–165.
4. Linscheid TR. Behavioral treatments for pediatric feeding disorders. *Behav Modif.* Jan 2006;30(1):6–23.
5. Burklow KA, Phelps AN, Schultz JR, McConnell K, Rudolph C. Classifying complex pediatric feeding disorders. *J Pediatr Gastroenterol Nutr.* Aug 1998;27(2):143–147.

6. Prasse, J. Kikano, G. An overview of pediatric dysphagia. *Clin Pediatrica*. 2009; 48: 247–251.

7. Hamilton BE, Miniño AM, Martin JA, Kochanek KD, Strobino DM, Guyer B. Annual summary of vital statistics: 2005. *Pediatrics*. Feb 2007;119(2):345–360.

8. Martin JA, Hamilton BE, Sutton PD, Ventura SJ, Menacker F, Munson ML. Births: final data for 2003. *Natl Vital Stat Rep*. Sep 2005;54(2):1–116.

9. Strauss D, Shavelle R, Reynolds R, Rosenbloom L, Day S. Survival in cerebral palsy in the last 20 years: signs of improvement? *Dev Med Child Neurol*. Feb 2007;49(2): 86–92.

10. Newman LA, Keckley C, Petersen MC, Hamner A. Swallowing function and medical diagnoses in infants suspected of dysphagia. *Pediatrics*. Dec 2001;108(6):E106.

11. Rommel N, De Meyer AM, Feenstra L, Veereman-Wauters G. The complexity of feeding problems in 700 infants and young children presenting to a tertiary care institution. *J Pediatr Gastroenterol Nutr*. Jul 2003;37(1):75–84.

12. Hawdon JM, Beauregard N, Slattery J, Kennedy G. Identification of neonates at risk of developing feeding problems in infancy. *Dev Med Child Neurol*. Apr 2000;42(4): 235–239.

13. Burklow KA, McGrath AM, Valerius KS, Rudolph C. Relationship between feeding difficulties, medical complexity, and gestational age. *Nutr Clin Pract*. Dec 2002;17(6): 373–378.

14. Jones HN, Muller CW, Lin M, et al. Oropharyngeal dysphagia in infants and children with infantile Pompe disease. *Dysphagia*. Dec 2010;25(4):277–283.

15. Field D, Garland M, Williams K. Correlates of specific childhood feeding problems. *J Paediatr Child Health*. 2003 May-Jun 2003;39(4):299–304.

16. Crelin E. *Functional Anatomy of the Newborn*. New Haven, CT: Yale University Press; 1973.

17. van der Meer A. Coordination of sucking, swallowing and breathing in healthy newborns. *J Ped Neonatal*. 2005;2: 69–72.

18. Laitman JT, Reidenberg JS. Specializations of the human upper respiratory and upper digestive systems as seen through comparative and developmental anatomy. *Dysphagia*. 1993;8(4):318–325.

19. Arvedson J. Assessment of pediatric dysphagia and feeding disorders: clinical and instrumental approaches. *Dev Disabil Res Rev*. 2008;14(2):118–127.

20. Laitman J. The evolution of the human larynx: nature's great experiment. In: Fried MP, Ferlito A, eds. *The Larynx*, 3rd ed. San Diego, CA: Plural; 2009:19–38.

21. Link DT, Willging JP, Miller CK, Cotton RT, Rudolph CD. Pediatric FEESST: fiberoptic endoscopic evaluation of swallowing with sensory testing. *Curr Gastroenterol Rep*. Jun 2005;7(3):240–243.

22. Heuschkel RB, Fletcher K, Hill A, Buonomo C, Bousvaros A, Nurko S. Isolated neonatal swallowing dysfunction: a case series and review of the literature. *Dig Dis Sci*. Jan 2003;48(1):30–35.

23. Jadcherla S. Characteristics of upper esophageal sphincter and esophageal body during maturation in healthy human neonates compared with adults. *Neurogastroenterol Motil*. 2005;17(5):663–670.

24. Jadcherla S, Gupta A, Coley BD, Fernandez S, Shaker R. Esophago-glottal closure reflex in human infants: a novel reflex elicited with concurrent manometry and ultrasonography. *Am J Gastroenterol*. 2007;102(10):2286–2293.

25. Jadcherla SR, Hogan WJ, Shaker R. Physiology and pathophysiology of glottic reflexes and pulmonary aspiration: from neonates to adults. *Semin Respir Crit Care Med*. Oct 2010;31(5):554–560.

26. Rudolph CD, Link DT. Feeding disorders in infants and children. *Pediatr Clin North Am*. Feb 2002;49(1):97–112, vi.

27. Jadcherla SR, Shubert TR, Golat IK, Jensen PS, Wei L, Shaker R. Upper and lower esophageal spincter kinetics are modified during maturation: effects of pharyngeal stimulusin premature infants. *Pediatr Res*. 2015; Jan. 77(1–1):99–106.

28. Kelly BN, Huckabee ML, Jones RD, Frampton CM. Nutritive and non-nutritive swallowing apnea duration in term infants: implications for neural control mechanisms. *Respir Physiol Neurobiol*. Dec 2006;154(3):372–378.

29. Schwarz SM, Corredor J, Fisher-Medina J, Cohen J, Rabinowitz S. Diagnosis and treatment of feeding disorders in children with developmental disabilities. *Pediatrics*. Sep 2001;108(3):671–676.

30. Reilly S, Skuse D, Poblete X. Prevalence of feeding problems and oral motor dysfunction in children with cerebral palsy: a community survey. *J Pediatr*. Dec 1996;129(6): 877–882.

31. Schanler RJ. Outcomes of human milk-fed premature infants. *Semin Perinatol*. Feb 2011;35(1):29–33.

32. Hwang YS, Lin CH, Coster WJ, Bigsby R, Vergara E. Effectiveness of cheek and jaw support to improve feeding performance of preterm infants. *Am J Occup Ther*. 2010 Nov–Dec 2010;64(6):886–894.

33. Shädler G, Süss-Burghart H, Toschke AM, von Voss H, von Kries R. Feeding disorders in ex-prematures: causes-response to therapy-long term outcomes. *Eur J Pediatr*. 2007;166(8):803–808.

34. Wiedmeier JE, Joss-Moore LA, Lane RH, Neu J. Early postnatal nutrition and programming of the preterm neonate. *Nutr Rev*. Feb 2011;69(2):76–82.

35. de Bildt A, Mulder EJ, Van Lang ND, et al. The visual rooting reflex in individuals with autism spectrum disorders and co-occurring intellectual disability. *Autism Res*. 2012;5(1):67–72 [Epub 2011 Sep 21].

36. Langmore SE, Schatz K, Olsen N. Fiberoptic endoscopic examination of swallowing safety: a new procedure. *Dysphagia*. 1988;2(4):216–219.

37. Aviv JE, Martin JH, Keen MS, Debell M, Blitzer A. Air pulse quantification of supraglottic and pharyngeal sensation: a new technique. *Ann Otol Rhinol Laryngol*. Oct 1993;102(10):777–780.

38. Shawker TH, Sonies BC, Stone M, Baum BJ. Real-time ultrasound visualization of tongue movement during swallowing. *J Clin Ultrasound.* 1983;11:485–490.

39. Geddes DT, Chadwick LM, Kent JC, Garbin CP, Hartmann PE. Ultrasound imaging of infant swallowing during breast-feeding. *Dysphagia.* 2010;Sep 25(3):183–191.

40. Burklow KA, Phelps AN, Schultz JR, McConnell K, Rudolph C. Classifying complex pediatric feeding disorders. *J Pediatr Gastroenterol Nutr.* 1998;27(2):143–147.

41. Arvedson J, Clark H, Lazerus C, Schooling T, Frymark T. Evidence-based systematic review: effects or oral motor interventions on feeding and swallowing in preterm infants. *Am J Speech Lang Path.* 2010;19(4):321–340.

42. Dahl M, Thommessen M, Rasmussen M, Seiberg T. Feeding and nutritional characteristics in children with moderate or severe cerebral palsy. *Acta Paediatr.* 1996;85:697–701.

43. Newman LA, Keckley C, Petersen MC, Hammer A. Swallowing function and medical diagnoses in infants suspected of dysphagia. *Pediatrics.* 2001;108, e106.

44. Stallings VA, Charney EB, Davies JC, Cronk CE. Nutritional status and growth of children with diplegic or hemiplegic cerebral palsy. *Dev Med Child Neurol.* 1993;35(11):997–1006.

45. Morgan AT, Mageandran SD, Mei C. Incidence and clinical presentation of dysarthria and dysphagia in the acute setting following paediatric traumatic brain injury. *Child Care Health Dev.* 2010 Jan;36 (1):44–45.

46. Waterman ET, Koltai PJ, Downey JC, Cacace AT. Swallowing disorders in a population of children with cerebral palsy. *Int J Pediatr Otorhinolaryngol.* 1992 Jul;24(1):63–71.

47. Taniguchi MH, Moyer RS. Assessment of risk factors for pneumonia in dysphagic children: significance of videofluoroscopic swallowing evaluation. *Dev Med Child Neurol.* 1994 Jun;36(6):495–502.

48. Kohr LM, Dargan M, Hague A, et al. The incidence of dysphagia in pediatric patients after open heart procedures with transesophageal echocardiography. *Ann Thorac Surg.* 2003 Nov;76(5):1450–1456.

49. Jones HN, Muller CW, Lin M, et al. Oropharyngeal dysphagia in infants and children with infantile Pompe disease. *Dysphagia.* 2010 Dec;25(4):277–283.

50. Dobbelsteyn C, Peacocke SD, Blake K, Crist W, Rashid M. Feeding difficulties in children with CHARGE syndrome: prevalence, risk factors, and prognosis. *Dysphagia.* 2008 Jun;23(2):127–135. Epub 2007 Nov 20.PMID:18027028.

51. Shah SS, Ohlsson A, Halliday H, Shah VS. Inhaled versus systemic corticosteroids for the treatment of chronic lung disease in ventilated very low birth weight preterm infants. *Cochrane Database Syst. Rev.* 2003; (2): CD002057. Update in: Cochrane Database Syst Rev. 2007; (4):CD002057. PMID:12804423.

52. Sullivan PB, Lambert B, Rose M, Ford-Adams M, Johnson A, Griffiths P. Prevalence and severity of feeding and nutritional problems in children with neurological impairment: Oxford Feeding Study. *Dev Med Child Neurol.* 2000 Oct;42(10):674–80.

53. Arvedson J, Rogers B, Buck G, Smart P, Msall M. Silent aspiration prominent in children with dysphagia. *Int J Pediatr Otorhinolaryngol.* 1994 Jan;28(2-3):173–81.

54. Stevenson RD, Allaire JH. The development of eating skills in infants and young children. In: Sullivan PB, Rosenbloom L, eds. *Feeding the Disabled Child.* London, UK: MacKeith Press; 1996:11–22.

Chapter 10

Treatment of Feeding and Swallowing Disorders in Infants and Children

A Look at the Chapter

In this chapter, we explore the feeding and swallowing treatment options for infants and children. Although swallowing safely is the underlying concern for all children, there are specific issues regarding feeding that must be taken into account. Children with birth disorders, genetic disorders, and developmental disorders require special attention in order to facilitate proper growth and nutrition needs. Various neonate and child syndromes and disorders will be presented with the focus on specific needs related to swallowing and feeding.

INTRODUCTION

In the adult patient with dysphagia, the majority of treatments are directed to safe swallowing. In the child, feeding and swallowing are two aspects that must be addressed in treatment. It is not uncommon for an infant to have feeding problems without swallowing problems, or vice versa. In this chapter, the principles and guidelines for feeding and swallowing will be reviewed with attention to individual groups of patients most commonly seen by the swallowing team.

Prior to treatment and following formal assessment, clinicians may want to use various assessment tools to determine the infant or child's level of readiness for treatment. Two tools that are appropriate for this are the Schedule for Oral-Motor Assessment (SOMA)[1] and the Dysphagia Disorder Survey.[2] Both tools are standardized for evaluating specific swallowing abilities in young children. The SOMA was developed for obtaining objective ratings of oral-motor skills in preverbal children in order to identify oral motor function. No special equipment is needed, and it can be done without a trained observer. Oral-motor function is assessed across a range of liquids and foods. The Dysphagia Disorder Survey is an observation tool that has been found to identify swallowing and feeding pathology from functionally competent swallowing behavior. It can

be used with adults and children who have developmental feeding disorders. Experienced clinicians may simply opt for informal treatment readiness assessment using their own developed checklists and trial swallow procedures.

Feeding disorders may be grouped into stages or phases related to function. Rudolph and Link[3] categorized these feeding phases in the following way:

Pre Oral Phase

Oral Phase

Pharyngeal Phase

Esophageal Phase

Gastroesophageal phase

Except for the pre-oral phase, these phases of swallowing are reviewed in detail in Chapter 2, and the caveats related to thinking of these as discrete phases have also been discussed. However, the phases as they relate to infants and children, especially the pre-oral and oral phases deserve additional consideration since they are relatively different in infants and children compared to adults.

Pre-oral Phase

The pre-oral phase involves the child's alertness, the selection of the appropriate food, and the proper manner of introducing the food into the oral cavity. Children are sensitive to various aspects of their environment, their food selection, and state of wakefulness/sleep. Thus, since the child may not be able to communicate this information to the caregiver, feeding success may fluctuate unrelated to the underlying cause dysphagia. Lack of proper behavior during feeding may be related to the taste and smell of the food/liquid, not only to the feeding/swallowing disorder itself.

Oral Phase

The oral phase of feeding consists of sucking or chewing and transfer. In the normal infant, sucking and mouthing motion may be normal, but it is not until some type of bolus is presented that the transfer aspect of this phase can be observed.

Children with poor oral motor function may have difficulty in each part of this phase with the result being poorly controlled management of the bolus after the transfer.

Pharyngeal Phase

In the pharyngeal phase, respiration temporarily ceases, the larynx elevates, the vocal folds close and the upper esophageal sphincter opens. This phase of swallowing is involuntary and in the normal child is triggered by the bolus in contact with the tonsillar pillars. Once the bolus clears the upper esophagus, respiration resumes. Since this phase is involuntary, coordination with the oral phase is important to prevent aspiration.

Esophageal Phase

The esophageal phase consists of esophageal transit and lower esophageal sphincter relaxation and opening. The upper esophageal sphincter relaxes in anticipation of the bolus reaching the esophagus. The lower esophagus relaxes to allow the bolus to enter the stomach. Various disorders of the esophagus may disrupt this activity, and the contents of the bolus may be regurgitated if not allowed into the stomach. The gastrointestinal phase involves the delivery of the bolus to the stomach and moving it to the small intestine for digestion.

Arvedson[4] stressed the importance of each stage of feeding noting that the preparatory feeding and oral stages, when not addressed carefully, may lead to refusal to eat due to the adverse sensations that may be developed in the presence of foods or liquids. Burklow et al[5] noted that in addition to the structural-medical-neurological status of the child, a behavioral component is often present that increases the complexity of management. In their evaluation of 103 children, the structural-neurological-behavioral paradigm was found to be

the most common classification of children with feeding problems. They concluded that complex feeding problems must be addressed as biobehavioral feeding disorders in order to achieve normal feeding.

FEEDING AND SWALLOWING BEHAVIORS

Feeding behavior is learned from the time the child begins the suck-swallow response. The complex interaction of the oral, pharyngeal, laryngeal, pulmonary, and gastrointestinal systems along with the awareness of the caregiver helps to ensure that normal feeding progresses as the child increases his or her demand for more and varied foods. Table 10–1 derived from various studies shows the major medical and behavioral conditions that may disrupt the

TABLE 10–1. Medical and Behavioral Problems That May Disrupt Normal Feeding

Neuromuscular/ Neurological	Anatomical/Congenital
Cerebral palsy	Cleft lip or palate
Bulbar palsy	Laryngomalacia
Myasthenia gravis	Subglottic stenosis
Arnold-Chiari malformation	Esophageal disorders
Poliomyelitis	Foreign body sensation
Down syndrome	Pierre Robin
Muscular dystrophy	
Inflammatory	**Behavioral**
Laryngopharyngeal reflux	Autism spectrum disorder
Gastroesophageal reflux	Depression
Caustic injection	
Adenotonsillitis	
Esophagitis	
Oncologic	**Trauma**
Various childhood cancers	Injury to head, neck, or torso
Radiation therapy sequelae	Burn

development and progression of normal feeding.[6–8] While it is generally accepted that a normal full-term-birth healthy infant will begin feeding and swallowing naturally, it is also possible that a preterm infant will also feed and swallow without any special needs.

When the child is immature, the feeding ability may be difficult and cause physiological distress, exhibited in many ways such as heart rate variations (**bradycardia)**, changes in respiratory patterns (**apnea)**, nasal flaring, or **hypoxemia**. Behavioral reactions to adverse feeding effects include fatigue, agitation, and disorganization. Oral motor intervention with **nonnutritive sucking** (NNS) is one way to improve the motor function for swallowing. Arvedson et al reviewed the evidence of the effects of oral motor interventions in preterm infants.[4]

Arvedson et al[4] found that NNS was consistently associated with significant positive changes on measures of swallowing physiology and reduced the number of days to reach total oral feeding in preterm infants. Oral stimulation alone was not found to have significant positive effects.

The importance of the initial feedings, whether by breast or bottle, set the pattern for future feeding development. Van der Meer et al[9] studied the coordination of sucking, swallowing, and breathing in healthy newborns, and they concluded that normal sucking precedes normal feeding. When there is no normal sucking pattern, a neurological reason must be identified. Table 10–2 summarizes their data related to coordination of sucking, swallowing, and breathing in newborns.

Even in the child born with structural or neurological problems, feeding and the development of normal feeding may progress without significant swallowing disorders, but the length of time at each stage of development may exceed the normal durations as described in Chapter 9.

The conditions that can affect the normal transition from sucking to swallowing to normal feeding may be grouped under the broad categories as shown in Table 10–3. Developmental delay can

TABLE 10–2. A Review of a Normal Coordinate Feeding Pattern Developed From the Onset of Sucking

1. A well-coordinated feeding pattern is characterized by coordination of sucking, swallowing, and breathing, where maximum sucking pressure is coordinated with breathing out, and swallowing takes place just before the onset of the next suck and between breathing out and breathing in.

2. An efficient sucking pattern is characterized by a relatively lower sucking pressure and longer duration of each suck.

3. When the coordination breaks down, breathing is typically the bottleneck, with infants being unable to maintain adequate ventilation while sucking and swallowing during nutritive feeding.

TABLE 10–3. Conditions That Can Affect the Transition to Normal Feeding and Swallowing in Infants

Condition
Developmental delay
Neurogenic diseases/disorders
Autism Spectrum Disorder
Oral-mechanical dysfunction

come from a number of conditions related to mental retardation. Children born with genetic syndromes may experience delay or inability to feed and progress to normal self-feeding depending on the syndrome and the accompanying issues.

For example, a child with **Prader-Willi syndrome** (mental retardation and hypotonia) may reach normal status in his or her self-feeding but at a slower rate than a normal child. Conversely, a child born with **Down syndrome (trisomy 21)** may continue to experience feeding and swallowing problems into adulthood. Many of these children have physical and mental limitations that require the child and the caregiver to pay close attention to their swallowing and eating behaviors long after childhood due to their limitations in motor control. Moreover, these children may have multiple problems that require a coordinated team to be involved in their long-term management.[10] Nonetheless, they can live independent and productive lives well into adulthood, but their swallowing problems may limit their ability to eat a regular diet in a normal time frame.

Mental retardation is a global health condition commonly associated with swallowing disorders. Table 10–4 modified from Right Diagnostics.com[11] lists common conditions that contribute to swallowing disorders when mental retardation is part or all of the diagnosis. Although each of these may involve a specific mode of treatment, the clinician should remember that 3 factors are important in the management of all infants and children with an underlying diagnosis of mental retardation. These are as follows:

1. Feeding and eating must be controlled based on the case history and clinical examination to avoid excessive rates of feeding/swallowing. Inappropriate foods may lead to choking or aspiration. The need for environmental adaptation to maximize feeding without distraction must be considered.

2. The clinician may need to structure the feeding schedule around the medication schedule to maximize alertness of the child.

3. Children with some aspect of mental retardation may experience aberrant behavior in certain conditions. They may be averse to eating due to discomfort associated with gastroesophageal reflux, poor bowel movement, or other conditions, even fatigue.

The caregiver must be aware that feeding and eating behaviors may vary from time to time based on these conditions.

TREATMENT OF SPECIFIC DISORDERS

Cerebral Palsy

Children with cerebral palsy (CP) may have spastic, ataxic, or hypotonic neuromuscular conditions, and the problem may be focused to one side (hemiplegia) or both. Children with CP have a variety of oral motor problems including abnormal bite, poor lip closure, weak sucking ability, and poor coordination of sucking with tongue movement. Sucking and swallowing problems are common in the first 12 months of life for the child with CP due primarily to oral motor dysfunction.[12] Drooling is one of the most common problems that children with CP have into later life. The clinician must be aware of how to place food in the child's mouth to limit the drooling. Special spoons, along with the proper size of bolus, will help in reducing the drooling (Figure 10–1).

The need for oral motor development in these children has been emphasized in programs that involve occupational therapists, physical therapists, and speech-language pathologists.[13] Eating and swallowing problems may extend into the teenage years. Dahl et al reported that at least 60% of CP children at 8 years of age remain undernourished and at nutritional risk.[14] Stallings et al report that approximately 30% of children with CP remain

Table 10–4. Causes of Swallowing Problems Related to Mental Retardation[a]

1. Epilepsy
2. Chromosome abnormalities
3. Diabetes insipidus, diabetes mellitus
4. Epileptic encephalopathy, early infantile
5. Infantile Gaucher disease
6. Hypertelorism with esophageal abnormality and hypospadias
7. Lead poisoning
8. Macrogyria, pseudobulbar palsy
9. Microcephaly
10. Various syndromes
11. Microcephaly
12. Myopathy
13. Niemann-Pick disease
14. Skeletal dysplasia associated with mental retardation
15. Tay-Sachs disease

[a]Modified from RightDiagnosis.com, September 7, 2011.

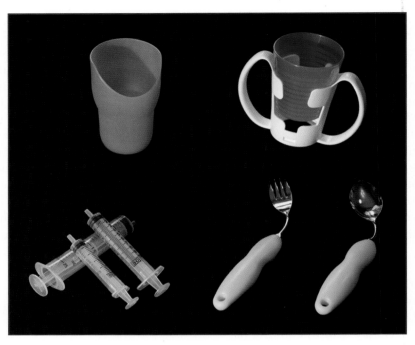

FIGURE 10–1. Spoon, fork, syringes, and cups used to aid in oral feeding problems.

undernourished and with stunted growth even into their late teenage years.[15]

Treatment of the child with CP focuses on the individual needs of the child identified in the clinical and instrumental assessments. These children may require extensive oral motor exercises, dietary modification, sensory stimulation with thermal or sour stimuli, brushing or stroking the oral structures to improve lip closure, and bolus movement in the oral cavity.

Down Syndrome

Down syndrome is a genetic disorder that causes mental retardation and physical defects. It is caused by the presence of an extra copy of chromosome number 21. This condition is called trisomy 21. Most children with Down syndrome have a large tongue with tongue protrusion and a small mouth that predisposes them to feeding and swallowing problems. One of the most common problems for infants with Down syndrome who are learning to feed is their low muscle tone (**hypotonia**). In addition, these children are predisposed to cardiac, respiratory,

and gastrointestinal problems. Furthermore, it is estimated up to 10% of children with Down syndrome also have celiac disease that usually requires a special diet.[10]

Swallowing behaviors seen in the child with Down syndrome include

Difficulty sucking or latching on

Taking longer than 30 minutes to feed a required amount of breast milk or formula

Spitting out everything you try to spoon feed

Not eating anything but baby food or refusing different textures beyond the appropriate age.

Coughing frequently on thin liquids

The treatments for dysphagia in the child with Down syndrome are oral motor exercises stimulation and, diet modification—maintaining thickened foods and liquids to reduce aspiration, and for the very young children, arrangement of positional feeding postures such as shown in Figure 10–2.

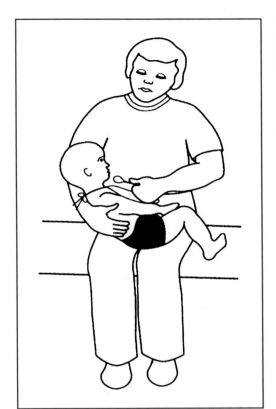
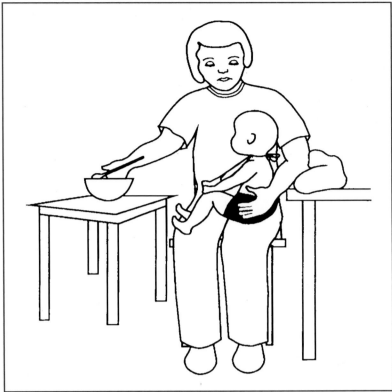

FIGURE 10–2. Feeding postures to reduce aspiration and gastroesophageal reflux.

Pierre Robin Sequence

Pierre Robin sequence (PRS) is a craniofacial anomaly that exists as an isolated condition characterized by cleft palate, micro/retrognathia, and **glossoptosis,** the latter of which is responsible for pharyngeal obstruction. Children with PRS are at high risk for respiratory insufficiency and prolonged hypoxia that, if left unrecognized, lead to impaired mental status. PRS may be part of other syndromes such as **velo-cardio facial** syndrome, **Treacher Collins** syndrome, and **Beckwith-Wiedemann** syndrome. Because of the anomalies in the nasal, oral, and pharyngeal cavities, the danger of airway obstruction is high in these children and should be diagnosed and treated with urgency. Dysphagia treatment in these children involves positioning the child to maintain a forward tongue, modifying the diet to prevent aspiration, and strengthening the velopharyngeal closure with tongue strength exercises. Surgical

procedures are often implemented to reduce the backflow of liquids into the nasopharynx.

Feeding the young child with PRS may involve having him or her lie on his side for oral feeding. Also, children may require supportive nasogastric feeding at early ages.[16] Eventually, when the issue of airway safety is no longer a problem, these children become self-feeders and learn to eat a regular diet.

Autism Spectrum Disorder

Autism spectrum disorder is a collision between behavioral patterns and feeding difficulties. For many children with autism, choking and aspiration of food or liquids are not the primary problems. Social and cognitive issues coupled with oral motor and gastroesophageal disorders often form a greater challenge to the swallowing rehabilitation team. To separate these four aspects of the autistic child's presentation is difficult since they interact with each other in feeding and swallowing as in other behaviors.

Treatment focuses on structuring the feeding and swallowing activities through a focused schedule. Treatment focus can be accomplished with the following:

Removing distractions from the feeding area

Limiting the utensils to those that are needed

Presenting food based on previous food selectivity choices

Using feeding "breaks" in the meal to prevent "shoveling, gulping, and stuffing"

Selecting proper feeding times based on other behavioral patterns of sleep and wakefulness

The use of charts and pictures to aid in the development of eating habits may also be helpful. Such charts and pictures can be found at the following two websites: **TEACCH:** Treatment and Education of Autistic and Related Communication Handicapped Children (http://www.teacch.com) and **PECS:** Picture Exchange Communication System (http://www.pecs-usa.com). The clinician should keep in mind that the child with autism spectrum disorder may present with multiple behaviors prior to feeding as well as during the mealtime. Recordkeeping by the caregiver/parent may offer indications as to when the child is ready to eat. In addition, a sequence of pre-eating activities may ultimately be developed to "usher in" the mealtime.

Fetal Alcohol Syndrome

Fetal alcohol syndrome (FAS) results when the pregnant mother uses alcohol during pregnancy. During pregnancy, alcohol poses extra risks to the fetus, especially during the first 3 months of pregnancy. When a pregnant woman drinks alcohol, it easily passes across the placenta to the fetus. Because of this, drinking alcohol can harm the baby's neurological and structural development.

Currently, there is no safe level of alcohol use during pregnancy.

The child born with FAS generally has multiple physical and mental anomalies, many of which are seen in the head and neck. In addition, the cardiovascular and nervous systems are at risk since alcohol reduces the oxygen that passes through the placenta to the developing child. A baby with fetal alcohol syndrome can be expected to have poor growth while in the womb and after birth; decreased muscle tone and poor coordination resulting in sucking difficulty and tongue manipulation; and delayed development in cognitive skills, oral motor control, speech, and movement. Structural deficits include narrow eyes, small head, small maxilla, and poor lip development.

The child at birth may be of low birth weight, have difficulty sucking, fatigue easily, and may need supportive nutrition through nasogastric feeding. The FAS child may progress to a completely oral diet, but this may take more than 1 year to accomplish. Moreover, the mental status of the child may limit his or her ability to learn feeding skills long after birth.

Rett Syndrome

Rett syndrome is a neurodevelopmental disorder that affects females almost exclusively. It is characterized by normal early growth and development followed by a slowing of development, loss of purposeful use of the hands, distinctive hand movements, slowed brain and head growth, problems with walking, seizures, and intellectual disability. Dr. Andreas Rett, an Austrian physician who first described it in a journal article in 1966, identified the disorder. It was not until after a second article about the disorder, published in 1983 by Swedish researcher Dr. Bengt Hagberg, as reported by Neul et al[17] that the disorder was generally recognized. Apraxia is perhaps the most severely disabling feature of Rett syndrome, interfering with every body movement, including swallowing, eye gaze, and speech.

Management of Rett syndrome is multidisciplinary in order to maximize the child's development. Because this disorder is progressive in nature, it may not be diagnosed at birth but requires clinical diagnosis with features similar to autism. Immature chewing patterns, weakness, and lack of control in the oral phase of swallowing and poor hand control causing self-feeding problems are present in Rett syndrome children.[18] Despite these issues, many of these children have voracious appetites, yet they have poor weight gain and poor nutrition. Many require antireflux medications as well as seizure medications.

Failure to Thrive

Normal infant growth and development tend to follow milestones, and pediatricians track these changes in newborns, infants, and children. However, in some cases, children do not reach the growth milestones. The milestones with regard to feeding were reviewed earlier in Chapter 9. It is safe to say that children with disorders such as Pierre Robin and Prader-Willi syndrome may be at risk for failure to thrive. In addition, children born prematurely or at low birth weight may also be at risk. Various syndromes as discussed above, have an acquired disease or disorder from the mother. In these children, the importance of an interdisciplinary team is critical to managing the infant.

Although neonatal and infant health care is generally very good in the United States, there are some countries where access to health care is limited, where mothers are not willing to report a child's failure to thrive, or where financial burdens limit care. In the United States, failure to thrive is generally related to the lack of prenatal care, unhealthy conditions in the mother, and environmental limitations.

Once the SLP knows the diagnosis, his or her role is to identify exercises for sucking, oral motor stimulation as discussed below, and trial feeding with various consistencies to maintain weight and continue to develop. At appropriate age levels, the SLP offers assessment of neural development, tracking of developmental milestones, and regular testing of oral motor abilities for growth. These results must be regularly reported to the pediatrician in charge.

OPTIONS AND CONSIDERATIONS IN TREATMENT OF FEEDING DISORDERS IN INFANTS AND CHILDREN

After careful assessments of the infant, the clinical team should be ready to manage the conditions they observed and documented. Children may refuse to eat for many reasons including behavioral problems not readily identified during the case history and objective assessments but only during the feeding activity. Therefore, the clinician and the caregiver must be acutely aware of behavioral changes that do not correlate with the findings during the assessment.

Oral Motor Interventions

Since feeding efficiency in the infant involves the strength and maintenance of sucking during the meal, the importance of oral motor strength and coordination are of prime importance in infant feeding.[4] Without the coordination of the suck-swallow-breathe sequence, aspiration, poor nutrition and failure to thrive will occur. Thus, the focus on oral motor strength and coordination begins in the neonatal care or intensive care unit following birth. Nonnutritive sucking and various forms of oral stimulation (brushing, thermal stimulation, and isometric stimulation) have become common as part of the treatment team's strategies. Special chairs such as those shown in Figure 10–3 may be useful in many situations.

Although outcomes assessment of oral motor strategies may be limited due to the clinical nature of the treatment and the number of people who may be involved in the treatments, clinical observation suggests that oral motor intervention is essential in treating the developing infant with feeding difficulties. Nonnutritive sucking (discussed below) appears to improve digestion of enteric feeding, may reduce the length of stay in the hospital and may help to

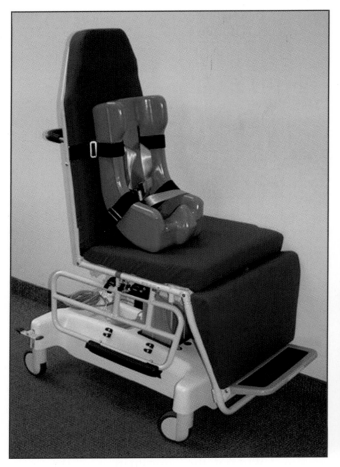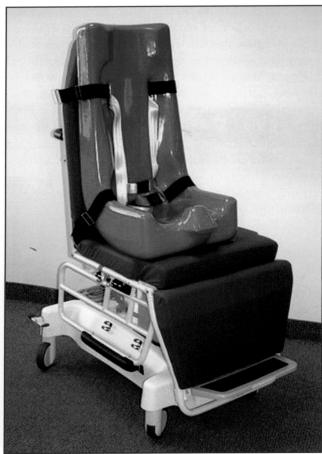

FIGURE 10–3. Special chairs used in feeding children with motor control difficulties.

establish maturity in the sucking pattern.[19,20] While the majority of studies of oral motor intervention have been done with preterm infants, these same strategies can be used with full-term infants when the clinician suspects short feeding times, refusal to eat, or other behaviors that cause the child to stop eating.

Oral motor interventions consist of techniques to create alertness and awareness of the need to swallow. These techniques consist of various types of brushing of the lips, tongue, or palate, ice placed on various oral structures, pressure massage, stimulation of the stretch reflexes by tapping with a pointed instrument and stimulation with a vibrator. The value of these will depend on the individual to produce a response (eg, the tongue should respond to a quick tap with a pointed instrument). A com-

plete program of oral motor intervention can be found at http://www.beckmanoralmotor.com. This program is applicable to the entire team working with preterm infants.

Nonnutritive Sucking (NNS)

Nonnutritive sucking, as its term implies, consists of having the infant suck on a pacifier, his or her thumb, and in some cases the mother's breast when not feeding. The goals of nonnutritive sucking are to improve the strength and coordination of sucking in the infant who is on gavage feeding or on a feeding tube and to help calm the infant. Sucking during gavage feeding is thought to further the development of the sucking reflex, stimulate sucking behavior in children who are lethargic in feeding, and improve digestion of the feeding. Others have found that NNS helps to calm infants who are hyperactive during the gavages feeding times. A study by Pinelli and Symington found evidence that hospital costs lowered, children were less defensive at eating, and transition to bottle feeding was improved in children who were subjected to nonnutritive sucking activities.[21] A recent study by Asadollahpour et al suggests that nonnutritive sucking prior to feeding was effective on oral feeding skills and weight gaining of the immature newborns. A NNS program was more effective than prefeeding oral stimulation on weight gain as well.[22]

NONORAL FEEDING

Nonoral feeding occurs in preterm infants who are too weak to suck; in infants born preterm, immature, or those with neurological disorders, syndromes, respiratory difficulties, and cardiac conditions; and/or with structural disorder such a cleft palate. Discharge from the neonatal intensive care unit (NICU) is often associated with ongoing feeding difficulties, resulting in increased financial costs and inability of the normal caregiver to be involved in daily care of the infant.

In infants requiring nonoral feeding, it is necessary to feed them through a nasogastric tube (NG) or oral gastric tube (OG). In cases where there are no structural problems in the oral cavity or oronasal cavity, the predominant feeding is via NG tube. However, there are no clear clinical guidelines currently in place to determine the route of feeding tubes in NICUs.[23] Physician preference or history of the institution appears to be the primary basis for selecting the route of feeding. Currently, many children who are born without the ability to obtain nourishment via the oral route will survive, and the need to manage the nonoral to oral transition becomes a major issue for nurses and other caregivers.

Oral feeding in the neonatal period requires precise coordination between sucking, swallowing, and breathing. Preterm infants and infants with various birth defects often have difficulty in establishing this key coordinative relationship. Hence, they are tube fed and remain hospitalized often in the NICU until they are able to safely meet their nutritional requirements orally. Issues related to cardiopulmonary stability must also be managed before the child is safely discharged.

Oral and tactile kinesthetic stimulation is often used to aid the preterm or otherwise compromised infant to improve the infant's suck-swallow-breathe pattern.[24] Gentle massaging of the oral structures, gums, and tongue along with nonnutritive sucking is often used and has been shown to be highly useful in many children, especially preterm children. Tactile stimulation to the head, neck, and arms may further improve the ability to move to oral feeding.

Several problems may occur in tube feeding that should be noted. Irritation of the tube itself may cause discomfort to the child. Stimulation to the nasopharynx and oropharynx may cause increases in irregular breathing or bradycardia due to the sensory stimulation. The SLP must be aware of the conditions in the NICU or hospital when encountering these children after discharge. In addition, selection of liquids for transitioning may be necessary for the child to not reject the new route of feeding.

ADDITIONAL FACTORS IN INFANT FEEDING AND SWALLOWING

Feeding in infants and children can be addressed in a number of ways. Postural adjustments using seating arrangements such as shown in Figure 10–2 are helpful since they offer support for the child, adjust the child to proper position for swallowing and prevent distractions by limiting movement.

Foods and Formulas

Types of foods and fluids that the infant swallows may also improve the nutritive aspect of feeding and swallowing. Feeding premature infants with human milk has the advantages of speeding up gastrointestinal maturation, reducing the duration of hospitalization, and may reduce the development of later metabolic syndromes that have been associated with formula feeds.[25]

In previous chapters, the swallowing maneuvers and postures have been discussed. These interventions should not be ignored in infants when appropriate. Although the maneuvers and postures require infant cooperation, applying a maneuver "game" with young children, especially with autistic children, may lead to improved nutrition.

Properly modified utensils and cups are now available from a number of sources. Table 10–5 inventories some of the common sources. Children with cleft palate, CHARGE syndrome, and trisomy 21

may require modified bottle nipples in early infancy, and later will need modified utensils, cups, and plates long after infancy to facilitate the easy manipulation of the food from plate to spoon/fork and from spoon/fork to mouth.

Many infants and children can adapt to a common nipple, but premature children need a nipple that can match the size of the oral cavity opening and also one that may require an improved seal to prevent leakage around the sides of the mouth in case the child has poor muscle tone.

TABLE 10–5. A Selection of Current Online Sources for Modified Feeding and Eating Utensils and Supplies (websites subject to change)

http://www.onestepahead.com/home.jsp (key word: feeding utensils) Flexible feeding utensils, suction bowls
http://www.alimed.com/alimed/rehabilitation/dining-aids/ Broad list of bottles, utensils, serving trays, color-coded supplies
http://www.equipmentshop.com/ Bowls, cups, seating support
Enfamil: http://www.infamil.com/ Pacifiers, nipples, feeding materials, parent information, formulas
Avent Bottles, sterilizers
Bionix Inc. https://www.Bionixmed.com Bottles, nipples, enteral feeding equipment, safe straws, infant drinking cups
http://www.pampers.com Feeding supplies, straws
http://www.happyfamilybrands.com Certified Organic Fruit and Veggie Purees to Introduce Solids To Baby
https://www.amazon.com/baby Feeding toys, supplies
http://www.lucieslist.com/ Spoons, cups, feeding supplies

Bottles for feeding come in various shapes and hardness. A hard plastic bottle may be sufficient for most children, and parents can maintain a better grip on a hard bottle. However, a soft bottle offers the feeder an opportunity to squeeze the bottle to keep the feeding ongoing.

Feeding Programs

Over the past 15 years, several individuals have developed specific feeding programs that encompass the work of the speech-language pathologist, the occupational therapist, and other developmental specialists. The Beckman program mentioned above is one program that focuses on oral motor training for infants and children with limitations in their ability to manage the fine motor control needed to feed and eat independently.

The feeding program developed by Toomey called the Sequential Oral Sensory Approach (SOS) integrates feeding training into a program for children with limitations in growth and development.[26] This program focuses on the acquisition of feeding skills based on the acquisition of other motor skills. In addition, the program focuses on desensitizing the child who will not eat using touch, smell, and finally taste. This popular program has yet to be tested rigorously, but those who follow the guidelines of the program speak highly of it. Since children slowly develop the sense of taste and smell, some foods that were tolerated early in life are no longer tolerated due to the smell, the taste, or even the consistency of the food.

Feeding programs have become multidisciplinary over the years, and the combined approaches of the speech-language pathologist, the occupational therapist, and the dietitian have shown that clinically, improvement in feeding in children with low birth weight, who are premature, or with neurological diseases occurs when the parent has help to diffuse the feeding program. Swallow specialists now focus on the need to develop changing consistencies as the child ages to meet his or her changing sensory system.

New Treatment Techniques

Early work on the use of expiratory muscle strength training (EMST) in adults for the treatment of swallowing may have implications for infants and children. Troche et al have shown that the use of EMST may help restore functional swallowing behavior in those patients with Parkinson's disease.[27] They explained that the reason for improvement in a group of Parkinson's disease patients was due to improved hyolaryngeal activity. Future work may find that for patients with poor motor control, EMST may offer additional improvement to the oral motor exercises that are currently available. Additional treatment techniques suggest that caregivers be aware of changes brought about by continued research in tongue strength and lip strength development.[28]

SUMMARY

Most importantly, children must not be considered simply as little adults. Normal children are in a constant state of neurological, neuromuscular, and behavioral development. They progress through the stages of feeding and swallowing as their bodies develop. When communication is normal, children understand the feeding and eating processes.

When developmental delays, prematurity, or diseases and disorders are seen in the newborn, a comprehensive program to address the developmental aspects of the child must include feeding and swallowing. Dysphagia in the infant is simply not a matter of preventing aspiration; rather, it is a program to ensure that the infant is getting enough nutrition to grow and overcome the challenges of eating regardless of mental retardation, preterm birth, or neurological disorders. Programs to stimulate oral motor control of the muscles needed to achieve safe self-feeding should be initiated as early as possible. Aggressive management of the child may ultimately allow him or her to reach a safe oral feeding behavior that provides proper nutrition to maximize physical development and growth.

DISCUSSION QUESTIONS

1. The feeding environment—How to prepare for the autistic child?
2. Search the literature and review the work of the occupational therapists who treat infants with swallowing disorders. In what ways do you see an overlap in their activities and the activities of the speech-language pathologist? How does this overlap benefit the child?

STUDY QUESTIONS

1. The phases of swallowing in the infant have been modified by Rudolph and Link to include
   A. Sucking phase
   B. Pre-oral phase
   C. The motor phase
   D. The delayed swallow phase

2. In the oral phase of infant feeding, the primary difficulty for the infant with poor oral motor function is
   A. Chocking
   B. Lip closure
   C. Bolus transfer to the pharyngeal phase
   D. Taste awareness

3. In an immature child, a common sign of physiological stress during feeding may be
   A. Bradycardia
   B. Apnea
   C. Agitation
   D. All of the above

4. In the child with Down syndrome, swallowing problems may be expected to return to normal
   A. At age 7
   B. At age 11
   C. At age 14
   D. Never

5. Social expectations, cognitive issues, oral motor delay, and one other condition challenge the swallowing therapist to understand the importance of scheduling feeding times for the child with autism spectrum disorder. What is it?
   A. Digestive disorders of the esophagus and stomach
   B. Child's weight
   C. Sleeping periods
   D. Selection of the proper foods

REFERENCES

1. Ko MJ, Kang MJ, Ko KJ, Ki YO, Chang HJ, Kwon JY. Clinical usefulness of Schedule for Oral-Motor Assessment (SOMA) in children with dysphagia. *Ann Rehabil Med.* 2011;35:477–484.
2. Sheppard JJ, Hochman R, Baer C. The dysphagia disorder survey: validation of an assessment for swallowing and feeding function in developmental disability. *Res Dev Disabil.* 2014;35:929–942.
3. Rudolph CD, Link, DT. Feeding disorders in infants and children. *Pediatr Clin North Am.* 2002;49(1):97–112.
4. Arvedson J, Clark H, Lazerus C, Schooling T, Frymark T. Evidence-based systematic review: effects or oral motor interventions on feeding and swallowing in preterm infants. *Am J Speech Lang Path.* 2010;19(4):321–340.
5. Burklow KA, Phelps AN, Schultz JR, McConnell K, Rudolph C. Classifying complex pediatric feeding disorders. *J Pediatr Gastroenterol Nutr.* 1998;27(2):143–147.
6. Thomas JA. Guidelines for bottle feeding your premature baby. *Adv Neonatal Care.* 2007;Dec 7(6):311–318.
7. Rudolph CD. Feeding disorders in infants and children. *J Pediatr.* 1994;125:5116–5124.
8. Arvedson JC, Rogers BT. Pediatric feeding and swallowing disorder. *Med Speech Lang Pathol.* 1993;1:202–203.
9. van der Meer A, Holden G, van der Weel R. Coordination of sucking, swallowing and breathing in healthy newborns. *J Ped Neonatal.* 2005;2(2):NT69–72.
10. Cooper-Brown L, Copeland S, Dailey S, Downey D, Petersen MC, Stimson C, Van Dyke DC. Feeding and swallowing dysfunction in genetic syndromes. *Dev Disabil Res Rev.* 2008;14(2):147–157. doi:10.1002/ddrr.19.
11. Right Diagnostics.Com. Sept. 7, 2011.
12. Reilly S, Skuse D, Poblete X. Prevalence of feeding problems and oral motor dysfunction in children with cerebral palsy: a community survey. *J Pediatr.* 1996;129(6):877–882.
13. Erasmus CE, van Hulst K, Rotteveel JJ, Willemsen MA, Jongerius PH. Clinical practice: swallowing problems in cerebral palsy. *Eur J Pediatr.* 2012 Mar;171(3):409–414.
14. Dahl M, Thommessen M, Rasmussen M, Seiberg T. Feeding and nutritional characteristics in children with moderate or severe cerebral palsy. *Acta Paediatr.* 1996;85:697–701.
15. Stallings VA, Charney EB, Davies JC, Cronk CE. Nutritional status and growth of children with diplegic or hemiplegic cerebral palsy. *Dev Med Child Neurol.* 1993;35(11):997–1006.
16. Marques IL, de Sousa TV, Carneiro AF, Peres SP, Barbieri MA, Bettiol H. Robin sequence: a single treatment protocol [in Portuguese]. *J Pediatr (Rio J).* 2005 Jan–Feb;81(1):14–22.
17. Neul JL, Zoghbi HY. Rett syndrome: a prototypical neurodevelopmental disorder. *Neuroscientist.* 2004;10(2):118–128.
18. Weaving LS, Ellaway CJ, Gecz J, Christodoulou J. Rett syndrome: clinical review and genetic update. *J Med Genet.* 2005;42:1–7.
19. Fucile S, Gisel E, Lau C. Effect of an oral stimulation program on sucking skill maturation in preterm infants. *Dev Med Child Neurol.* 2005;47:158–162.
20. Bernbaum JC, Pereira GR, Watkins JB, Peckham GJ. Nonnutritive sucking during gavage feeding enhances growth and maturation in premature infants. *Pediatrics.* 1983;71:41–45.
21. Pinelli J, Symington AJ. Non-nutritive sucking for promoting physiologic stability and nutrition in preterm infants. *Cochrane Database Syst Rev.* 2005;(4).
22. Asadollahpour F, Yadegari F, Soleimani F, Khalesi, N. The effects of non-nutritive sucking and pre-feeding oral stimulation on time to achieve independent oral feeding for preterm infants. *Iran J Pediatr.* 2015 Jun;25(3):e809. doi:10.5812/ijp.25(3)2015.809 [Epub 2015 Jun 27].
23. Birnbaum R, Limperopoulos C. Nonoral feeding practices for infants in the neonatal intensive care unit. *Adv Neonatal Care.* 2009 Aug;9(4):180–184.
24. Fucile S, McFarland DH, Gisel EG, Lau C. Oral and nonoral sensorimotor interventions facilitate suck-swallow-respiration functions and their coordination in preterm infants. *Early Hum Dev.* 2012; June 88(6):345–350.

25. Schanler RJ. Outcomes of human milk-fed premature infants. *Semin Perinatol.* 2011;35(1):29–33.

26. Toomey K. *Understand Why Children Won't Eat and How to Help. Feeding Strategies for Older Infants and Toddlers.* Essay, Fall 2001:100.

27. Troche MS, Okun MS, Rosenbek JC, et al. Aspiration and swallowing in Parkinson disease and rehabilitation with EMST: a randomized trial. *Neurology.* 2010 Nov 23; 75(21):1912–1919.

28. Lazarus C. Tongue strength and exercise in healthy individuals and in head and neck cancer patients. *Semin Speech Lang.* 2006 Nov;27(4):260–267.

Chapter
11

Surgical Treatment and Prosthetic Management of Swallowing Disorders

A Look at the Chapter

The clinician treating swallowing disorders is always working within a team of rehabilitation specialists. Included in the team are surgeons and prosthodontists. The role of the surgeon is limited to improving the valving of different sphinters within the upper aerodigestive tract (eg glottic closure) to provide a way to aid with the airways toilette (eg tracheostomy) or to facilitate enteric nutrition (eg gastrostomy tube) when diseases or neurologic conditions render the vocal folds, the larynx, and the food and liquid passageways unsafe for swallowing or for those organs to hinder swallowing. Part one of this chapter deals with the surgical options in the treatment of swallowing disorders. Part two examines prosthodontic appliances to aid in the act of swallowing when vital organs such as the tongue are missing or partially missing.

Because surgery is used in combination with swallowing rehabilitation, nutrition and prosthodontics applications, the multidisciplinary team approach offers the patient the highest advantage to achieve a functional swallowing mechanism.

INTRODUCTION

Surgery may help to palliate select swallowing disorders by improving the sphincteric mechanisms of the velopalatine, glottic, or upper esophageal sphincters, reducing obstruction (intra- or extraluminal), providing the means for pulmonary toilette, or bypassing the upper aerodigestive tract to enhance enteric nutrition, hydration, and the administration of medications. Surgery does not restore lost function; however, patients in whom conservative treatment (ie, diet adjustments and direct swallowing therapy/maneuvers) fail to achieve a safe swallow, surgery may help compensate neuromuscular deficits by optimizing the remaining function, improving the valving mechanism, or expanding the mechanical conduit. Surgery is most often used in combination with other forms of swallowing rehabilitation, frequently resulting in the return to oral intake.

The use of enteric tubes, such as a gastrostomy, jejunostomy, or gastrojejunostomy, surgically placed, provide additional means to maintain hydration and nutrition for patients who are unable to swallow by mouth.

Oral prosthodontics is the discipline that deals with providing a substitute for lost structures of the oral cavity (ie, congenital or acquired). Congenital oral defects include cleft lip, cleft palate, cleft mandible, and bifid uvula. Acquired oral defects are those primarily related to surgical treatment of diseases, sharp or blunt trauma, or burns.

Oral prosthodontists design prosthetic appliances (dental, palatal, or tongue prostheses), provide medical therapy, and adjust or modify environmental factors (eg, design utensils to improve and control feeding) to aid in the rehabilitation of swallowing disorders. In general, the prosthetic rehabilitation team is led by a prosthodontist; however, its implementation and function require continual input from the head and neck surgeon and speech-language pathologist. Ideal dietary characteristics, including bolus size, consistency, and viscosity, must be considered in patients who are being fitted with a prosthetic appliance. Therefore, communication among the care team members, including the nutritionist, is critical to optimize the outcomes. A speech-language pathologist must assess the swallowing function before, during, and following the fitting of the prosthesis to evaluate its effectiveness. Furthermore, most prostheses require several fittings to achieve optimal placement and bulk, and the speech-language pathologist may have to assess speech and swallowing after every adjustment. Pressure measurement using the Iowa Oral Performance Instrument (IOPI) is useful to estimate the ideal location and bulk of the prosthetic appliance, thus fulfilling both speech and swallowing needs. Once a device is fitted, the speech-language pathologist devises a rehabilitation program that maximizes the value of the prosthesis.

Oral prosthetics are advocated to improve speech intelligibility following extirpative surgery of the mandible, maxilla, tongue, or palate, and to improve the oral preparatory and oral phases of swallowing (ie, chewing, bolus formation, decreasing the tongue-palate distance, and increasing the propulsive pressure on the bolus). The incidence and severity of speech and swallowing problems following surgery are related to the size and location of the tumor; the structures involved in the surgery, radiation, or chemotherapy; and the amount of remaining functional tissue. Patients with large tumors (cancer stages III and IV), often suffer both speech (64%) and swallowing problems (75%).[1] Furthermore, instruments that measure quality-of-life issues, such as the SWAL-QOL, suggest that oral cancer and its consequences lead to significant deterioration of quality of life. This chapter will focus on oral prosthodontics as it relates to defects resulting from oncologic surgery and how oral and oropharyngeal prostheses help to compensate deficits by optimizing the remaining function by improving the valving mechanism and the bolus propulsion.

REHABILITATIVE SURGICAL PROCEDURES

Vocal Fold Medialization

Vocal fold medialization improves the closure of the glottis, thus improving swallowing efficiency and safety.[2,3] It aims to close any remaining glottic gap on vocal fold adduction, thus providing a secure closure to the vocal folds. This effectively separates the lower airways from the foodway during the passage of the bolus, thus reducing the possibility of aspiration and improving phonation.

Medialization of the vocal folds may be achieved by transendoscopic, transoral, or transcutaneous injection or by open transcervical laryngeal framework techniques.[2–10] Table 11–1 summarizes

TABLE 11–1. Vocal Fold Medialization Procedures, Substances, and Origin of Substances

Injection	
Gelfoam Surgifoam	Gelatin powder
Radiesse voice gel	Carbomethylcellulose
Cymetra	Cadaveric dermis
Teflon	Human engineered
Autologous tissue	
Fat	Human
Fascia	Human
Collagen	Human or animal
Hyaluronic acid gels (various)	Bacterial engineered
(GAG-polysaccharide)	Calcium hydroxyapatite
Radiesse	
Laryngeal framework surgery	
Medialization laryngoplasty	
Silastic	Human engineered
Gore-Tex	Human engineered
Hydroxyapatite	Calcium hydroxyapatite
Cartilage	Human
Adjunctive procedure	
Arytenoid adduction/ repositioning	

the current options for vocal fold medialization. Contraindications for medialization of a vocal fold include a compromised airway (eg, bilateral vocal fold paralysis) and/or lack of evidence that the dysphagia is secondary to a paralyzed vocal fold.

Vocal Fold Injection

A lateral vocal fold injection (VFI) can medialize a vocal fold affected by atrophy, paresis, or immobility especially if improvement or return of function is expected.[11–13] Figure 11–1 shows a patient with vocal fold atrophy who may be a suitable candidate for injection. The vocal folds show a glottic gap (bowing) that persists during phonation or swallowing.

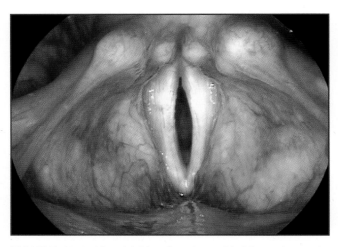

FIGURE 11–1. Vocal folds of patient with bilateral atrophy prior to undergoing vocal fold injection.

Vocal fold injection has the advantage of avoiding open surgery, but, despite the apparent simplicity of the procedure, it is technically challenging and associated with multiple complications (Table 11–2).

VFI is most effective when the arytenoid cartilage is not subluxated anteriorly (there is no vertical level disparity between the vocal folds) and the vocal fold is at a paramedian position. VFI is not entirely effective when the paralyzed vocal fold is in the extreme lateral position (ie, cadaveric position), as a significant posterior gap persists, even when there appears to be adequate closure of the anterior glottis. Contraindications for vocal fold injection include coagulation disorders or anticoagulation therapy, a compromised airway, and/or lack of evidence that the paralyzed vocal fold contributes to the dysphagia.

Vocal fold injection has grown in popularity for both correction of voice and swallowing disorders due to the new and improved injectable materials, increased use of the procedure, and laryngological training to help in selecting the proper patients and the proper techniques for achieving maximum vocal fold approximation. Sulica et al outlined the indications and complications of vocal fold injection.[12] While vocal fold injection augments the closure of the vocal folds, it alone may not be sufficient to curb aspiration.[13]

A paste or gel comprising gelatin powder (eg, Gelfoam, Johnson & Johnson, New Jersey), hyaluronic

TABLE 11–2. Complications of Vocal Fold Injection

1. **Overinjection:** Improper vocal fold closure (early anterior contact); airway obstruction
2. **Misplaced injection:** Inappropriate segmental glottis closure
3. **Underinjection:** Lack of vocal fold closure

acid, or acellular dermis may be used as a temporary treatment of vocal fold paralysis. Injection of the vocal fold with gelatin paste can result in improved glottic closure, and henceforth, improved swallowing; therefore, it is an excellent, cost-effective option for the treatment of dysphagia due to vocal fold paralysis when the recovery of the vocal fold paralysis is expected. Hyaluronic acid and acellular dermis are available in commercial preparations and are adequate, albeit more expensive options. Reabsorption of these materials is variable, but overall they offer a medialization effect for 6 to 12 weeks. Calcium hydroxyapatite is also available as gel form, and its effect tends to last longer (6 to 18 months).

Autologous fat has been injected to treat both voice and swallowing disorders. Its reabsorption is extremely variable, thus making the final result unpredictable. In a typical injection, the vocal fold is overinjected, creating a convex vocal fold to account for the initial reabsorption of fat. However, the initial convexity causes early anterior contact and a posterior gap, which may increase the risk of aspiration as well as cause a temporary change in voice quality.

Teflon injection is effective in improving vocal function, particularly if the vocal fold is not too far from the midline. Teflon lost favor as an injectable material for the larynx due to the occurrence of Teflon (foreign-body) granulomas. However, this is not a concern when treating patients with terminal diseases (e.g., advanced lung cancer presenting with a vocal fold palsy). The complications and advantages of Teflon are shown in Table 11–3.[14] While Teflon injection may lead to an inflammatory foreign body reaction, it is not unique in this respect. This type of reaction can also occur with any of the other injectable materials; albeit not as marked as with the Teflon. Teflon is rarely used in medialization procedures; other materials have been found to be more adaptable to laryngeal closure.

TABLE 11–3. Intracordal Teflon Injection[a]

Problems and Complications
Difficult surgical exposure (eg, cervical spine limited range of motion)
Nonreversible
Technically challenging
Inconsistent postoperative vocal quality
Does not close posterior glottis gap
Teflon migration
Teflon granuloma
Advantages
Does not require surgery
May be performed in an office setting (selected cases)

[a]Adapted from Andrews, Netterville, and Mercati.[14(p291)]

Laryngeal Framework Surgery

In our opinion, laryngeal framework surgery should be considered the gold standard for the treatment of aspiration due to glottic insufficiency. Our own data, and that of others, suggest that more than 80% of patients with glottic insufficiency can be rehabilitated using these procedures and adjunct swallowing therapy.[2,3–9,13]

Medialization Laryngoplasty. Medialization laryngoplasty involves inserting an implant, between the ala of the thyroid cartilage and the vocal fold, thus displacing the vocal fold medially. In select cases, it may even displace a subluxated arytenoid posteriorly into a more anatomical position. Commonly used implants are made of silicone, Gore-Tex (WL Gore & Assoc., Flagstaff, Arizona), or calcium hydroxyapatite.

A medialization laryngoplasty is adjustable to the patient's needs, reversible, and does not interfere with neuromuscular recovery. It leads to a more competent glottis sphincter, thus improving the safety of swallowing and the effectiveness of the cough protective mechanism.[7–9] Figure 11–2 shows the typical position of the vocal fold silicone implant.

Table 11–4 lists the most common indications and advantages of medialization laryngoplasty.

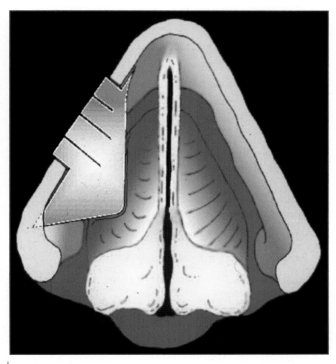

FIGURE 11–2. The implant should have smooth contours that gently displace the entire paraglottic space as needed. The maximum plane of medialization can be placed at any level, either within the window or below the level of the window, as determined by the depth gauge.

Table 11–5 lists common complications and limitations of medialization laryngoplasty.

Hendricker et al[15] reported on the value of medialization laryngoplasty using Gore-Tex for the treatment of aspiration. The authors presented the outcomes of 121 procedures performed in 113 patients. The main outcome measures included the discontinuation of gastrostomy tube (g-tube), avoidance of g-tube, and subjective improvement ratings. Their study included 20 patients with dysphagia, who required g-tubes for alimentation. Eleven of these 20 (55%) patients were able to stop using the g-tube after a medialization laryngoplasty with Gore-Tex. Five additional patients avoided the placement of a g-tube after medialization laryngoplasty. Patients with penetration reported less penetration and improved swallow function.

Arytenoid Adduction or Medialization. Arytenoid adduction or arytenoidopexy are techniques that

TABLE 11–4. Indications and Advantages of Medialization Laryngoplasty[a]

Indications
Glottic incompetence secondary to unilateral vocal fold paralysis
Sacrifice of or injury to cranial nerve X during skull base surgery
Incomplete glottis closure secondary to vocal fold paresis or atrophy
Selected traumatic or postsurgical defects

Contraindications
Relative
Fibrosis resulting from laryngeal radiation
Loss of external framework (ie, vertical hemilaryngectomy)
Prior Teflon injection
Absolute
Impaired contralateral vocal fold abduction (ie, airway compromise)

Advantages
Well tolerated under local anesthesia
Reversible and adjustable
Reproducible vocal results (does not interfere with mucosal wave)
Can be performed in conjunction with arytenoid adduction (closes posterior gap)
Implant does not migrate, change shape, or produce a foreign body reaction

Disadvantages
Learning curve
May extrude if ventricular mucosa is violated
Requires "open" transcervical approach
Unknown long-term effect

[a]Adapted from Andrews, Netterville, and Mercati.[14(p292)]

TABLE 11–5. Medialization Laryngoplasty: Complications and Limitations[a]

Undermedialization secondary to intraoperative vocal fold edema
Implant contamination from entry into the laryngeal ventricle
Intracordal hematoma
Transient stridor from postoperative edema
Overmedialization of anterior one-third of the true vocal fold resulting in a strained voice
Posterior glottis gap requiring addition of an arytenoid adduction for closure
Modest improvement with bilateral medialization for presbylaryngis

[a]Adapted from Andrews, Netterville, and Mercati.[14(p294)]

arytenoid muscle.[5] Therefore, the arytenoid rotates internally, in an oblique axis, relocating the vocal process medially and caudally, and adducting the vocal fold.

During the arytenoid medialization surgery, the body of the arytenoid is sutured in a medial position over the cricoid. Furthermore, the arytenoid, which is frequently subluxated anteriorly (due to the paralysis of the posterior and lateral cricoarytenoid muscles that insert into its muscular process) is retracted posteriorly and fixed in a more anatomic position. This corrects the vocal fold foreshortening and places the affected vocal fold at the same level as the "functioning" vocal fold as shown in Figure 11–3.

An arytenoid repositioning procedure is effective closing a wide posterior glottal gap that is commonly associated with an increased risk of aspiration.

Hypopharyngeal Pharyngoplasty. A hypopharyngeal pharyngoplasty involves the plication or removal of redundant mucosa of the piriform sinus that is often associated with a paralyzed hypopharynx, thus reducing the "ballooning" and the pooling of secretions often observed during a MBS and FEES.[17]

Cricopharyngeal Myotomy. Cricopharyngeal myotomy should be considered for patients with incomplete relaxation of the upper esophageal sphincter (UES) or those with abnormal muscular contrac-

specifically aim to close a posterior glottis gap in patients with unilateral adduction paralysis of the vocal fold.[7] The arytenoid adduction procedure applies traction on the muscular process of the arytenoid, emulating the activity of the lateral crico-

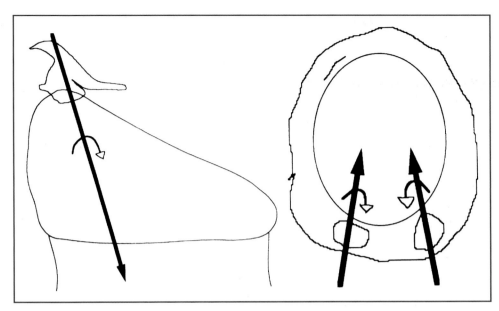

FIGURE 11–3. Axis of rotation in arytenoid adduction. Adapted with permission from Newman, Hengesteg, Lepage, Kaufman, and Woodson.[16(p269)]

tions during the relaxation period. Common clinical scenarios include patients with laryngeal paralysis due to pathology of the central nervous system or proximal vagus nerve that also produce pharyngeal motor or sensory deficits or patients with Zenker diverticulum. Pharyngeal propulsion in patients presenting with a brainstem stroke or a high-vagal paralysis (proximal lesion) is often inadequate to propel the bolus past a dysfunctional cricopharyngeal sphincter.[10,11] This leads to pharyngeal "pooling" of the swallowed material and spillage over the arytenoids/aryepiglottic folds into an insensate larynx ("postswallow" aspiration). In such patients, restoration of glottic closure may not be sufficient to correct the dysphagia and aspiration. Patients with a Zenker diverticulum present with a dysfunctional opening of the upper esophageal sphincter and accumulation of secretions and food in the diverticulum.[18–20] These can be regurgitated and aspirated. Transoral cricopharyngeal myotomy offers the advantage of avoiding a cervical scar and diminishing the possibility of injuring the recurrent laryngeal nerve (RLN).[21]

Cricopharyngeal myotomy is a useful adjunct to vocal fold medialization. Table 11–6 presents the common indications for cricopharyngeal myotomy.

Table 11–7 presents the pitfalls and complications of this procedure. Cricopharyngeal myotomy is contraindicated in patients with significant gastropharyngeal reflux and is ineffective in patients with poor laryngeal elevation (anterosuperior axis). In addition, patients with poor pharyngeal propulsion do not benefit from a CP myotomy.[23] Alternatively, a botulinum toxin injection to the cricopharyngeus muscle may provide a "medical myotomy" and may confirm the diagnosis of C-P spasm.[23,24]

Palatopexy

Acquired velopalatine incompetence (VPI) can result from partial or complete loss of the soft palate, or from neuromuscular dysfunction. A unilateral palatal adhesion (palatopexy) is indicated for patients with permanent unilateral palatal paralysis that does not respond to conservative measures. A synechia is surgically created at the level of Passavant ridge, the site of "normal" closure of the velopalatine valve.[25] Even patients with very mild liquid reflux often have moderate to severe nasal quality to their speech, which dramatically improves after a palatal adhesion. Figure 11–4 shows the adhesion location.

TABLE 11–6. Cricopharyngeal Myotomy[a]

Indications
Dysphagia secondary to
Central nervous system disorders
Peripheral nervous system disorders
Vagal injury (laryngeal/pharyngeal paralysis)
Diabetic/peripheral neuropathy
Muscular disease
Oculopharyngeal dystrophy
Steinert myotonic dystrophy
Polymyositis
Myasthenia gravis
Hyperthyroidism/hypothyroidism
Postsurgical
Total laryngectomy
Oral cavity/oropharyngeal resection
Zenker diverticulum
Cricopharyngeal achalasia

Contraindications
Severe weakness of the pharyngeal muscles (unable to propel bolus)
Severe/uncontrolled GERD
Pharyngeal varices
Postbilateral neck injections
Thoracic outlet syndrome

[a]Adapted from Pou.[22(p300)]

TABLE 11–7. Cricopharyngeal Myotomy: Pitfalls and Complications[a]

Patient Factors/Poor Patient Selection
Severe/uncontrolled GERD resulting in postoperative aspiration and pneumonia
Extreme pharyngeal muscle weakness with inability to propel bolus

Surgical Errors
Injury to the recurrent laryngeal nerve
Accidental pharyngotomy
Pharyngocutaneous fistulae

[a]Adapted from Pou.[22(p308)]

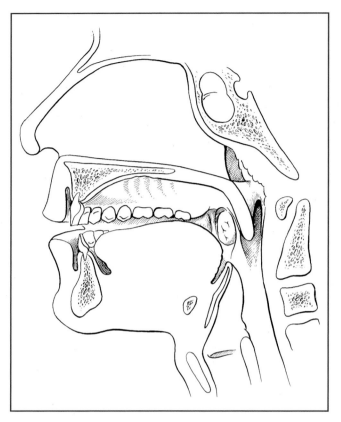

FIGURE 11–4. The adhesion is at the level of Passavant ridge to allow closure of the contralateral normal velopharynx. Adapted from Netterville.[25(p311)]

Dysfunction of the soft palate resulting in either unilateral or bilateral paralysis of the soft palate creates varying degrees of VPI. During the process of swallowing, VPI is manifested by the regurgitation of liquids, and rarely solids, into the nasopharynx and nasal cavity.

Pharyngoesophageal Dilatation

Pharyngoesophageal dilatation involves the use of tapered bougies of increasing diameter that are inserted sequentially to expand a stenotic segment, or the insertion of balloons that are sequentially inflated to a desired diameter, thus expanding the lumen. Its use is increasing due to the increased incidence of pharyngoesophageal stenosis associated with chemoradiotherapy.[26,27]

Surgical Closure of the Larynx

Patients who continue to aspirate despite the use of conservative measures and adjunctive surgical procedures may require surgical closure of the larynx. In patients with intractable aspiration, a surgical separation of the airway from the foodway provides palliation, thus stopping the aspiration and, in some, allowing oral intake.

Most commonly, patients requiring a laryngotracheal separation are those with neurologic disorders such as cerebrovascular accidents (CVAs) and amyotrophic lateral sclerosis (ALS). Laryngotracheal diversion, known as the standard Lindeman procedure, involves the creation of an anastomosis between the subglottic trachea and the esophagus, and a permanent stoma from the distal trachea. A laryngotracheal separation, or modified Lindeman procedure, involves the closure of the proximal subglottic trachea as a blind pouch and the opening of

a permanent tracheostoma, as shown in Figure 11–5. This latter technique best meets the desired criteria of simplicity, reliability, and reversibility. Table 11–8 shows various surgical procedures used to separate the esophagus from trachea in patients with intractable aspiration.

In the rare clinical scenario where a patient suffers intractable aspiration but still has a fair prognosis, one must consider a tracheotomy and the use of a laryngeal stent to close the proximal airway.[29,30]

PALLIATIVE SURGICAL PROCEDURES

Gastrostomy Tube (GT)

Percutaneous endoscopic gastrostomy (PEG) or open gastrostomy tubes provide a temporary or permanent route for nutrition, hydration, and administration of

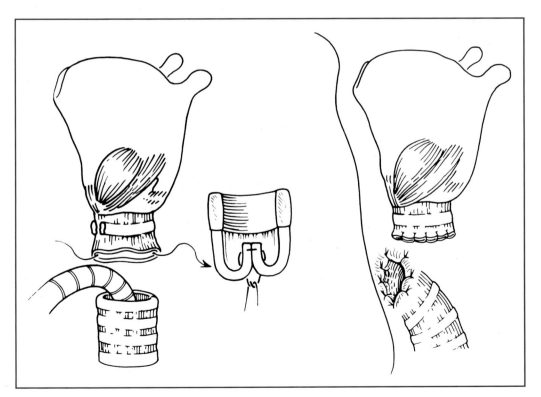

FIGURE 11–5. With laryngotracheal separation (modified Lindeman procedure), the proximal subglottic trachea is closed as a blind pouch and a permanent stoma is created from the distal trachea. Adapted from Snyderman.[28(p314)]

TABLE 11–8. Surgical Procedures Used to Separate Esophagus From Trachea[a]

Procedure	Control of Aspiration	Preservation of Speech	Reversibility
Tracheostomy	–	+	+
Laryngeal stent	+/–	+/–	+
Laryngotracheal separation	+	–[b]	+
Total laryngectomy	+	–[b]	–

[a]Adapted from Snyderman.[28(p315)]

[b]Alaryngeal speech—either tracheoesophageal speech or esophageal speech, is possible.

medications. GT should, however, be reserved for patients in whom all other alternatives have been unsuccessful, and/or those patients with severe nutritional deficiencies, who cannot meet their protein/caloric requirements with an oral diet. It should be noted, however, that the GT does not necessarily prevent aspiration and in patients with diminished reflexes may even increase the risk of aspiration pneumonia (i.e., reflux aspiration). Therefore, it appears that while G-tubes may benefit some dysphagic patients, such as those receiving chemoradiotherapy, they may not help and, indeed, may be a source of complications in other patient populations, such as those with dementia.[31–35] Alternative enteric tubes such as jejunostomy or gastro jejunostomy tubes may be superior options in select patients. Long-term monitoring of patients with GT and repeated testing as indicated is prudent as they may recover swallowing function even years after the primary event.[36]

Tracheotomy

Tracheostomy implies the placement of a tube into the trachea through a transcervical incision. The most common indication for the procedure is the need for prolonged mechanical ventilation. Other factors influencing a recommendation for tracheotomy are shown in Table 11–9. A tracheotomy does not enhance the ability of the patient to swallow,

TABLE 11–9. Factors Influencing the Recommendation for a Tracheotomy in Chronic Ventilator-Dependent Patients[a]

1. Need for prolonged mechanical ventilation
2. Primary diagnosis
3. Comorbidities
4. Nasal versus oral tube
5. Patient comfort
6. Ease of endotracheal suction
7. Expected duration of ventilator support
8. Effect of reducing "dead space"
9. Patient motion
10. Complications of endotracheal tube
11. Perceived risk of laryngeal complications

[a]Adapted from Eibling and Carrau.[38(p260)]

and in fact will result in greater swallowing dysfunction and aspiration.[37] Therefore, devices such as expiratory valves or fenestrated tubes, and decannulation are commonly advocated to aid swallowing in patients with a tracheotomy.

Expiratory Speaking Valve

An expiratory speaking valve is a removable one-way valve that opens to permit inhalation, but closes during expiration to divert the airflow through the larynx. Its advantages and contraindications are shown in Tables 11–10 and 11–11. Figure 11–6 shows examples of expiratory speaking valves. The valve fits over the open tracheotomy tube to improve subglottic pressure when talking or swallowing.

It is important to monitor the patient when trying a speaking valve for the first time. Signs and symptoms of difficulty using a speaking valve are shown in Table 11–11.

TABLE 11–10. Advantages of Expiratory Valve Use[a]

1. The patient can communicate verbally
2. Airflow provides proprioceptive cues during swallowing exercises and learning of maneuvers
3. True vocal fold adduction exercises will be minimalized because of subglottic air pressure buildup
4. Improved pressure to aid in bolus propulsion

[a]Adapted from Gross and Eibling.[39(p255)]

TABLE 11–11. Contraindications for the Use of a Speaking Valve

1. Unconscious/comatose patients.
2. Severe behavior problems.
3. Patients with cognitive disorders.
4. Severe medical instability, especially pulmonary failure.
5. Severe tracheal stenosis or edema.
6. Any airway obstruction above the tube that precludes expiration through the glottis.
7. Thick and copious secretions that persist after valve placement.
8. Foam-filled tracheotomy tube cuff (Bivona).
9. Total laryngectomy or laryngotracheal separation.
10. Insufficient passage for air around the tube, either with the cuff down or with a cuffless tube.
11. Inability to maintain adequate ventilation with cuff deflation in ventilator dependent patient.
12. If valve is already placed, remove it if skin color changes.
13. Remove valve if the patient shows increased restlessness, stridor, grunting, head bobbing, or other signs of anxiousness.

Fenestrated Tracheostomy Tube

A fenestrated tracheostomy tube has a large single or multiple small openings to permit air to pass into the upper airway and oral cavity. Long-term use of fenestrated tubes is ill advised, as the friction of the fenestra against the tracheal walls produces exuberant granulation tissue, which has been associated with bleeding and/or life-threatening airway compromise. Figure 11–7 shows examples of fenestrated tracheostomy tubes.

Decannulation

The patient's ability to tolerate decannulation can be estimated by the amount of oral and tracheal secretions and by the patient's tolerance of tube capping. Decannulation is the most effective single intervention to enhance swallowing in patients with a tracheotomy.

Cricothyrotomy

Cricothyrotomy is an incision made through the skin and the cricothyroid membrane most commonly performed for the relief of airway obstruction. Most commonly, it is used in lieu of tracheotomy in emergency situations. Electively, it may be used in select patients undergoing surgery that requires a median sternotomy (eg, cardiac bypass surgery), as it is less likely to infect the sternotomy wound than a standard tracheotomy.

Conclusions

Surgical procedures are more commonly used as adjuncts to rehabilitative and compensatory therapy. They strive to improve the swallow by upgrading the function of the different valving mechanisms. In patients with severe swallowing disorders and/or malnutrition, they provide an avenue to maintain an adequate hydration and proteo-caloric intake as well as to provide the means for tracheopulmonary toilette. A surgical separation of the airway and foodway is recommended for patients with intractable aspiration with a poor prognosis for recovery.

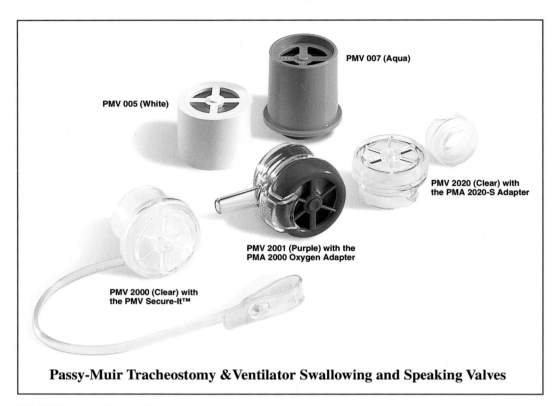

Passy-Muir Tracheostomy & Ventilator Swallowing and Speaking Valves

FIGURE 11–6. Passy-Muir valves. The valve fits over the open tracheotomy tube to restore subglottic pressure when talking or swallowing.

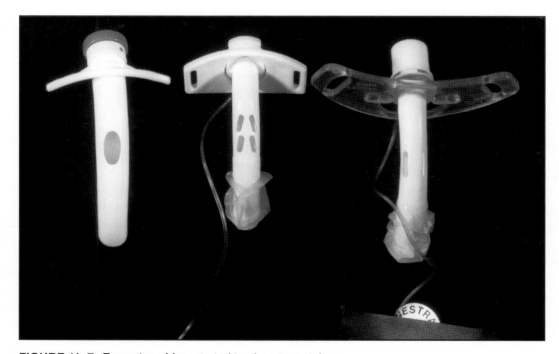

FIGURE 11–7. Examples of fenestrated tracheostomy tubes.

PROSTHESES

Oral Prosthodontics and Dentures

The presence of teeth to grind food to a soft consistency is a major determinant of the types of food one can swallow. Many patients without normal dentition or a prosthetic dental appliance can manage more than a liquid consistency; however, a properly fitted dental prosthesis speeds up the meals and increases the variety of food texture and firmness that a person can swallow safely. For some, an adequate dentition may be the difference between a liquid-only diet and an unrestricted diet that includes solid consistencies.

An oral prosthesis may consist of dentures only or may be a combined dental and palatal reshaping. A palatal reshaping prosthesis like that shown in Figure 11–8 is used to provide a framework for dentition and lower the palatal vault, thus creating a contact area with the tongue to provide the necessary propulsion for the bolus. Dentures may be incorporated into the palatal reshaping prosthesis.

Dentures may be of 1 or 2 types: (1) fixed or implanted dentures or (2) removable dentures. Implants are significantly more expensive; however, they offer greater stability than removable dentures, which eventually may not fit properly due to a change in tissue structure, damage to the denture, or atrophy of tissue that may occur after radiation therapy or chemotherapy. Implantable dentures, however, may not be an option in all patients due to surgical removal of tissue or bone. A full upper and lower dental arch ensures improved mastication even when oral muscles are weak or partially missing following oral cancer surgery.

In any case, proper dentures aid in modifying diet consistencies, increase the rate of eating, and help to improve the efficiency of tongue motion during swallowing.[40–42]

Dental implants have led to improved subjective assessments, such as appearance, masticatory improvement, and denture retention. However, functional impairment cannot be fully compensated by implant-supported prosthodontics, but such treatment contributes essentially to general well-being and relief of disease-related social restrictions.[43]

Teoh et al[44] measured functional outcomes using 4 individual assessments (nutritional status, swallowing, masticatory performance, and speech) and 1 measure that combined the information from these assessments, the global measure of functional outcome (GMFO), in 2 groups of patients with at least 6 months of postoperative convalescence after mandibular resection and reconstruction for head and neck cancer. The group that received prosthetic intervention scored significantly higher in the GMFO than the comparison group. The use of prosthesis was associated with a higher GMFO score even after controlling for other significant factors such as xerostomia, number of remaining mandibular teeth, number of tooth-to-tooth contacts, type of reconstruction, flap interference, and tongue defect.

However, the use of dental implants has been questioned by several authors,[45,46] suggesting that there may be a risk factor for developing cancer. Eguia del Valle et al[45] found cancer cells in the inflamed tissue surrounding osseointegrated dental implants and Kwok et al[46] reported cancer in the periphery of dental implants in 3 patients.

Palate Lowering Prostheses

Palate lowering prostheses, sometimes referred to as maxillary prostheses, are devices that help to complement the palatal vault. They are similar to palate reshaping prostheses but generally do not

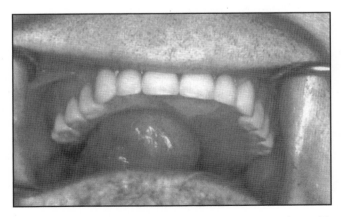

FIGURE 11–8. Prosthesis for palatal augmentation with anterior dental prosthesis attached to permanent dentition.

include dentures. They help to increase bolus transit to the posterior oral cavity and increase tongue palate contact pressures to propel the bolus into the oropharynx. They are designed by the maxillofacial prosthodontist with the help of the speech-language pathologist to maximize both speech and the oral preparatory and oral phases of swallowing.[47]

Prosthetic restoration for swallowing disorders related to hard palate defects should begin intraoperatively with the placement of a temporary obturating prosthesis. The obturator restores oronasal separation, thus facilitating oral feeding and improving speech intelligibility. In addition, restoring the oronasal separation reduces the likelihood of wound infection from residual food particles collecting in spaces above the maxillary arch and helps to prevent food from being packed into the defect by separating the oral from the nasal cavity.

The design and application of a hard palate prosthesis is enhanced if the surgical device is created with the intention to fit a temporary device. Five to 7 days after surgery, the surgical obturator is removed and remodeled to fit the surgical defect. The temporary palatal prosthesis is substituted by a permanent device several months after surgery. With adequate retention and stability, the prosthesis will provide important contouring to aid the tongue in oral phase manipulation of food boluses. Various types of materials have been advanced in the treatment of hard palate defects such as **polymethylmethacrylate** and other polymers.[48] Titanium-based obturators have also been proposed and may offer less bacteria buildup than other devices.[49]

Soft Palate Prostheses

Following proper fitting of a hard or soft palate prosthesis, it is expected that the oral preparatory and oral phases of swallowing will improve. Improvement is based on shaping the oral cavity to maintain maximal control of the bolus in the oral cavity without spillage, proper mastication of the bolus, directing the bolus to the posterior oral cavity, slowing down the transit of liquids, and increasing the force of propulsion.

Soft palate prostheses are designed primarily to reduce the distance between the palate and posterior tongue. If the defect is large, the prosthesis is extended into the pharyngeal region to facilitate the sphincteric action of the lateral and posterior pharyngeal wall, as shown in Figure 11–9. Oral exercises

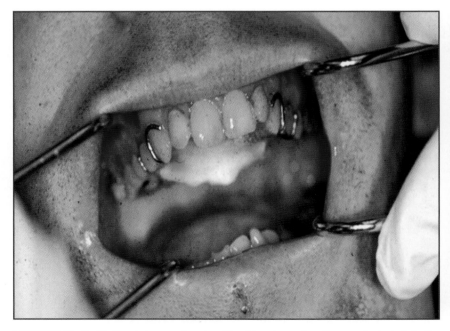
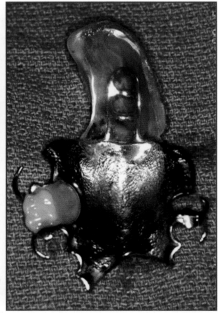

FIGURE 11–9. Soft palate prosthesis with obturator extending posteriorly into the pharyngeal area to improve contact during swallowing.

to complement prosthetic restoration are presented in Chapter 7

Restoration of the soft palate for improved swallowing is indicated when there are large defects involving the posterior border of the soft palate, when there is a nonfunctional band of tissue posteriorly in the soft palate, or when lateral pharyngeal defects affect sphincteric action of the palate in conjunction with the tongue and pharynx.

Velopharyngeal incompetence is typically addressed using the soft palate prosthesis. This prosthesis pushes or lifts the palate posteriorly to promote contact of the soft palate with the posterior and lateral pharyngeal walls. Use of this device requires adaptation by the patient, because initially the patient may feel discomfort or the prosthesis may stimulate the gag reflex. Shifman and colleagues[50] developed a speech and swallowing prosthesis for the management of velopharyngeal incompetence that relies on nasopharyngeal obturation instead of palatal elevation. Although the device was developed primarily for speech improvement, it may also aid in swallowing. Other devices have been proposed, although they are mostly for improvement of speech. The nasal speaking valve (NSV) developed by Suwaki and colleagues[51,52] is a valve that is placed through the nose to reduce the nasal air flow and increase oral pressure. Patients report that it is less uncomfortable than oral obturators such as a palatal lift, and it provides improvement in oronasal separation. Therefore, the NSV can be worn for a longer period of time. As it is inserted into the nostrils (it relies on clips to hold it in place), this device can be used by edentulous patients.

A systematic review of speech and swallowing following surgical treatment of advanced oral and oropharyngeal carcinoma by Kreeft et al[53] found that the use of palatal obturators generally improved speech production to a level of intelligible speech in most settings, but swallowing deficits remain even with the most advanced and customized devices.

Lingual Prostheses

The tongue is the primary means of transporting foods and liquids to the oropharynx. When the tongue is removed surgically, either partially or completely, the patient relies on dietary modifica-tions (various liquid consistencies), modified postures (head tilted back), or, most often, an enteral feeding tube to get the food into the stomach.

Partial or total resection of the tongue (glossectomy) results in significant swallowing and speech disorders over a long period of time.[54–56] Total glossectomy results in a large oral space where pooling of saliva and liquids can occur, eventually leading to postswallow (i.e., postprandial) aspiration. Although speech may be intelligible, articulation disorders persist and reflect the degree of tongue removed. Leonard and Gillis[57] presented results of improved control of food bolus using a tongue prosthesis. However, problems often remain even after prosthetic management.

Table 11–12 lists the goals of prosthetic rehabilitation after total glossectomy. A properly fitted tongue prosthesis reduces the oral cavity size, thus reducing the possibility of retained secretions that might later be aspirated. Guidance of oral intake by a speech-language pathologist helps to obtain maximum benefits. This may require the use of a syringe to place food posteriorly or may involve having the patient monitor the placement of the food in front of a mirror. Table 11–13 summarizes the goals of prosthetic rehabilitation after partial glossectomy. Feeding devices may be needed to aid in the oral preparatory and oral phases of swallowing.

Physical and Environmental Adjustments

Physical or environmental factors may interfere with a safe and successful nutrition. Therefore, physical and occupational therapists play a significant

TABLE 11–12. Major Goals in Prosthetic Rehabilitation After Total Glossectomy[a]

1. To reduce the size of the oral cavity, which will minimize the degree of pooling of saliva and improve resonance.
2. To develop surface contact with the surrounding structures during speech and swallowing.
3. To protect the underlying fragile mucosa.
4. To direct the food bolus into the oropharynx.
5. To improve appearance and psychosocial adjustment.

[a]Adapted from Zaki.[58(p252)]

TABLE 11–13. Adjunctive Treatments to Improve Swallowing Following Partial Glossectomy[a]

1. Tilt head posteriorly if anterior-posterior tongue movement is impaired. This increases the speed of oral transit.

2. Tilt head to the side least affected to control movement of bolus.

3. Thermal stimulation may assist in activating the pharyngeal swallow by increasing sensation near the anterior faucial pillars.

4. Tongue palate contact exercises with specific placement goals may strengthen the posterior tongue movement or increase the range of posterior tongue motion.

5. Chewing exercises manipulating wet gauze or chewing gum to practice manipulating the bolus.

6. Practicing speech sounds such as /d/, /t/, /g/, and /k/ to improve range of motion of remaining structures.

[a]Adapted and updated from Gross and Eibling.[39(p258)]

role in the management of patients with swallowing disorders.

The following physical and environmental factors must be considered for the complete management of the dysphagic patient:

1. Balance—chair height or proper positioning in bed
2. Head support
3. Tray positioning
4. Adaptable syringes
5. Lighting
6. Plates and bowls—not breakable, with deep retaining walls
7. Adaptable utensils—custom-designed eating utensils
8. Handrails in kitchen and eating areas

SUMMARY

The goals of prosthetic management are to improve both speech and swallow function; restore esthetics to the head and neck areas; provide comfort in breathing, swallowing, and speaking; and improve

the quality of life. Therefore, prosthetic management offers an alternative to surgical management of defects following surgery, radiation, or chemotherapy for head and neck cancer in select patients. New materials, the use of dental implants, and reduced time frames in prosthetic management all provide the clinician with tools that contribute to swallow safety. Computer-assisted models using 3-dimensional CT scans provide the maxillofacial prosthodontist with the ability to shape prostheses more accurately at the first fitting. Ultimately, preoperative modeling may allow the prosthesis to be fitted directly after surgery, thus speeding up the rehabilitation process and improving the quality of life.

STUDY QUESTIONS

1. A paralyzed vocal fold may lead to
   A. Dysphonia
   B. Prandial aspiration
   C. Weak cough
   D. Atelectasis
   E. All of the above

2. Surgery for a patient with dysphagia and a paralyzed vocal fold would most likely be
   A. Botulinum toxin injection to the true vocal folds
   B. Vocal fold augmentation
   C. Palatal prosthesis
   D. Thyroplasty type 1

3. Improvement in chewing can best be accomplished by a
   A. Dental prosthesis
   B. Palatal prosthesis
   C. Nasal prosthesis
   D. Lingual prosthesis

4. Soft palate prostheses are designed primarily
   A. To improve nasopharynx approximation
   B. To reduce the distance between the palate and posterior tongue
   C. To strengthen the remainder of the soft palate
   D. To fill in the lateral walls of the oral cavity

5. The preferred surgical procedure to close the posterior glottis is

A. Vocal fold augmentation

B. Pharyngoplexy

C. Arytenoid adduction

D. Tracheotomy

REFERENCES

1. Conqueiro MM, Schramm A, Schoen R, et al. Speech and swallowing impairment after treatment for oral and oropharyngeal cancer. *Arch Otolaryngol Head Neck Surg.* 2008;134:1299–1304.

2. Pou A, Carrau RL, Eibling DE, Murry T. Laryngeal framework surgery for the management of aspiration in high vagal lesions. *Am J Otolaryngol.* 1998;19:1–7.

3. Carrau RL, Pou A, Eibling DE, Murry T, Ferguson BJ. Laryngeal framework surgery for the management of aspiration. *Head Neck.* 1999;21:139–145.

4. Lacoureye O, Paczona R, Ageel M, Hans S. et al. Intracordal autologous fat injection for aspiration after recurrent laryngeal nerve paralysis. *Eur Arch Otorhinolaryngol.* 1999;256:458–461.

5. Mastronikolis NS, Remacle M, Kiagiadaki D, Lawson G, Bachy V, Van Der Vorst S. Medialization thyroplasty for voice restoration after transoral cordectomy. *Eur Arch Otorhinolaryngol.* 2013 Jul;270(7):2071–2078. doi:10.1007/s00405-013-2462-8.

6. Zeitels SM, Hillman RE, Desloge RB, Bunting GA. Cricothyroid subluxation: a new innovation for enhancing the voice with laryngo plastic phonosurgery. *Ann Otol Rhinol Laryngol.* 1999;108:1126–1131.

7. Zeitels SM, Hochman I, Hillman RE. Adduction arytenopexy: a new procedure for paralytic dysphonia with implications for implant medialization. *Ann Otol Rhinol Laryngol.* 1998;173(suppl):2–24.

8. Maragos NE. The posterior thyroplasty window: anatomical considerations. *Laryngoscope.* 1999;109:1228–1231.

9. Link DT, Rutter MJ, Liu JH, Willgiung JP. Pediatric type I thyroplasty: an evolving procedure. *Ann Otol Rhinol Laryngol.* 1999;108:1105–1110.

10. Perie S, Coifier L, Laccourreye L, Hazebroucq V, Chaussade S, St Guily JL. Swallowing disorders in paralysis of the lower cranial nerves: a functional analysis. *Ann Otol Rhinol Laryngol.* 1999;108:606–611.

11. Shama L, Connor NP, Ciucci MR, McCulloch TM. Surgical treatment of dysphagia. *Phys Med Rehabil Clin North Am.* 2008 Nov;19(4):817–835, ix.

12. Sulica L, Rosen CA, Postma GN, Simpson B, Amin M, Courey M, Merati A. Current practice in injection augmentation of the vocal folds: indications, treatment principles, techniques, and complications. *Laryngoscope.* 2010 Feb;120(2):319–325.

13. Damrose EJ. Percutaneous injection laryngoplasty in the management of acute vocal fold paralysis. *Laryngoscope.* 2010 Aug;120(8):1582–1590.

14. Andrews RJ, Netterville JL, Mercati AL. Laryngeal framework surgery: medialization laryngoplasty. In: Carrau RL, Murry T, eds. *Comprehensive Management of Swallowing Disorders.* San Diego, CA: Plural Publishing; 2006:291–296.

15. Hendricker RM, deSilva BW, Forrest LA. Gore-Tex medialization laryngoplasty for treatment of dysphagia. *Otolaryngol Head Neck Surg.* 2010 Apr;142(4):536–539.

16. Newman TR, Hengesteg A, Lepage RP, Kaufman KR, Woodson GE. Three-dimensional motion of the arytenoid adduction procedure in cadaver larynges. *Ann Otol Rhinol Laryngol.* 1994;103:265–270.

17. Mok P, Woo P, Schaefer-Mojica J. Hypopharyngeal pharyngoplasty in the management of pharyngeal paralysis: a new procedure. *Ann Otol Rhinol Laryngol.* 2003 Oct;112(10):844–852.

18. Ferreira LE, Simmons DT, Baron TH. Zenker's diverticula: pathophysiology, clinical presentation, and flexible endoscopic management. *Dis Esophagus.* 2008;21(1):1–8.

19. Oh TH, Brumfield KA, Hoskin TL, Kasperbauer JL, Basford JR. Dysphagia in inclusion body myositis: clinical features, management, and clinical outcome. *Am J Phys Med Rehabil.* 2008 Nov;87(11):883–889.

20. Lang RA, Spelsberg FW, Winter H, Jauch KW, Hüttl TP. Transoral diverticulostomy with a modified Endo-Gia stapler: results after 4 years of experience. *Surg Endosc.* 2007 Apr;21(4):532–536 [Epub 2006 Dec 20].

21. Jacobs JR, Logemann J, Pajak TF, Pauloski BR, Collins S, Casiano RR. Failure of cricopharyngeal myotomy to improve dysphagia following head and neck cancer surgery. *Arch Otolaryngol Head Neck Surg.* 1999;125:942–946.

22. Pou A. Cricopharyngeal myotomy. In: Carrau RL, Murry T, eds. *Comprehensive Management of Swallowing Disorders.* San Diego, CA: Plural Publishing; 2006:305–308.

23. Alberty J, Oelerich M, Ludwig K, Hartmann S, Stoll W. Efficacy of Botulinum toxin A for treatment of upper esophageal sphincter dysfunction. *Laryngoscope.* 2000;110:1151–1156.

24. Ashan SE, Meleca RJ, Dworkin JP. Botulinum toxin injection of the cricopharyngeal muscle for the treatment of dysphagia. *Otolaryngol Head Neck Surg.* 2000;22:691–695.

25. Netterville JL. Palatal adhesion/pharyngeal flap. In Carrau RL, Murry T, eds. *Comprehensive Management of Swallowing Disorders.* San Diego, CA: Singular Publishing; 1999:309–312.

26. Tang SJ, Singh S, Truelson JM. Endotherapy for severe and complete pharyngo-esophageal post-radiation stenosis using wires, balloons and pharyngo-esophageal puncture. *Surg. Endosc.* 2010 Jan;24(1):210–214.

27. Nguyen NP, Smith HJ, Moltz CC, et al. Prevalence of pharyngeal and esophageal stenosis following radiation for head and neck cancer. *J Otolaryngol Head Neck Surg.* 2008 Apr;37(2):219–224.

28. Snyderman CH. Laryngeal closure. In: Carrau RL, Murry T, eds. *Comprehensive Management of Swallowing Disorders*. San Diego, CA: Plural Publishing; 2006:313–320.

29. Takano Y, Suga M, Sakamoto O, et al. Satisfaction of patients treated surgically for intractable aspiration. *Chest*. 1999;116:1251–1256.

30. Qu SH, Li M, Liang JP, Su ZZ, Chen SQ, He XG. Laryngotracheal closure and cricopharyngeal myotomy for intractable aspiration and dysphagia secondary to cerebrovascular accident. *ORL J Otorhinolaryngol Relat Spec*. 2009;71(6):299–304 [Epub 2009 Nov 24].

31. Klor BM, Milianti FJ. Rehabilitation of neurogenic dysphagia with percutaneous endoscopic gastrostomy. *Dysphagia*. 1999;14:162–164.

32. Nakajoh K, Nakagawa K, Sekizawa T, Arai MH, Sasaki H. Relation between incidence of pneumonia and protective reflexes in post-stroke patients with oral or tube feeding. *J Int Med*. 2000;247:19–42.

33. Finucane TE, Christmas C, Travis K. Tube feeding in patients with advanced dementia. A review of the evidence. *JAMA*. 1999;282:1365–1370.

34. McCann R. Lack of evidence about tube feeding—food for thought. *JAMA*. 1999;282(14):1380–1381.

35. James A, Kapur K, Hawthorne AB. Long-term outcome of percutaneous endoscopic gastrostomy feeding in patients with dysphagic stroke. *Age Aging*. 1998;27:671–676.

36. Rehman HU, Knox J. There is a need for a regular review of swallowing ability in patients after PEG insertion to identify patients with delayed recovery of swallowing. Letter to the Editor. *Dysphagia*. 2000;15:48.

37. Leder SB, Ross DA. Investigation of the causal relationship between tracheotomy and aspiration in the acute care setting. *Laryngoscope*. 2000;110:641–644.

38. Eibling DE, Carrau RL. Tracheotomy. In: Carrau RL, Murry T, eds. *Comprehensive Management of Swallowing Disorders*. San Diego, CA: Plural Publishing; 2006:265–278.

39. Gross RD, Eibling DE. Passy-Muir valve/decannulation. In: Carrau RL, Murry T, eds. *Comprehensive Management of Swallowing Disorders*. San Diego, CA: Plural Publishing; 2006:255–262.

40. Irish J, Sandhu N, Simpson C, et al. Quality of life in patients with maxillectomy prostheses. *Head Neck*. 2009; 31(6):813–821.

41. Liedberg B, Norten P, Owall B, Stoltze K. Masticatory and nutritional aspects of fixed and removeable partial dentures. *Clin Oral Invest*. 2004;8:11–17.

42. Hattori F. The relationship between wearing complete dentures and swallowing function in elderly individuals: a videofluorographic study. *Kokubyo Gakkai Zasshi*. 2004;71;102–111.

43. Muller F, Schadler M, Wahlmann U, Newton JP. The use of implant supported prostheses in the functional and psychosocial rehabilitation of tumor patients. *Int J Prosthodont*. 2004;17(5):512–517.

44. Teoh KH, Patel S, Hwang F, Huryn JM, Verbel D, Zlotolow IM. Prosthetic intervention in the era of microvascular reconstruction of the mandible—a retrospective analysis of functional outcome. *Int J Prosthodont*. 2005 Jan–Feb; 18(1):42–54.

45. Eguia del Valle A, Martinez-Condo Llamosas R, López Vicente J, et al. Primary oral squamous cell carcinoma arising around dental osseointegrated implants mimicking peri-implantitis. *Med Oral Patol Oral Cir Bucal*. 2008; 13:489–491.

46. Kwok J, Eyeson J, Thompson I, McGurk M. Dental implants and squamous cell carcinoma in the at-risk patient: report of three cases. *Br Dent J*. 2008;205:543–545.

47. Wheeler R, Logemann JA, Rosen M. Maxillary reshaping prostheses: effectiveness in improving speech and swallowing of post surgical oral cancer patients. *J Prosthet Dent*. 1980; 43:313–319.

48. Ortegon SM, Martin JW, Lewin JS. A hollow delayed surgical obturator for a bilateral subtotal maxillectomy patient: a clinical report. *J Prosthet Dent*. 2008;99:14–18.

49. Depprich RA, Handaschel JG, Meyer U, Meissner G. Comparison of prevalence of microorganisms on titanium and silicone/polyethyl methacrylate obturators used for rehabilitation of maxillary defects. *J Prosthet Dent*. 2008;99:400–405.

50. Shifman A, Finkelstein Y, Nachmani A, Ophir D. Speech-aid prostheses for neurogenic velopharyngeal incompetence. *J Prosthet Dent*. 2000;83(1):99–106.

51. Suwaki M, Nanba K, Ito E, Kumakkura I, Minagi S. The effect of nasal speaking valve on the speech under experimental velopharyngeal incompetence condition. *J Oral Rehabil*. 2008;35(5):361–369.

52. Suwaki M, Nanba K, Ito E, Kumakkura I, Mingi S. Nasal speaking valve: a device for managing velopharyngeal incompetence. *J Oral Rehabil*. 2008 Jan;35(1):73–78.

53. Kreeft AM, Van der Molen L, Hilgers FJ, Balm AJ. Speech and swallowing after surgical treatment of advanced oral and oropharyngeal carcinoma: a systematic review of the literature. *Eur Arch Otorhinolaryngol*. 2009;266: 1687–1698.

54. Reiger JM, Zalmanowitz JG, Li SY, et al. Functional outcomes after surgical reconstruction of the base of tongue using a radial forearm free flap in patients with oropharyngeal carcinoma. *Head Neck*. 2007;29:1024–1032.

55. Zuydam AC, Lowe D, Brown JS, Vaughan ED, Rogers SN. Predictors of speech and swallowing function following primary surgery for oral and oropharyngeal cancer. *Clin Otolaryngol*. 2007;30:428–437.

56. Furia CLB, Kowalski LP, Latoarre MD, et al. Speech intelligibility after glossectomy and speech rehabilitation. *Arch Otolaryngol Head Neck Surg*. 2001;127:877–883.

57. Leonard R, Gillis R. Effects of a prosthetic tongue on vowel intelligibility and food management in a patient with total glossectomy. *J Speech Hear Dis*. 1982;47:25–32

58. Zaki HS. Dental prosthetics. In: Carrau RL, Murry T, eds. *Comprehensive Management of Swallowing Disorders*. San Diego, CA: Plural Publishing. 2006:249–255.

Case Studies

A Look at the Chapter

In this chapter, the authors present a series of cases in which the key members of the swallowing team, the speech-language pathologist and the otolaryngologist, work together to improve the patient's quality of life. Since swallowing involves the organs of mastication, articulation, phonation, and respiration, the case studies address the functions of these systems as they relate to swallowing. Often, they also involve the vocal folds and cases are presented where it is equally important to address vocal fold function. First, we present the basic needs of a comprehensive swallowing center. This information is valuable to students, clinicians, and administrators who are planning to develop new comprehensive swallowing centers. This is followed by case studies with examples of how different members of the swallowing center are involved in the management of swallowing disorders.

INTRODUCTION

Swallowing relies on the muscles of the head, neck, and respiratory muscles. When swallowing disorders are suspected, the clinician often encounters patients with concerns about their voice and their breathing. The lips, tongue, teeth, nasopharynx, velopharynx, oropharynx, and larynx and respiratory system are all involved in swallowing as well as speaking. Swallowing requires the manipulation of food in the oral cavity followed by transmission to the esophagus while protecting the airway by closing the vocal folds. Speech and voice production require use of many of the same neuromuscular systems to accomplish communication. Anatomically, physiologically, and functionally, there is a significant overlap between the production of speech, voice, and swallowing functions. Clinicians who treat disorders of swallowing should have specific knowledge of the structures and their

functions as they relate to breathing, speech, and voice production.

From a practical point of view, there are many reasons for unifying the personnel and facilities to manage swallowing disorders. Those with expertise in swallowing and voice disorders often staff a comprehensive swallowing center. Patients in a comprehensive swallowing center can express their needs regarding swallowing disorders and also about concerns about their speech or voice to individuals who have a keen interest and understanding of the entire problem. The development of a comprehensive center that brings together those who have a special interest and expertise in the diagnosis and treatment of problems affecting the organs of swallowing, voice, and breathing eliminates the need for a patient to travel from place to place to address these concerns.

The concept of a comprehensive swallowing center is not new. The management of speech, voice, and swallowing disorders in patients with head and neck cancer dates back over 100 years ago when the first laryngectomy was reported by Billroth and Gussenbauer in 1874, and reviewed by Fasching[1] who also included a report of fitting a patient with a pneumatic artificial larynx. This device introduced sound into the pharynx through a surgically created fistula. Although the fistula aided the patient in communication, it also reduced the propelling force associated with swallowing and was eventually abandoned. However, since that time, the emphasis on postsurgical rehabilitation of swallowing and communication has been reflected in the advent of numerous surgical procedures designed to preserve voice and speech after head and neck cancer followed by rehabilitation by speech-language pathologists, physical and occupational therapists, and dietitians. This group of specialists staff a comprehensive voice and swallowing center.

The modern era of dysphagia management began with the publication of Logemann's text on the evaluation and treatment of swallowing disorders in 1983.[2] In that early work, clinicians were introduced to the importance of diagnosing and treating swallowing problems that arose from surgical procedures to treat head and neck cancers, as well as neurological events such as stroke and degenerative neuromuscular diseases.

Many of the current conservative surgical procedures, as well as the organ preservation protocols requiring radiation and chemoradiation to treat cancer of the head and neck, alter the natural swallowing patterns or compound the preexisting problems of speech and swallowing.

Moreover, organ preservation procedures may also contribute to voice and/or speech disorders such as hoarseness, vocal weakness, disrupted resonance, and dysarthria. The state-of-the-art comprehensive swallowing center is composed of a team that understands the anatomy and physiology of the organs of the speech, voice, and swallowing mechanisms, the physiology of swallowing and brings together a unified program to maximize recovery of communication and swallowing functions.

In this chapter, the organization of a voice and swallowing center is described. The functional basis for a specialized voice and swallowing center will be shown with case studies of typical patients seen by the specialists in the center. In addition, the diagnostic equipment and space needed to maintain a functional voice and swallowing center are presented.

DIAGNOSIS

The oral cavity, pharynx, and larynx share the responsibility and burden of channeling expiratory airflow and voice upward and outward and propelling foods, liquids, and medications downward into the esophagus and stomach. Because of this shared passage, speech-language pathologists (SLPs) and otolaryngologists who are both uniquely trained in the anatomy, physiology, and neurology of the head, neck, and upper aerodigestive tract are ideal professionals to develop and lead the team in the management of patients with swallowing, voice, and speech problems. The SLPs who treat swallowing problems in head and neck cancer patients are usually trained to treat voice and speech disorders in these patients. SLPs who treat language and speech disorders in the acute and long-term stroke and neu-rologically disordered populations are also involved in the treatment of swallowing disorders. Regardless of the underlying condition, the role of the SLP is to assess the patient's functional communication needs and safety of swallowing.

Once the assessment is made, the SLP and the otolaryngologist propose a plan of rehabilitation to the patient that may include pre- and postoperative treatments, cognitive therapy, and/or voice therapy.

The personnel of the swallowing center work together with the patient to achieve a safe and functional swallow and maximize the patient's communication needs to improve overall quality of life.

The important elements for the SLP to consider include the conditions at the onset of the problem, prior illnesses (including those related to birth or occurring at birth), genetic or inherited disorders and diseases, and the patient's family history of diseases, especially those related to the current condition. Currently prescribed and over-the-counter medications should also be noted as well as the patient's prior level of function. Rehabilitation specialists should remember that treatment of swallowing requires a general level of cognition that allows the patient to follow commands, some of which may be complex. For infants and children with swallowing problems, psychologists, occupational therapists, and cognitive specialists may be involved to facilitate the patient's needs.

The role of the otolaryngologist is to conduct a comprehensive head and neck examination, to recommend special tests, and to propose and manage medical or surgical intervention. The oral-motor assessment examines the motor functions of the cranial nerves involved in swallowing, and the ability of the vocal folds to function in voice production and swallowing. Specific tests of voice and swallowing are done by the otolaryngologist and with other team members of the swallowing center as discussed in Chapters 5 and 9. Special tests such as magnetic resonance imaging or pulmonary function tests may be ordered by the otolaryngologist or neurologist and reviewed by the swallowing team.

The SLP who treats swallowing disorders must have an understanding of the cranial nerve functions. He or she must also recommend and conduct the proper tests and, along with the other members of the treatment team, offer a plan of rehabilitation. Table 12–1 summarizes major conditions and disorders routinely seen in a comprehensive swallowing center. Some of these conditions are primarily related to swallowing disorders, while others may be initially related to voice, speech, and airway disorders. A coordinated treatment team whose members understand that speech and swallowing disorders may require specialized treatment ideally sees patients for all of these related conditions.

The members of a comprehensive swallowing center determine the diagnosis and develop a plan of treatment using the patient's complaints and the documentation from proper examinations, such as laryngeal imaging during swallowing or results of radiological studies of swallowing.

The rehabilitation specialists (occupational therapist, speech-language pathologist, physical therapist) must obtain the medical diagnosis prior to treatment for swallowing, speech, and/or voice disorders. The otolaryngologist, neurologist, or the pediatric otolaryngologist make the diagnosis and rely on the combined test results and the patient's history.

Prior to instrumental assessment or imaging, the clinician will want to document the patient's problems using case history information and appropriate self-assessment tools whenever possible. During the bedside assessment, trial swallows may be given to observe patient behaviors. Proper tests, either the flexible endoscopic evaluation of swallowing (FEES) or modified barium swallow, may be selected based on the trial swallows. Thus, diagnosis in the state-of-the-art swallowing center will include the use of patient self-assessment tools such as those listed in the Appendices or perhaps special tests of motor speech functions.

INSTRUMENTATION

Special diagnostic and treatment equipment play an important role in the swallowing center. Specifically, systems that allow the visualization of the upper aerodigestive tract structures under dynamic conditions guide clinicians in making the diagnosis

TABLE 12–1. Common Conditions, Disorders, and Diseases That May Have Components of Speech, Voice, and Swallowing Disorders

Vocal fold paralysis	Laryngopharyngeal reflux
Vocal fold paresis	Gastroesophageal reflux
Superior laryngeal nerve paralysis	Dehydration
Vocal fold atrophy	Long-term intubation
Bilateral vocal fold paralysis	Tracheostomy
Chronic cough	Medications
Shortness of breath	Early postradiation dysphagia
Parkinson disease	Long-term radiation dysphagia
Cerebral vascular accident	Lingual, oral, and oropharyngeal cancers
Amyotrophic lateral sclerosis	Larynx preservation surgeries
Myasthenia gravis	Benign tumors of the head and neck
Vocal fold granuloma	Autism
Mental retardation	Autoimmune diseases

and developing treatment plans. Transnasal flexible laryngoscopy (TFL) with a video camera attached to allow recording is used for the assessment of the nasopharynx, oropharynx, and larynx. The larynx and vocal folds may be observed during breathing, speaking, swallowing, and other vegetative activities during a TFL examination. TFL with video recording allows the clinician to perform and review FEES examinations with the patient as well as to archive the exams for comparison after treatment.

Videostrobolaryngoscopy (VSL) with video recording is also a key instrument in the voice and swallowing center. VSL provides the clinician with a tool to observe the vocal folds under stroboscopic light for the purpose of assessing vocal fold movement, closure, and symmetry, all of which can have an effect on swallowing. Some clinics may also employ a high-speed digital imaging video recording system, a relatively new tool for the diagnostician to examine details of vocal fold vibration. Recording at speeds of 2000 frames per second and above, high-speed imaging captures the real-time motion of the vocal folds.

A typical scenario in a swallowing center may begin with a patient coming with a complaint of "something sticking in my throat and occasional hoarseness." Following a detailed case history, the FEES examination may be the appropriate starting point. Likely, the patient will have significant laryngeal edema and erythema. If the remainder of the FEES examination is normal, one possible initial treatment is medication for the edema and erythema. If the patient is also complaining of pain or regurgitation, an esophagram may be ordered at that time. Following the FEES exam, medical treatment can begin while the esophagram is being done. Depending on the results of the esophagram and if swallowing and hoarseness are still complaints, the team may wish to combine a FEES examination with a videofluoroscopic swallow study (VFSS) or a stroboscopic (VSL) examination depending on the specific complaint. Based on the diagnosis, treatment by the SLP as well as continued follow-up by the otolaryngologist may be ordered. Both team members working in the same center will usually have access to each other's records as well as the records of others involved in the diagnosis, through electronic medical records. The likelihood of complete communication is enhanced in a comprehensive swallowing and voice center. A video record and clinical notes that are maintained in an efficient archiving system allow all members of the treatment team to review the patient's progress and plan further treatment, if necessary, during subsequent visits.

Many swallowing centers now offer a transnasal esophagoscopy (TNE), a procedure to examine the esophagus and entrance to the stomach for esophageal disorders. This procedure described by Bush and Postma provides a look into the esophagus without the need for sedation or radiation.[3]

Acoustic analysis systems may also be used by swallowing specialists when there is a need to assess speech intelligibility, speech amplitude, or rate of speaking. Although these systems are used more commonly for primary complaints of voice and speech disorders, patients with many of the disorders listed in Table 12–1 may eventually require treatment for speech and/or voice problems once the swallowing problem has been diagnosed and treated, allowing the patient to have a safe swallow. These systems allow the clinician to obtain a baseline measure of all aspects related to the organs of swallowing.

Analysis of airflow and air pressure is reserved primarily for problems related to the voice; however, the same measures may also be important in assessing vocal fold closure, improving vocal fold closure, and monitoring breathing function during swallowing. Subsequent measurements of these parameters should be documented as the patient progresses in rehabilitation. Martin-Harris and colleagues[4] described a system for observing and recording apnea during swallowing. Observations of the respiratory patterns provide an understanding of the coordination of the respiratory and phonatory systems during swallowing.

> *Other systems such as those described by Pitts et al[5] and Laciuga et al[7] are now well known to improve both swallowing and vocalization.*

Electromyography (EMG) is becoming more important in the diagnosis and treatment of swallowing and voice disorders. Although it is not critical to have

EMG equipment available in the voice and swallowing center, its availability eliminates the need for a second trip to a specialist's office. With EMG in the office and a consulting neurologist available, information regarding nerve function can be obtained during the same visit, avoiding further delays to the start of treatment.

PERSONNEL

The development of a voice and swallowing center brings together specialists who have a special interest in the speech and swallowing organs and expertise in the diagnosis and treatment of problems affecting these organs. SLPs who are engaged in the diagnosis and treatment of voice and swallowing disorders should maintain contact with the American Speech-Language-Hearing Association's Special Interest Divisions 3 and 13. Each division offers special courses at the organization's annual convention as well as maintains websites with access to resources, special programs, and continuing education. In the United States, not all SLPs treat swallowing or voice disorders on a regular basis. In some countries, the SLP is considered the voice therapist or phoniatrician, the voice clinician, or the dysphagia therapist, indicating special training or extensive expertise in these areas. The American Academy of Otolaryngology-Head and Neck Surgery has a speech and swallowing subcommittee to monitor regulations and propose standards to improve patient safety and clinical compliance with existing diagnostic and treatment codes. Many of the otolaryngologists who are fellowship trained in voice often provide the medical and surgical leadership of the comprehensive swallowing center. Students (both speech-language pathology and medical) are encouraged to observe in a swallowing clinic.

> *Nothing is as valuable as shared real-time experience.*
>
> —*Anonymous*

In a comprehensive swallowing center, communication between clinicians and patient and among clinicians is ongoing and direct. Using this clinical service delivery model, the key members are in close proximity and interact in the testing and treatment phases of patient care. The rationale for having all specialists in close proximity is that individuals with different professional backgrounds can see the same patient, conduct their tests and assessments within the same day, and communicate the results to each other without delay. The nonsurgical therapeutic aspects of swallowing disorders provide unparalleled continuity of care for the patient if all of the specialists are "in the loop." The digital or analog media of a particular swallowing examination allows all members of the therapeutic team to see the same examination but attend to different aspects as they relate to the presenting symptoms. Having the specialists in close proximity adds to efficient use of everyone's time, especially the patient's, and allows for shared real-time experiences during and after the examination.

Physicians and other health care professionals with specific areas of expertise in swallowing in addition to an understanding of the neurophysiology of swallowing are integral to the comprehensive care of patients seen in a swallowing center. In particular, the following physician specialties are necessary: gastroenterology, pulmonology, neurology, psychiatry, and radiology. In addition to the SLP, other nonphysician health care professionals are also vitally important to deliver complete care to patients with voice and swallowing disorders. They include nurses, registered dieticians, physical therapists, occupational therapists, and social workers.

FACILITIES

A defined space is necessary to house the medical and rehabilitation staff and the special equipment used by the individuals involved in the management of patients with swallowing disorders. Treatment rooms should be well lit and have a decor that fits the mission of the center. The waiting area and treatment rooms should be designed for patient comfort. Reading materials or brochures that focus on voice, communication, and swallowing should be available in the waiting areas. These may be obtained from the American Speech-Language-Hearing Association and from the Academy of Otolaryngology-Head and Neck Surgery.

Rooms should be large enough to accommodate the specialists, the patients, and significant others as well as consultants who will come to participate in specific portions of the examinations. Although the swallowing center is usually located in a medical setting, the need for patient comfort and convenience of a treatment center should not be overlooked.

CASE STUDIES FROM VOICE AND SWALLOWING CENTERS

It is not always obvious to a patient or to the referring internist if the patient's underlying problem will involve treatment for swallowing only or for the speech and voice problems that may coexist. The value of a comprehensive swallowing center to the referring physician is that she or he will know that by referring the patient to a place where a group of individuals have expertise in both areas, the diagnostic workup will be comprehensive. The clinicians will evaluate the patient's complaints and suggest an orderly treatment approach. The internist will not have to find additional resources and will only need to maintain contact with one group. The following cases are common examples of the types of patients seen in a comprehensive swallowing center.

Parkinson's Disease

Parkinson's disease provides an excellent example of a medical condition that illustrates the value of a center where dysphagia, voice, and communication disorders are managed. A neurologist usually refers these patients because either changes in the voice or difficulty swallowing certain food consistencies, usually solid foods, are the symptoms. Over time, the patients with Parkinson's disease develop vocal weakness, dysarthria, and ultimately begin to cough and choke when swallowing. The patient often reports a change in her or his voice coinciding with the diagnosis of Parkinson's disease, but may not notice changes in swallowing other than an increase in throat clearing, excess mucus, globus sensation,

and increased cough. However, on questioning, they may note that the cough is more pronounced after eating lunch and dinner. If the Reflux Symptom Index (RSI) is used, it is usually above normal and the Voice Handicap Index and the Voice Handicap Index-10 may also be above normal.[8,9] Weight loss may be reported.

The patient is a 55-year-old male with a 2-year history of Parkinson's disease. He reported a history of vocal weakness to his primary care physician. Based on the patient's symptoms of choking, weak cough, voice change, dysphagia, coughing after meals and his EAT-10 score of 35, a FEES examination was appropriate. In some centers, this is done by the SLP; in others, the otolaryngologist does it. After increased difficulty in talking and then several months later experiencing dysarthria and choking on liquids, his primary physician referred him to a neurologist who diagnosed Parkinson's disease and referred him to the swallowing and voice center. His primary complaint at that first visit was related to his voice. Because of the diagnosis, the complaint of both voice and swallowing, the FEES exam was administered. Figure 12–1 was taken after swallowing a bolus consisting of a cracker. Evidence of the remaining bolus is present along with secretions,

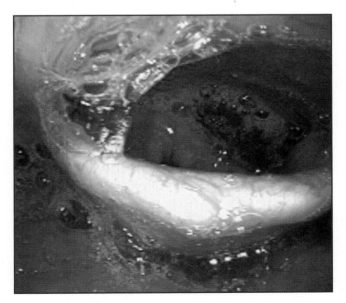

FIGURE 12–1. Patient with diagnosis of Parkinson's disease. The examination photo was taken after eating a small piece of cracker coated with green food coloring. The patient noted that he swallowed it completely but coughed afterward.

which the patient did not report feeling prior to the test. Video 1–3 is a FEES examination of a patient with a history of dysphagia. Note that the bolus fails to completely pass into the esophagus. The problem is due to weakness in the muscles. The patient was prescribed a proton-pump inhibitor (PPI), referred to the SLP for swallowing and voice therapy to improve vocal fold closure and manage the dysarthria. The SLP also recommended following solid foods with a sip of water ("liquid wash-down"). The Lee Silverman Voice Treatment, a special voice therapy for patients with Parkinson's disease,[10] was also discussed and treatment recommended.

Video 3–5 is a FEES examination of a patient with advanced Parkinson's disease. Note the sluggish movements, the attempts of laryngeal elevation, and eventually the penetration that begins to

occur. Video 12–1 is an example of a patient with early Parkinson's disease reporting the feeling of food remaining in his throat. He shows slow upper esophageal opening (UES). Note how the bolus moves in almost slow motion compared to the normal subject in Video 1–2.

In Chapter 6, we introduced expiratory muscle strength training (EMST). This exercise technique involves exhaling against a resistance, usually a small device containing some type of resistance. Although it has been used mostly for improving speech, several investigations have suggested that it has promise for improving swallowing as well. Rationale for the use of strength training was outlined by Burkhead et al[11] and suggests that strength training will increase functional muscle reserve, stimulate recruitment of additional motor units, and prepare the swallow organs for the rapid series of events that will follow. Given that the patients with Parkinson's disease have both a slow-acting neuromuscular system and weakness in that action, strength training may be a reasonable approach to improving both swallowing and voice in these patients.

Video 12–2 shows a patient with Parkinson's disease who is being treated with breathing exercises using a breath trainer. Note the early penetration and aspiration and then the cough that helps to clear the aspirate material.

The visit to a voice and swallowing center by a patient with Parkinson's disease enables clinicians to maximize the value of the patient's visit and diag-

nose and offer a comprehensive plan of treatment for the major problems of voice and swallowing in one visit. The otolaryngologist and the SLP send one report back to the referring physician that includes the results of the history, medical examination, test outcomes, and treatment plans.

The organization of swallowing and voice specialists under one roof facilitates a comprehensive diagnostic examination followed by a plan for the necessary treatments. There is no need for time-consuming referrals, loss of valuable examination data, or confusion about who is treating what aspect of the problem.

Cough and Hoarseness

Cough is a common complaint of patients seen by an otolaryngologist. The patient may associate the cough with eating, talking, or no specific activity. When the cough is related to mealtimes, the personnel at a comprehensive swallowing center are knowledgeable and equipped to treat the patient. The referring physician can feel assured that by referring the patient to a comprehensive center, the issues related to swallowing, coughing, and hoarseness will be addressed.

RC is a 48-year-old attorney who reported increased throat clearing and cough following surgery for gall bladder removal. At first, he noted a raspy voice, but then his cough increased. The cough happened mostly when talking, although more recently, the cough was occurring when he swallowed liquids and even at random times. His family physician prescribed an antacid that did not improve the cough or the voice after 4 weeks. Initially, he was sent for a modified barium swallow at an outpatient center. The report was normal swallow with no penetration or aspiration on any of the consistencies. His physician then referred him to a comprehensive swallowing center. His VHI-10 was 16, above the normal value, and his RSI was 18, also above normal. Notable also was the rating of 5 for hoarseness on the RSI. Given that his symptoms were related to his voice and also to his swallowing, the FEES was selected as the diagnostic test of choice.

Figure 12–2 shows the vocal folds of the 48-year-old male attorney. A left vocal process granuloma

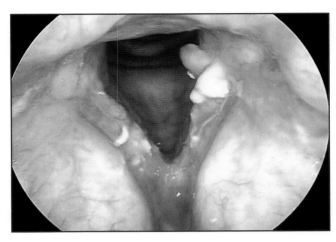

FIGURE 12–2. Vocal folds of a patient with left vocal process granuloma. The white areas seen may be related to the extensive use of antibiotics, which were prescribed prior to his current examination.

was diagnosed. The FEES was administered by the ENT and SLP and revealed normal swallow followed by throat clearing. When given several consistencies of foods to swallow—applesauce, cracker, and an apple—he showed no penetration, no aspiration, and no obvious delay or residual bolus in the piriform sinus or valleculae. The FEES was reported as normal swallow function.

The patient was diagnosed with a vocal process granuloma, chronic inflammation, and laryngopharyngeal reflux (LPR) (see Figure 12–2). The results of the diagnosis and plan of treatment were sent to the referring physician. At the first visit, he was asked to go on voice rest for a 5-day period since he was nearly aphonic. A modified diet eliminating highly acid liquids and foods (caffeine, chocolate, alcohol, pepper, spicy foods, mints, and carbonated beverages) was also started.

Based on the findings of the FEES and the Reflux Finding Score (RFS) (Appendix 2), the patient's antacid medicine was stopped and a PPI was prescribed twice daily, to be taken 30 to 60 minutes before breakfast and dinner. Because of his hoarseness, he was also referred to the SLP for vocal hygiene and voice therapy. The SLP saw him 4 times beginning after his voice rest period, working mostly on reducing the hard glottal onset in his speaking pattern and counseling him as to temporary diet and lifestyle changes necessary to treat the vocal fold

granuloma and the laryngopharyngeal reflux. This included an increase in water consumption.

When he returned 3 months later, he noted that his coughing associated with talking was substantially reduced. His VHI-10 was now a 5. The vocal folds were examined via transnasal flexible laryngoscopy and the granuloma was no longer visualized. His FEES exam was normal with no penetration or aspiration. Figure 12–3 shows the vocal folds at the 3-month follow-up examination. He remained on the PPI medication once a day and continued with 4 additional therapy sessions.

Although this type of patient is often seen in the swallowing center, the diagnosis and treatment may not always be obvious. For example, a patient who initially seemed similar to the patient described in the previous paragraph was concerned about his increasing hoarseness, which had been present for 8 to 10 months. His wife noted that he often coughed, but it was primarily after eating or drinking or on waking up. An 8-pound weight loss over the past 6 months was reported. His internist referred him for evaluation of his voice. The SLP noted the presence of a nasal quality in his speech. A complete FEES was done. Figure 12–4 shows the result following the swallow of a nectar consistency. There was penetration to the level of the vocal folds. Based on

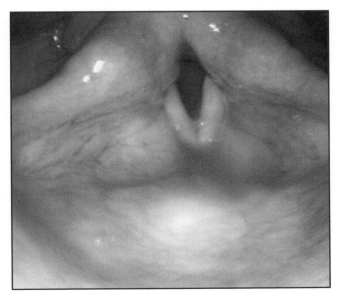

FIGURE 12–3. The vocal folds at 3-month follow-up of the patient with the vocal process granuloma.

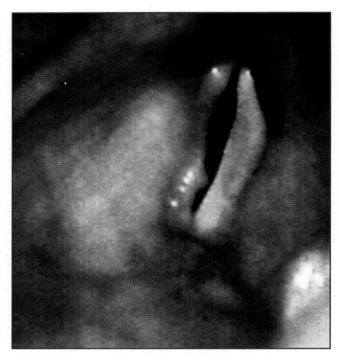

FIGURE 12–4. Patient with significant vocal fold edema and vocal fold atrophy. Note the food coloring down to the level of the vocal folds, indicating penetration of blue-colored water.

the results of the SLP (nasal speech quality) and the swallowing examination (penetration), this patient was sent for a neurological consultation. He was ultimately diagnosed with amyotrophic lateral sclerosis (ALS). This case points out the importance of obtaining a thorough case history, selecting the proper examinations and knowing the signs and symptoms of related neurological diseases and then consulting other specialists when there is a need for more answers.

In this case, the multiple findings obtained by the SLP and ENT combined to suggest a neurological disorder, specifically ALS. The neurologist confirmed the diagnosis, and the patient was referred back to the SLP for treatment of his swallowing and referred to the ALS self-help group located in the city.

Zenker Diverticulum

A 64-year-old man in otherwise good health complained to his primary physician of occasional hoarseness, throat clearing, occasional burping, recently a "gurgling" sound in his throat, and often the taste of food after swallowing. Following the case history and examination of the patient, the primary physician offered him a 4-week course of a popular PPI and dietary modifications. After 6 to 8 weeks, the problem had increased in severity, his hoarseness and throat clearing were more regular, and he indicated several episodes of regurgitation. The primary physician referred him to a voice and swallowing center, indicating in the referral letter that the patient was hoarse and not improving despite twice-daily PPI medication, a modest 7-pound weight loss, and discomfort due to the burping.

At the swallowing center, the patient completed the Reflux Symptom Index, scoring 31, and the Voice Handicap Index-10 with a score of 17 and the EAT-10 score of 12. Given the report from the family physician and the ratings of reflux and voice handicap index, it was decided to start the examination with a transnasal flexible laryngoscopy. On exposure of the larynx and vocal folds, there was clear evidence of regurgitation. Mucus was seen in the piriform sinus. A few sips of water were given to the patient. Although he swallowed all without penetration or aspiration, there were clear signs of regurgitation. At that point, the examination was ended, and the patient was sent for a barium esophagram to determine if a Zenker diverticulum was present. Figure 12–5 shows the radiographic view of the Zenker diverticulum. His PPI medication was resumed and increased to twice daily, 30 minutes before breakfast and dinner. Because of his hoarse voice quality, he was referred to the SLP for a program of vocal hygiene and voice therapy. Voice therapy was an appropriate referral, as this was his original complaint to his internist and continued to be a complaint of his at the swallowing center.

Ultimately, the patient was taken to surgery for a Zenker diverticulotomy and cricopharyngeal myotomy. His follow-up visit included a transnasal flexible laryngoscopy in which the piriform sinus areas were found to be clear of mucus. The noise associated with his swallow was also gone, and he no longer complained of regurgitation. His RSI was now 12. At a 6-month follow-up visit, the patient was experiencing no swallowing problems and only occasional hoarseness. His VHI-10 was a 3, and no further treatment was planned.

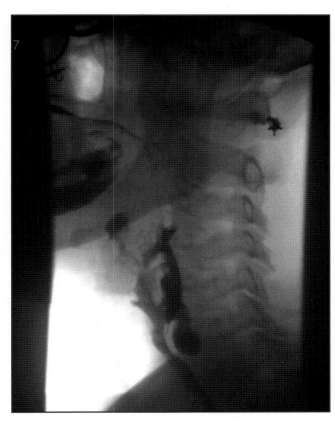

FIGURE 12–5. Radiographic image of Zenker diverticulum obtained during the barium esophagram.

Early Laryngeal Cancer

A 49-year-old male accountant was sent to a swallowing center by his family physician after a 4-month history of hoarseness, a 2-month history of throat pain while swallowing, and a 6-pound weight loss over the previous 3 months. He saw an otolaryngologist in his hometown who prescribed an antacid and suggested voice therapy for the hoarse voice quality. However, when the SLP conducted a thorough clinical history and review of his symptoms, she learned that he also complained of throat pain and difficulty swallowing grainy foods. His history revealed that he had smoked cigarettes for 15 years and quit 7 years ago. The SLP suggested that he seek a second opinion. He was referred to the Swallowing Center by the SLP. However, because the patient was very busy, he did not schedule the appointment immediately. In fact, it was 10 weeks after the first ENT visit before he was seen in the swallowing center.

In the center, it was decided to address the main complaint of hoarseness with a rigid strobovideolaryngoscopic examination following a review of his history and the VHI-10, which was 24. Video 12–3 shows the exam with the lesion on the right vocal fold. Significant edema was present, and a lesion was found on the right true vocal fold. Vocal fold motion was normal, as were abduction and adduction. A direct laryngoscopy and biopsy was scheduled, and a diagnosis of a T1 vocal fold cancer was made by the pathologist (Figure 12–6). The FEES exam was negative for penetration and aspiration, but the patient noted pain when swallowing a large cracker bolus. The patient opted for radiation therapy. He was also referred to the SLP for vocal hygiene counseling during the radiation treatment. Three weeks following treatment, he remained hoarse, with a VHI-10 of 11. He continued voice therapy sessions for 6 weeks. When he was seen in the voice and swallowing center 3 months after radiation treatment finished, the vocal folds were free of lesions. His VHI-10 was 4. He noted that he could now return to full-time practice without vocal fatigue or significant hoarseness. Regular follow-up examinations were scheduled in the swallowing center.

This case highlights the importance of the need for a comprehensive examination when a patient who is currently smoking or who has smoked in the past complains of hoarseness lasting more than 2 weeks. The SLP was correct in sending the patient back to his primary care doctor for a referral for a

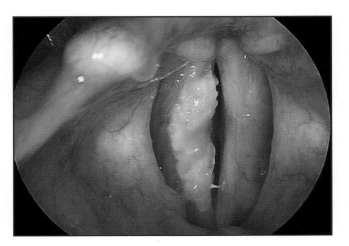

FIGURE 12–6. A 49-year-old male patient following biopsy of right true vocal fold. The diagnosis was T1 vocal fold cancer.

second opinion from a comprehensive swallowing and voice center. Small lesions on the vocal folds may not be apparent on direct observation. With the proper equipment to observe, record, and archive the examination, the otolaryngologist, the SLP, and the patient together can review the details of the examination and develop a plan of treatment without delay. In this case, there was considerable delay from the first visit to the internist followed by referral to an otolaryngologist, then the SLP, and finally the voice and swallowing center. Because of schedules and, to some extent, procrastination, it took nearly 3 months to obtain a definitive diagnosis.

Dysphagia and Vocal Fold Paralysis

The onset of vocal fold paralysis may follow surgery or may develop along with multiple neuropathies. The patient may complain of weak voice, vocal fatigue, difficulty swallowing, or occasional cough after swallowing. Figure 12–7 shows the vocal folds of a 67-year-old male with a 14-month history of vocal fatigue following coronary bypass surgery. Prior to his surgery, he spoke extensively as a trial lawyer. For the 3 months prior to his visit he reported an increase in coughing and occasional choking on liquids. He had been previously seen for 2 sessions of swallowing therapy in a rehabilitation center, which he noted had been helpful, but he still complained of vocal fatigue. His voice was

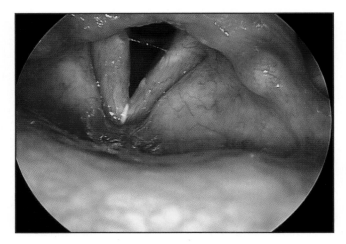

FIGURE 12–7. A 67-year-old male with a left vocal fold paralysis.

breathy and his maximum phonation time was 9.5 seconds. A modified barium swallow and a FEES test were done at previous institutions. Neither exam revealed penetration or aspiration, according to the written reports. He noted that when he was "careful," he could swallow small amounts of liquid without difficulty. During the current FEES examination, the patient also swallowed small amounts of liquids without difficulty; however, when challenged with repeated swallows, he began to cough. Trace amounts of liquid were seen at the level of the vocal folds. He indicated that on both previous tests, he was never challenged with repeated sips of liquid. Both previous tests were stopped after small amounts of liquid were swallowed successfully.

This patient was diagnosed with vocal fold paresis by the otolaryngologist. Because the patient had a weak voice and was experiencing aspiration, the recommended treatment for this patient was a vocal fold augmentation. This was done in the office with calcium hydroxyapatite. The goal was to increase his overall voice production and reduce penetration and aspiration through vocal fold approximation. Following his surgery, he reported improved swallowing and little or no coughing. He was seen for 4 sessions of swallowing therapy that included exercises to improve vocal fold closure and to continue to use safe swallowing techniques. Three months after surgery, his maximum phonation time increased to 15.5 seconds, and he was no longer coughing on liquids or solid food.

This case is an example of a team approach for both diagnosis and combined surgical and behavioral treatments. The SLP was part of the overall assessment process and realized that long-term voice or swallowing therapy would not be sufficient to treat the patient based on the findings of the voice and swallowing assessments. Following vocal fold augmentation, voice use improved and swallowing was no longer an issue for him.

Late Effects of Radiation Therapy in the Head and Neck Region

Radiation therapy (XRT) has been increasing in frequency for the treatment of cancer in the head and neck region. It is used as a single treatment in many cases, such as nasopharyngeal cancer, but it is more commonly used as a secondary treatment in other regions of the head and neck. During the course and for several weeks following radiation therapy, patients experience fatigue, mucositis, dysphagia, dysarthria, and dysphonia. This results in a decrease in quality of life following treatment. These changes are well known, and with adequate care, proper nutrition, and rest, recovery from the XRT treatment regimen slowly occurs. Of course, depending on whether or not surgery preceded the XRT, some problems related to swallowing and speech may remain for a lifetime. Video 12–4 shows a patient following radiation therapy for an oral pharyngeal cancer. Note the vocal folds and the lack of mobile tissue in the exam. He can no longer elevate the vocal folds due to the fibrosis effect of the radiation treatments

Recently, patients who have undergone XRT only for tumors of the oral cavity, larynx, and pharynx have been reporting increasing problems swallowing 3 to 5 years after successful treatment of their primary disease. Several studies have examined late effects of XRT. Suarez-Cunqueiro and colleagues[12] studied 851 patients and reported speech problems in 63.8%, and swallowing problems were reported by 75.4% of the group studied. The variables that presented a significant association with speech and swallowing impairment were gender, tumor location, stage of tumor, treatment modality, and reconstruction type. For patients who underwent XRT only, Langendijk[13] examined the later effects of treatment for various head and neck tumors and found that late radiation-induced toxicity, particularly in swallowing and xerostomia, have a significant impact on the more general dimensions of quality of life. These findings suggested that the development of new radiation-induced delivery techniques should focus on reduction of the dose not only to the salivary glands, but also to the anatomical structures that are involved in swallowing.

JW is a 65-year-old male who underwent radiation therapy for an early stage oral cancer tumor in 2006. He completed 30 sessions of radiation therapy over a 6-week period, a total of 70 cGy, considered a standard dose in the approximate period of time it usually takes for this amount of treatment. Over the course of treatment, he suffered minor mucosi-

tis and a 9-pound weight loss. His speech was only mildly distorted and gradually improved over the next 6 weeks. He maintained his nutrition on liquid supplements. Approximately 6 weeks following the completion of radiation therapy, he underwent a FEES examination that was reported to be normal, with no penetration or aspiration of liquids or foods. Eventually, JW went back to work as an accountant. He maintained his regular visits with his oncologist and his otolaryngologist at 6-month intervals. At 3 years postradiation, he was seen for a regular visit with his oncologist, who noted a 5-pound weight loss since his last visit. Also noted was excessive throat clearing. The patient reported that he was having some difficulty swallowing foods even when he chewed carefully. He completed the RSI, with a rating 14, and the EAT-10 with a score of 22, above the normal range and suggestive of laryngopharyngeal reflux. In addition, he was given the MDADI (see Chapter 5) and the results showed that his swallowing was having an impact on his quality of life. He subsequently was seen by his otolaryngologist and following a comprehensive head and neck examination, a FEES examination was ordered. When the SLP and the otolaryngologist saw him for the FEES examination, there was mild dysarthria (distortions of /k, g, l, r/, and posterior vowels). His cough was strong and his voice was loud but he remained with severe hoarseness and moderately severe breathiness. Figure 12–8 shows a still photo of the exam following a 10-cc bolus of honey-thickened liquid. The FEES examination was interpreted as penetration, minimal aspiration followed by a cough, and pooling of the material in the piriform sinus and the valleculae. On 4 subsequent swallows, a chin tuck, a Mendelsohn maneuver, a head tilt backward, and a smaller bolus were tried. Only the Mendelsohn maneuver improved the swallow, showing less residual material in the piriform sinus with 2 swallows. A subsequent CT scan failed to identify additional cancer, and JW was told that he was experiencing late-stage toxicity from radiation that he completed 3 years before.

The swallowing problem that JW was now experiencing is due primarily to radio necrosis. There may also be loss of taste, continually decreasing salivary function, and dehydration.[14] Laryngeal radio necrosis is a difficult late complication of radiation

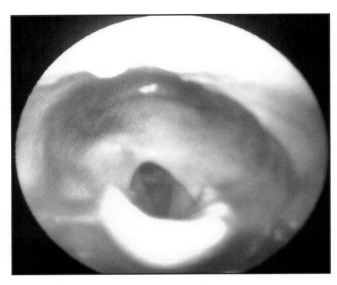

FIGURE 12–8. This photo shows the late effects of radiation therapy toxicity in Patient, JW.

therapy. It is associated with hoarseness, edema, pain, weight loss, and upper airway obstruction. The medical treatment options are limited, and in severe cases, the patient may require tracheostomy or laryngectomy. It is not uncommon for the patient to feel "better" 6 to 8 weeks after the completion of XRT and thus want to go on with his or her life away from day-to-day medical involvement; however, it is necessary to confront the issues of late toxicity and consider a long-term program of speech and swallow management. There is little data to suggest that a long-term program of speech and swallow exercises will help, but patients should be encouraged to continue to practice exercises that improve speech and swallowing. These exercises include tongue and jaw range-of-motion exercises and chewing exercises. A hygiene program of brushing teeth 3 times daily, maintaining hydration, avoiding drying foods and liquids, and of course avoiding cigarette smoking is recommended.

The role of the SLP has not yet been fully outlined for these patients; however, as more and more patients with late effects of radiation are seen, a greater awareness is building in the long-term care of patients who have undergone XRT. We cannot say if JW would be speaking and swallowing better if he continued range-of-motion exercises and regular follow-up appointments with his SLP, but additional research may lead to evidence to support this type of treatment.

This case describes the late effects of XRT, which includes both severe speech and swallowing problems. It remains to be seen how these cases will be treated in the future, but based on general principles of muscle physiology and exercise, it might be expected that patients can experience less severe late complications of radiation therapy if an aggressive exercise program for speech and swallowing is undertaken shortly after recovery from the XRT treatment toxicity and continued for a longer period of time. Newer radiation treatment protocols that were described in Chapter 4, specifically image guided radiation therapy (IMRT), may help to reduce the side effects of the treatment.

Failure to Thrive in an Autistic Child

A 31-month-old child was taken to a pediatrician because he was refusing to eat. An extensive history revealed that the child had a history of refusing to eat in the past but eventually began to eat. His mother described several interesting new behaviors. For approximately 6 months, he has pushed his food away from the table, spitting it out when he did eat it, and would run away from the table when his mother tried to place him in a high chair. He would often go to his room or another room in the house and start stacking books in a neat pile or taking his toys out of his toy box and lining them up on the floor and then replacing them in the toy box. The mother reported that recently, he would not answer her with yes or no responses. He would no longer smile when his father came home from work; he kept his head down and looked away from people when they talked to him. The pediatrician referred the child to the SLP because his language and speech also seemed inappropriate for his age. Table 12–2 reports the child's profile as reported by his parents.

The child was not cooperative when the SLP attempted to do an oral-motor examination. However, when the child was shown a series of pictures of animals, he began to stack the pictures in the cor-

TABLE 12–2. Patient Characteristics Reported by Parents

Age (months)	Weight (pounds)	Speech	Other Behavior Noted
18	22	Single-word responses	Occasional smile
24	24	Repeated single-word responses	Rare 2-word sentences
30	25	No 2-word responses	No smiles
31	25	Single-word responses	Shrieks; no eye contact

ner of the room. The therapist then began to show him pictures of various parts of the body—face, hands, and so forth. When she showed him a picture that emphasized the stomach, the child turned the picture over and ran out of the room. A picture of a dog brought him back into the room. So the therapist began again to show him pictures and they made 2 stacks—animals on one side and pictures of faces on the other side. When she showed him the picture emphasizing the stomach, again the boy turned the picture over, but this time he went to the stack of animal pictures and lined them up in a row. The therapist engaged the boy to repeat the names of several pictures, but when she showed him the picture that emphasized the stomach, he said "no" instead of repeating "belly." The FEES video of this child is shown in Video 12–5.

A pediatric psychologist ultimately diagnosed this child as having autism spectrum disorder (ASD). Because of the unusual behavior with the pictures reported by the SLP, the child was put on a mild medication for reflux disease. A plan for eating was developed by the SLP and the pediatric psychologist. One task that seemed to help in the feeding and eating program was to have the child use various pictures of food to feed his favorite pictures of animals. Ultimately, that group of foods that he selected to feed the dog and the horse were introduced into his diet.

The child began to gain weight. However, ASD has many unusual behaviors and the child continued to have other autistic behaviors related to communication and socialization. He continued to receive treatment by the pediatrician, the pediatric psychologist, and the SLP. His parents were introduced to the problems of ASD and joined a self-help group. After 6 months, the child maintained his weight and actually gained several pounds. Eating, although still a problem because of food selection and distractions while eating, substantially improved.

This case is unusual in that ASD is often diagnosed earlier than 31 months of age. In addition, the fact that the lack of weight gain and growth was present diminished the other signs, although they were still present. The parents just associated the communication and socialization changes with the abnormal eating behaviors. Importantly, once the SLP identified that eating was only a part of the problem, the child was diagnosed appropriately, and the nutritional aspects of the underlying problem were addressed.

SUMMARY

Having all specialists involved in diagnosis and treatment of swallowing, speech, and voice disorders available in a comprehensive swallowing and voice center allows patients to receive diagnoses and treatment plans in a more timely manner than the multiple referrals necessary when specialists are in different facilities. In addition, it allows members of the team to review the same diagnostic tests and to consult, when necessary, to develop the most timely and optimal treatment plan for a patient.

DISCUSSION QUESTIONS

1. Discuss the options, benefits, and drawbacks for the swallowing team to be a virtual team rather than a team working together in one location. Under what conditions could a virtual team be considered an integral part of the swallowing center?
2. Write out 1 to 2 sentences of the responsibilities of all members of a comprehensive swallowing team. Include as many specialists as you feel are necessary to address all types of swallowing problems.

STUDY QUESTIONS

1. In the treatment of a patient with a swallowing problem, the voice and communication needs of the patient should
   A. Take precedence over the swallowing problem, because it is important for the patient to give a thorough case history
   B. Be equally important as the swallowing problem
   C. Be addressed after the safety of the swallowing problem is determined
   D. Be of little importance until a swallowing treatment program is begun

2. A swallowing treatment team consisting of an otolaryngologist and an SLP should
   A. Maintain regular communication and report changes in the patient's medical and swallowing status even if they do not work in the same center
   B. Not share records of the patient's care, because there are patient privacy rules that must be maintained
   C. Each do the same instrumental test of the patient's swallowing problem in order to compare results
   D. Avoid repeating tests done by previous examiners due to insurance costs

3. Instrumental tests of swallowing are repeated
   A. At intervals following radiation therapy
   B. When a patient complains of a change in his or her swallowing
   C. After a treatment change is noted by the SLP
   D. All of the above

4. Hoarseness for 3 weeks in a patient who comes to the swallowing clinic is a sign of
   A. Voice disorder
   B. Reflux disease
   C. Dysphagia
   D. Possibly all three (A, B, and C)

5. If a patient reports that his modified barium swallow test was stopped after 3 separate swallows of liquid and no penetration or aspiration was seen,
   A. A diagnosis of a normal swallow should be put in the medical record
   B. The speech-language pathologist should ask to continue the examination
   C. The examination should be stopped and the patient put on a liquid diet
   D. The examination should be stopped and a diet should be prepared by the swallow team

REFERENCES

1. Fasching W. The contribution made by the 2nd Department of Surgery, Vienna University, to the treatment of colorectal cancer (author's transl) [in German]. *Wien Klin Wochenschr.* 1979 Feb 2;91(3):68–74.
2. Logemann JA. *Evaluation and Treatment of Swallowing Disorders.* San Diego, CA: College-Hill Press; 1983.
3. Bush CM, Postma GN. Transnasal esophagoscopy. *Otolaryngol Clin North Am.* 2013 Feb;46(1):41–52.
4. Martin-Harris B, Brodsky MB, Mickel Y, Ford CL, Walters B, Heffner J. Breathing and swallowing dynamics across the adult lifespan. *Arch Otolaryngol Head Neck Surg.* 2005:131(9):762–770.
5. Pitts T, Troche M, Mann G, Rosenbek J, Okun MS, Sapienza C. Using voluntary cough to detect penetration and aspiration during oropharyngeal swallowing in patients with Parkinson disease. *Chest.* 2010 Dec;138 (6): 1426–1431.

6. Pitts T, Bolser D, Rosenbek J. Impact of expiratory muscle strength training on voluntary cough and swallow function in Parkinson Disease. *Chest*. 2009;135(5):1301–1308.

7. Laciuga H, Rosenbek JC, Davenport PW, Sapienza CM. Functional outcomes associated with expiratory muscle strength training: narrative review. *J Rehabil Res Dev*. 2014;51(4):535–546.

8. Belafsky PC, Postma GN, Koufman, JA. Validity and reliability of the Reflux Symptom Index (RSI). *J Voice*. 2002; 16:274–277.

9. Rosen CA, Lee AS, Osborne J, Zullo T, Murry T. Development and validation of the Voice Handicap Index-10. *Laryngoscope*. 2004;114:1549–1556.

10. Ramig L, Gray S, Baker K, et al. The aging voice: a review: treatment data and familial and genetic perspectives. *Folia Phoniatr Logop*. 2001;53(5):252–265.

11. Burkhead LM, Sapienza CM, Rosenbek JC. Strength training exercise in dysphagia rehabilitation: principles, procedures and directions for future. *Dysphagia*. 2007; 22:251–265.

12. Suarez-Cunqueiro MM, Schramm A, Schoen R, et al. Speech and swallowing impairment after treatment for oral and oropharyngeal cancer. *Arch Otolaryngol Head Neck Surg*. 2008 Dec;134(12):1299–1304.

13. Langendijk JA, Doornaert P, Verdonck-de Leeuw IM, Leemans CR, Aaronson NK, Slotman BJ. Impact of late treatment-related toxicity on quality of life among patients with head and neck cancer treated with radiotherapy. *J Clin Oncol*. 2008 Aug 1;26(22):3770–3776.

14. Givens DJ, Karnell LH, Gupta AK, et al. Adverse events associated with concurrent chemoradiation therapy in patients with head and neck cancer. *Arch Otolaryngol Head Neck Surg*. 2009 Dec;135(12):1209–1217.

Glossary

Achalasia: a disorder of the esophagus that prevents normal swallowing. In achalasia, which means "failure to relax," the esophageal sphincter remains contracted. Achalasia affects the esophagus, the tube that carries swallowed food from the back of the throat down into the stomach. A ring of muscle called the lower esophageal sphincter encircles the esophagus just above the entrance to the stomach. Normal peristalsis is interrupted and food cannot enter the stomach. Achalasia is caused by degeneration of the nerve cells that normally signal the brain to relax the esophageal sphincter. The ultimate cause of this degeneration is unknown. Autoimmune disease or hidden infection is suspected.

Acini: small, saclike dilations composing a compound gland.

Akathisia: a movement disorder characterized by inner restlessness and the inability to sit or stand still. Akathisia may appear as a side effect of long-term use of antipsychotic medications, Lithium, and some other psychiatric drugs. Persons with akathisia typically have restless movements of the arms and legs such as tapping, marching in place, rocking, crossing and uncrossing the legs. They may feel anxious at the thought of sitting down.

Amyotrophic lateral sclerosis (ALS): often referred to as "Lou Gehrig's disease," ALS is a progressive neurodegenerative disease that affects nerve cells in the brain and the spinal cord. Motor neurons reach from the brain to the spinal cord and from the spinal cord to the muscles throughout the body. With voluntary muscle action progressively affected, patients in the later stages of the disease may become totally paralyzed. Dysphagia is progressive in ALS.

Anaerobic pneumonia: see aspiration pneumonia.

Anterior faucial arches: the arches that separate the mouth from the pharynx.

Aphagia: the inability or refusal to swallow. It is related to **dysphagia** which is difficulty swallowing, and odynophagia, painful swallowing. Aphagia may be temporary or long term, depending on the affected organ. It is an extreme, life-threatening case of dysphagia. Depending on the cause, untreated dysphagia may develop into aphagia.

Aphasia: an acquired communication disorder that impairs a person's ability to process language but does not affect intelligence. Aphasia impairs the ability to speak and understand others, and most people with aphasia experience difficulty reading and writing.

Apnea: a period of time during which breathing stops or is markedly reduced. There are 3 forms of apnea: blockage of the airways, cessation of respiratory effort (usually brain related and referred to as "central"), and a combination of airways blockage and central apnea. Apneas usually occur during sleep as well as briefly during a normal swallow.

Aspiration: the inhalation of either oropharyngeal or gastric contents into the airway below the vocal folds.

Aspiration pneumonia: also known as anaerobic pneumonia, this is inflammation of the lungs and airways to the lungs (bronchial tubes) from breathing in foreign material. Aspiration pneumonia is caused by breathing foreign materials (usually food, liquids, vomit, or fluids from the mouth) into the lungs. This may lead to:

- A collection of pus in the lungs (lung abscess)
- An inflammatory reaction
- A lung infection (pneumonia)

Atrophy: muscle atrophy is the wasting or loss of muscle tissue. There are 2 types of muscle atrophy. Disuse atrophy occurs from a lack of physical exercise. In most people, muscle atrophy is caused by not using the muscles enough. The most severe type of muscle atrophy is neurogenic atrophy. It occurs when there is an injury to, or disease of, a nerve that connects to the muscle. This type of muscle atrophy tends to occur more suddenly than disuse atrophy.

Examples of diseases affecting the nerves that control muscles:

- Amyotrophic lateral sclerosis (ALS or Lou Gehrig's disease)
- Guillain-Barré syndrome
- Polio (poliomyelitis).

Autoimmune diseases: a varied group of more than 80 serious, chronic illnesses that involve almost every human organ system. This group includes diseases of the nervous gastrointestinal and endocrine systems as well as skin and other connective tissues, eyes, blood, and blood vessels. In all of these diseases, the underlying problem is similar—the body's immune system becomes misdirected, attacking the very organs it was designed to protect.

Baclofen: a muscle relaxer and an antispastic agent. Baclofen is used to treat muscle symptoms caused by multiple sclerosis, including spasm, pain, and stiffness.

Barium: a radiopaque element that allows visualization of the boluses in fluoroscopy.

Barrett's esophagus: a serious complication of gastroesophageal reflux disease (GERD). In Barrett's esophagus, normal tissue lining the esophagus changes to tissue that resembles the lining of the intestine. About 10% of people with chronic symptoms of GERD develop Barrett's esophagus. Barrett's esophagus does not have any specific symptoms, although patients with Barrett's esophagus may have symptoms related to GERD. It does, though, increase the risk of developing esophageal adenocarcinoma, a serious, potentially fatal cancer of the esophagus.

Beckwith-Wiedemann syndrome: a condition that affects many parts of the body. It is classified as an overgrowth syndrome, which means that affected infants are considerably larger than normal (macrosomia) and tend to be taller than their peers during childhood. Growth begins to slow by about age 8, and adults with this condition are not unusually tall. In some children with Beckwith-Wiedemann syndrome, specific parts of the body on one side or the other may grow abnormally large, leading to an asymmetric or uneven appearance. This unusual growth pattern, which is known as hemihyperplasia, usually becomes less apparent over time. Some infants with Beckwith-Wiedemann syndrome have an abnormally large tongue (macroglossia), which may interfere with breathing, swallowing, and speaking.

Benzodiazepines: among the most commonly prescribed depressant medications in the United States today. More than 15 different types of benzodiazepine medications exist to treat a wide array of both psychological and physical maladies based on dosage and implications. Commonly prescribed benzodiazepines include Xanax (alprazolam), Librium (chlordiazepoxide), Valium (diazepam), and Ativan (lorazepam) and flunitrazepam, trade name Rohypnol. Many of these drugs slow down the motion of the esophagus.

Beta-agonist: an agent, chemical, or chemical reaction that tends to null another.

Bifid uvula: A bifid uvula is a uvula that is forked or split in appearance. The uvula is a structure in the rear middle of the mouth, located in front of the tonsils, which forms part of the soft palate.

Bile: a yellow-green fluid that is made by the liver, stored in the gall bladder, and passes through the common bile duct into the duodenum where it helps digest fat. The principal components of bile are cholesterol, bile salts, and the pigment bilirubin.

Bipolar electrocautery: an electrocautery in which both active and return electrodes are incorporated into a single, handheld instrument, so that the current passes between the tips of the two electrodes and affects only a small amount of tissue.

Bite reflex: a swift, involuntary biting action that may be triggered by stimulation of the oral cavity. The bite can be difficult to release in some cases, such as when a spoon or tongue depressor is placed in a patient's mouth.

Bolus: a rounded mass that can be hard (pill) or soft (chewed food or liquids) that is given or taken and delivered to the swallowing organs of the body.

Botulinum toxin: (botulin) a neurotoxin made by *Clostridium botulinum*; causes paralysis in high doses but is used medically in small, localized doses to treat disorders associated with involuntary muscle contraction and spasms.

Botulism: a rare but serious illness. The cause is a toxin (poison) made by a bacterium called *Clostridium botulinum*. It occurs naturally in soil. There are several kinds of botulism. Foodborne botulism comes from eating foods contaminated with the toxin. Wound botulism happens when a wound infected with the bacteria makes the toxin. It is more common in heroin users. Infant botulism happens when a baby consumes the spores of the bacteria from soil or honey. All forms can be deadly and are medical emergencies. Symptoms include double or blurred vision, drooping eyelids, slurred speech, difficulty swallowing, dry mouth, and muscle weakness. Treatment may include antitoxins, intensive medical care, or surgery of infected wounds.

Brachytherapy: an advanced cancer treatment. Radioactive seeds or sources are placed in or near the tumor itself, giving a high radiation dose to the tumor while reducing the radiation exposure in the surrounding healthy tissues.

Bradycardia: a slower than normal heart rate. The heart usually beats between 60 and 100 times a minute in an adult at rest. A heart with bradycardia beats fewer than 60 times a minute. Bradycardia can be a serious problem if the heart does not pump enough oxygen-rich blood to the body. For some people, however, bradycardia does not cause symptoms or complications. An implanted pacemaker and other treatments may correct bradycardia and help the heart maintain an appropriate rate.

Brainstem stroke: a stroke that originates in the brainstem. Because the brainstem handles many of the body's basic life support functions, such as swallowing, breathing, and heart rate, a brainstem stroke can be fatal. As with other strokes, early treatment is essential.

Bruxism: the habit of clenching and grinding the teeth. It most often occurs at night during sleep, but it may also occur during the day. It is an unconscious behavior, perhaps performed to release anxiety, aggression, or anger.

Candida: a yeast infection of the esophagus caused by the same fungus that causes vaginal yeast infections. The infection develops in the esophagus when the body's immune system is weak (such as in people with diabetes or HIV). It is usually very treatable with antifungal drugs. Like *Candida*, this viral infection can develop in the esophagus when the body's immune system is weak. It is treatable with antiviral drugs.

Candidiasis: a fungal infection caused by yeasts that belong to the genus *Candida*. There are over 20 species of *Candida* yeasts that can cause infection in humans, the most common of which is *Candida albicans*. *Candida* yeasts normally live on the skin and mucous membranes without causing infection; however, overgrowth of these organisms can cause symptoms to develop. Symptoms of candidiasis vary depending on the area of the body that is infected. Candidiasis that develops in the mouth or throat is called "thrush" or oropharyngeal candidiasis.

Celiac disease: a condition that damages the lining of the small intestine and prevents it from absorbing parts of food that are important for staying healthy. The damage is due to a reaction to eating gluten, which is found in wheat, barley, rye, and possibly oats.

The exact cause of celiac disease is unknown. The lining of the intestines contains areas called villi, which help absorb nutrients. When adults and children with celiac disease eat foods or use products that contain gluten, their immune system reacts by damaging these villi. This damage affects the ability to absorb nutrients properly. A person becomes malnourished, no matter how much food he or she eats.

The disease can develop at any point in life, from infancy to late adulthood.

People with celiac disease are more likely to have:

- Autoimmune disorders such as rheumatoid arthritis, systemic lupus erythematosus, and Sjögren syndrome
- Addison disease
- Down syndrome
- Intestinal cancer
- Intestinal lymphoma
- Lactose intolerance
- Thyroid disease
- Type 1 diabetes

Central pattern generators (CPGs): biological neural networks that produce rhythmic patterned outputs without sensory feedback. CPGs have been shown to produce rhythmic outputs resembling normal "rhythmic motor pattern production" even in isolation from motor and sensory feedback from limbs and other muscle targets.

To be classified as a rhythmic generator, a CPG requires (1) 2 or more processes that interact such that each process sequentially increases and decreases, and (2) that, as a result of this interaction, the system repeatedly returns to its starting condition. CPGs have been found in practically all vertebrate species investigated, including human.

Cervical osteophyte: a bony outgrowth or protuberance on the cervical vertebrae. Unless, the osteophyte is exceptionally large, it will not interfere with swallowing even when it can be observed on radiological exams.

Cervical spondylosis: common, age-related changes in the area of the spine at the back of the neck. With age, the vertebrae (the component bones of the spine) gradually form bone spurs, and their shock-absorbing disks slowly shrink. These changes can alter the alignment and stability of the spine. They may go unnoticed, or they may produce problems related to pressure on the spine and associated nerves and blood vessels. This pressure can cause weakness, numbness, and pain in various areas of the body.

Chagas disease: called also American or South American trypanosomiasis. An acute, subacute, or chronic form of trypanosomiasis seen widely in Central and South America, caused by *Trypanosoma cruzi*, and transmitted by the bites of reduviid bugs. The acute form, prevalent in children, is marked initially by an erythematous nodule (chagoma) at the site of inoculation; high fever; unilateral swelling of the face with edema of the eyelid (Romaña's sign); regional lymphadenopathy; hepatosplenomegaly; and meningoencephalic irritation. The subacute form may last for several months or years and is characterized by mild fever, severe asthenia, and generalized lymphadenopathy. The chronic form, which may or may not be preceded by an acute episode, is characterized principally by cardiac manifestations (myocarditis) and gastrointestinal manifestations (including megaesophagus and megacolon).

Charcot-Marie-Tooth disease: a genetic disease of nerves characterized by progressively debilitating muscle weakness, particularly of the limbs. The foremost feature is marked wasting of the distal extremities, particularly the peroneal muscle groups in the calves, resulting in "stork legs." The disease usually weakens the legs before the arms. Charcot-Marie-Tooth is one of the more frequent genetic diseases and the most common genetic disease of peripheral nerves. Physical therapy can help to delay somewhat the wasting of limbs. The disease is genetically heterogeneous. It can be inherited as an autosomal dominant, autosomal recessive, or X-linked trait. There are also sporadic cases with no family history of the disease that are due to new dominant mutations. Abbreviated CMT.

CHARGE syndrome: a recognizable (genetic) pattern of birth defects that occurs in about one in every 8,000 to 10,000 births worldwide. It is an extremely complex syndrome, involving extensive medical and physical difficulties that differ from child to child. The vast majority of the time, there is no history of CHARGE syndrome or any other similar conditions in the family. Babies with CHARGE syndrome are often born with life-threatening birth defects, including complex heart defects and breathing problems. Swallowing and breathing problems make life difficult even when they come home. All are likely to require special feeding arrangements. Despite these seemingly insurmountable obstacles, children with CHARGE syndrome often far surpass their medical, physical, educational, and social expectations.

Community-acquired pneumonia (CAP): develops in people with limited or no contact with medical institutions or settings. The most commonly identified pathogens are *Streptococcus pneumoniae*, *Haemophilus influenzae*, atypical bacteria (i.e., *Chlamydia pneumoniae*, *Mycoplasma pneumoniae*, *Legionella*), and viruses. Symptoms and signs are fever, cough, sputum production, pleuritic chest pain, dyspnea, tachypnea, and tachycardia. Diagnosis is based on clinical presentation and chest x-ray. Treatment is with empirically chosen antibiotics. Prognosis is excellent for relatively young or healthy patients, but many pneumonias, especially when caused by *S. pneumoniae*, *Legionella*, *Staphylococcus aureus*, or influenza virus, are serious or even fatal in older, sicker patients.

Cortical regulation: refers to the direct regulation by the brain of physiological functions including cellular functions. This regulation occurs through the autonomic nervous system exerting direct innervation of body organs and tissues that starts in the brainstem. Lower brain areas are under control of cerebral cortex.

Corticosteroids: any of the class of drugs of steroid hormones made by the cortex or the adrenal gland. Used regularly in treating inflammation.

Coughing: a cough is a forceful release of air from the lungs that can be heard. Coughing protects the respiratory system by clearing it of irritants and secretions.

Craniotomy: a surgical operation in which an opening is made in the skull.

Cricopharyngeal myotomy: a surgical operation that divides the cricopharyngeal muscle by cutting or slicing parts of the muscle to weaken or relax it. Thus, when an individual swallows, the small muscle is relaxed and does not prevent the flow of the bolus from passing into the esophagus. Prior to performing this operation, the surgeon may elect to dilate the muscle in hopes that dilation will achieve passage of the bolus.

Decannulation: the removal of a cannula or tube that may have been inserted during a surgical procedure.

Deep tendon reflex: reflexes that involve muscle contractions when tendons are stimulated.

Dehydration: lack of proper fluids in the body. Dehydration is a dangerous condition that may cause tissue breakdown or even shock. Once diagnosed, the patient may require hospitalization and intravenous fluid support until stable.

Dementia: significant loss of intellectual abilities such as memory capacity, severe enough to interfere with social or occupational functioning. Criteria for the diagnosis of dementia include impairment of attention, orientation, memory, judgment, language, motor and spatial skills, and function. By definition, dementia is not due to major depression or schizophrenia. Dementia is reported in as many as 1% of adults 60 years of age. It has been estimated that the frequency of dementia doubles every 5 years after 60 years of age. Alzheimer disease is the most common cause of dementia. There are many other causes of dementia, including (in alphabetical order) AIDS (due to HIV infection), alcoholism (the dementia is due to thiamine deficiency), brain injury, brain tumors, Creutzfeldt-Jakob disease, dementia with Lewy bodies (tiny round structures made of proteins that develop within nerve cells in the brain), drug toxicity, encephalitis, meningitis, Pick disease (a slowly progressive deterioration of social skills and changes in personality leading to impairment of intellect, memory, and language), syphilis, thyroid disease (hypothyroidism), and vascular dementia (damage to the blood vessels leading to the brain).

Diazepam: a benzodiazepine used as an antianxiety agent, sedative, antipanic agent, antitremor agent, skeletal muscle relaxant, anticonvulsant, and in the management of alcohol withdrawal symptoms.

Diplopia: the perception of two images of a single object.

Diverticula: A gut diverticulum (singular) is an outpouching of the wall of the gut to form a sac. Diverticula (plural) may occur at any level from esophagus to colon. A true diverticulum includes all three layers of the gut; the lining mucosa, the muscularis, and the outer serosa. False diverticula are missing the muscularis and are therefore very thin walled. Colonic diverticula are typically false.

Dopamine: a monoamine neurotransmitter formed in the brain by the decarboxylation of dopa and essential to the normal functioning of the central nervous system. Dopamine is classified as a catecholamine (a class of molecules that serve as neurotransmitters and hormones). Dopamine is formed by the decarboxylation (removal of a carboxyl group) from dopa. A reduction in its concentration within the brain is associated with Parkinson's disease.

Down syndrome: see Trisomy 21.

Dysgeusia: an unpleasant alteration of taste sensation, often with a metallic taste.

Dysphagia: difficulty swallowing. The condition results from impeded transport of liquids, solids, or both from the pharynx to the stomach. Dysphagia should not be confused with globus sensation, a feeling of having a lump in the throat, which is unrelated to swallowing and occurs without impaired transport.

Dystonia: a movement disorder characterized by sustained, irregular, muscle contractions that result in writhing or twisting movements and unusual body postures.

Eaton-Lambert syndrome: a disease seen in patients with lung cancer; characterized by weakness and fatigue of hip and thigh muscles and an aching back; caused by antibodies directed against the neuromuscular junctions.

Electrocautery: the cauterization of tissue by means of an electrode that consists of a red hot piece of metal, such as a wire, held in a holder, and is heated by either direct or alternating current. The term "electrocautery" is used to refer to both the procedure and the instrument used in the procedure.

Electromyography (EMG): a diagnostic procedure to assess the health of muscles and the nerve cells that control them (motor neurons).

Motor neurons transmit electrical signals that cause muscles to contract. An EMG translates these signals into graphs, sounds, or numerical values that a specialist interprets.

An EMG uses tiny devices called electrodes to transmit or detect electrical signals.

During a needle EMG, a needle electrode inserted directly into a muscle records the electrical activity in that muscle.

A nerve conduction study, another part of an EMG, uses electrodes taped to the skin (surface electrodes) to measure the speed and strength of signals traveling between 2 or more points.

EMG results can reveal nerve dysfunction, muscle dysfunction, or problems with nerve-to-muscle signal transmission.

Emphysema: a chronic respiratory disease where there is overinflation of the air sacs (alveoli) in the lungs, causing a decrease in lung function, and often, breathlessness.

Empyema: a condition in which pus (fluid filled with immune cells) accumulates in the area between the lungs and the inner surface of the chest wall. This area is known as the pleural space. Empyema, also called pyothorax or purulent pleuritis, usually develops after pneumonia, which is an infection of the lung tissue. Pus in the pleural space cannot be coughed out. Instead, it needs to be drained by a needle or surgery.

Endoluminal (intraluminal): related to the interior space of tubular structures in the body, e.g., esophagus, intestines.

Enteral nutrition: a way to provide food through a tube placed in the nose, the stomach, or the small intestine. A tube in the nose is called a nasogastric tube or nasoenteral tube. A tube that goes through the skin into the stomach is called a gastrostomy or percutaneous endoscopic gastrostomy (PEG) tube. A tube into the small intestine is called a jejunostomy or percutaneous endoscopic jejunostomy (PEJ) tube. Enteral nutrition is often called tube feeding.

Epidemiology: classical—The study of populations in order to determine the frequency and distribution of disease and measure risks.

Clinical—Epidemiology focused specifically upon patients. Epidemiology is the study of populations in order to determine the frequency and distribution of disease and measure risks.

Epiglottitis: a potentially life-threatening condition that occurs when the epiglottis swells, blocking the flow of air into the patient's lungs. A number of factors can cause the epiglottis to swell—burns from hot liquids, direct injury to the throat, and various infections. The most common cause of epiglottitis in children in the past was infection with *Haemophilus influenzae* type b (Hib), the same bacterium that causes pneumonia, meningitis, and infections in the bloodstream. Epiglottitis can occur at any age.

Esophageal body: the body of the esophagus is composed of 2 muscle types. The proximal esophagus is predominantly striated muscle, while the distal esophagus and the remainder of the gastrointestinal tract contain smooth muscle. The mid-esophagus contains a graded transition of striated and smooth muscle types. The muscle is oriented in 2 perpendicular opposing layers: an inner circular layer and an outer longitudinal layer, known collectively as the muscularis propria. The longitudinal muscle is responsible for shortening the esophagus, while the circular muscle forms lumen-occluding ring contractions.

Esophageal diverticulum: an outpouching of mucosa through the muscular layer of the esophagus. It can be asymptomatic or cause dysphagia and regurgitation. Diagnosis is made by barium swallow; surgical repair is rarely required.

Esophagectomy: a surgical procedure to remove a portion of the esophagus and then reconstruct it using part of another organ, usually the stomach or large intestine. Esophagectomy is a common treatment for esophageal cancer, and less common for Barrett esophagus and achalasia (a swallowing disorder).

Esophagitis: an inflammation that may damage tissues of the esophagus, the muscular tube that delivers food from the mouth to the stomach. Esophagitis can cause painful, difficult swallowing, and chest pain. Causes of esophagitis include stomach acids backing up into the esophagus, infection, oral medications, and allergies. Treatments for esophagitis depend on the underlying cause and the severity of tissue damage. If left untreated, esophagitis can damage the lining, interfere with normal function, and lead to complications such as scarring, stricture, and difficulty swallowing.

Esophagoduodenoscopy: an endoscopic test of the esophagus and stomach usually done by a gastroenterologist. Now known as EGD.

Esophagram: a series of x-rays of the esophagus. The x-ray pictures are taken after the patient drinks a solution that coats and outlines the walls of the esophagus. It is also called a *barium swallow*.

Exophytic tumor: a tumor that grows outward beyond the surface epithelium from which it originates.

External beam radiation therapy (EBRT): uses high-energy rays (or particles) to destroy cancer cells or slow their rate of growth. A carefully focused beam of radiation is delivered from a machine outside the body. External beam radiation therapy usually involves treatments 5 days a week for about 6 weeks. The treatment itself is painless and much like getting a regular x-ray. Each treatment lasts only a few minutes, although the setup time—getting the patient into place for treatment—usually takes longer. EBRT has effects on swallowing, mainly related to inflammation.

Fasciculation: involuntary muscle twitches.

Fetal alcohol syndrome: the sum total of the damage done to the child before birth as a result of the mother drinking alcohol during pregnancy. Fetal alcohol syndrome (FAS) always involves brain damage, impaired growth, and head and face abnormalities. Fetal alcohol syndrome is one of the leading causes of mental retardation in the United States. FAS is an irreversible, lifelong condition that affects every aspect of a child's life and the lives of the child's family. However, FAS is 100% preventable if a woman does not drink alcohol while she is pregnant. There is no cure for FAS. Children born to mothers who drink alcohol demonstrate failure to thrive. As the child begins to mature, signs of mental retardation begin to appear. However, with early identification and diagnosis, children with FAS can receive services such as special feeding, modified diets, and ultimately special education that can help increase their potential.

Flexible endoscope: endoscopy with flexible cabling that allows examination of labyrinthine structures in the body.

Fibrosis: the formation of fine scar-like structures that cause tissues to harden and reduces the flow of fluids through these tissues. The formation of fibrous tissue, as in repair or replacement of parenchymatous elements. Tissue that has lost its normal elasticity due to scarring.

Full-term newborn: retained in the uterus for the normal period of gestation before birth.

Gag reflex or pharyngeal reflex: a reflex contraction of the back of the throat, evoked by touching the soft palate. It prevents something from entering the throat except as part of normal swallowing and helps prevent choking. Different people have different sensitivities to the gag reflex.

Gastroesophageal reflux: return of stomach contents back up into the esophagus. This frequently causes heartburn because of irritation of the esophagus by stomach acid.

Gastroparesis: also called *delayed gastric emptying*, this is a disorder in which the stomach takes too long to empty its contents. Normally, the stomach contracts to move food down into the small intestine for digestion. The vagus nerve controls the movement of food from the stomach through the digestive tract. Gastroparesis occurs when the vagus nerve is damaged and the muscles of the stomach and intestines do not work normally.

Gastrostomy: a surgical procedure for inserting a tube through the abdomen wall and into the stomach. The tube, called a "g-tube," is used for feeding or drainage. Gastrostomy is performed because a patient temporarily or permanently needs to be fed directly through a tube in the stomach. Gastrostomy is also performed to provide drainage for the stomach when it is necessary to bypass a long-standing obstruction of the stomach outlet into the small intestine.

Gelfoam: a substance that is used to improve vocal fold bulk. Gelfoam is injected into paralyzed or partially paralyzed vocal folds to increase bulk and improve closure of the vocal folds.

Globus sensation: a subjective feeling of a lump or foreign body in the throat. It is sometimes called globus pharyngeus. The term "globus hystericus" was previously used because of the belief that psychogenic factors were involved and that globus sensation was just a type of somatization disorder presenting with pseudoneurological symptoms. However, it is now widely considered that globus sensation can have underlying physiological or anatomical causes and there are thought to be a number of potential etiologies.

Glossitis: a condition in which the tongue is swollen and changes color. Finger-like projections on the surface of the tongue (called papillae) are lost, causing the tongue to appear smooth. Changes in the appearance of the tongue may be a primary condition or it may be a symptom of other disorders such as dehydration. Glossitis occurs when there is acute or chronic inflammation of the tongue.

Glossodynia: also known as burning mouth syndrome (BMS), "burning tongue" and "orodynia," is a condition characterized by a burning or tingling sensation on the lips, tongue, or entire mouth.

Glossopharyngeal nerve: the ninth cranial nerve (CN IX). Problems with the glossopharyngeal nerve result in trouble tasting and swallowing.

Halitosis: the condition of having stale or foul-smelling breath.

Hematoma: an abnormal localized collection of blood in which the blood is usually clotted or partially clotted and is usually situated within an organ or a soft tissue space, such as within a muscle; caused by a break in the wall of a blood vessel. The break may be spontaneous, as in the case of an aneurysm, or caused by trauma.

Hemiparesis: muscle weakness on only one side of the body. When hemiparesis happens as a result of a stroke, it commonly involves muscles in the face, arm, and leg. Swallowing is often seen being done in one side of the mouth.

Herpes simplex virus (HSV): an infection that causes herpes. Herpes can appear in various parts of the body, most commonly on the genitals or mouth. There are 2 types of the herpes simplex virus. HSV-1, also known as oral herpes, can cause cold sores and fever blisters around the mouth and on the face. HSV-2 is generally responsible for genital herpes outbreaks.

Human immunodeficiency virus (HIV): a virus that gradually attacks the immune system, which is the body's natural defense against illness. If a person becomes infected with HIV, he or she will find it harder to fight off infections and diseases. The virus destroys a type of white blood cell called a T-helper cell and makes copies of itself inside them. T-helper cells are also referred to as CD4 cells.

Huntington disease: a hereditary disorder with mental and physical deterioration leading to death. Although characterized as an "adult-onset" disease, it can affect children as well. Huntington disease describes an autosomal dominant pattern of inheritance with high penetrance (a high proportion of persons with the gene develop the disease). The characteristic findings of Huntington disease are caused by loss of neurons (nerve cells) in the brain. The disease is due a gene in chromosome band 4p16.3. The gene, called HD, contains an unstable repeating sequence of 3 nucleotide bases (CAG) in the DNA. Normal people have an average of 19 CAG repeats and at most 34 such repeats while virtually all patients with Huntington disease have more than 40. The Huntington disease gene codes for a protein that has been named (confusingly) huntingtin whose function is unknown. The elevated numbers of CAG repeats in the Huntington disease gene lead to the production of an elongated huntingtin protein that appears to correlate with the loss of neurons in the disease. Mood disturbance is usually the first symptom seen, with bipolar disorder–like mood swings that may include mania, depression, extreme irritability or angry outbursts, and psychosis. Other symptoms include dysphagia, chorea (restless, wiggling, turning movements), muscle stiffness and slowness of movement, and difficulties with memory and other cognitive processes. The HD gene is located on chromosome 4, and is an autosomal dominant gene. Only one copy need be inherited to cause the illness. Diagnosis is by genetic testing, and family members of people with Huntington disease may also want to know if they carry the HD gene. At this time, there is no cure for HD, although medication may be used to control symptoms of the illness, such as mood swings and chorea.

Hypokinesia: slow or diminished movement of body musculature. It may be associated with basal ganglia diseases, mental disorders, and prolonged inactivity due to illness.

Hypothyroid: deficiency of thyroid hormone that is normally made by the thyroid gland, which is located in the front of the neck.

Hypotonia: decreased muscle tone. It can be a condition on its own, called benign congenital hypotonia, or it can be indicative of another problem where there is progressive loss of muscle tone, such as muscular dystrophy or cerebral palsy. It is usually detected during infancy.

Hypoxemia: a below-normal level of oxygen in the blood, specifically in the arteries. Hypoxemia is a sign of a problem related to breathing or circulation, and may result in various symptoms, such as shortness of breath. Hypoxemia is determined by measuring the oxygen level in a blood sample taken from an artery (arterial blood gas). It can also be estimated by measuring the oxygen saturation of the blood using a pulse oximeter—a small device that clips to the finger. Normal arterial oxygen is approximately 75 to 100 millimeters of mercury (mm Hg). Values under 60 mm Hg usually indicate the need for supplemental oxygen. Normal pulse oximeter readings usually range from 95% to 100%. Values under 90% are considered low.

Hypoxia: a reduction of oxygen supply to a tissue below physiological levels despite adequate perfusion of the tissue by blood.

Insensate: (1) Lacking sensation or awareness; inanimate. (2) Lacking human feeling or sensitivity; brutal; cruel. (3) Lacking sense; stupid; foolish.

Intensity-modulated radiation therapy (IMRT): an advanced type of radiation therapy used to treat cancer and noncancerous tumors. IMRT uses advanced technology to manipulate photon and proton beams of radiation to conform to the shape of a tumor. The goal of IMRT is to conform the radiation dose to the target and to avoid or reduce exposure of healthy tissue to limit the side effects of treatment.

Intubation: insertion of a tube into the trachea for the purpose of aided ventilation.

Ischemia: inadequate blood supply (circulation) to a local area due to blockage of the blood vessels to the area.

Isokinetic neck exercises: head exercises performed with a specialized apparatus that provides variable resistance to a movement, so that no matter how much effort is exerted, the movement takes place at a constant speed. Such exercise is used to improve muscular strength and endurance, especially after injury.

Isometric neck exercises: head exercises that only require the hands for strengthening the neck muscles. Isometric exercises are the very basic strengthening exercises to help build endurance to the muscle. Isometric exercises recruit muscles in order to strengthen without pain or movement.

Jejunostomy tube: a feeding jejunostomy tube, also called a *J-tube*, is a tube inserted through the abdomen and into the jejunum (the second part of the small bowel) to assist with feeding and to provide nutrition.

Killian triangle: a triangular area in the wall of the pharynx between the oblique fibers of the inferior constrictor muscle, and the transverse fibers of the cricopharyngeus muscle through which the Zenker diverticulum occurs.

Laryngeal penetration: material entering the laryngeal vestibule during the act of swallowing.

Laryngopharyngeal Reflux (LPR): a condition that occurs in a person who has gastroesophageal reflux disease (GERD). Acid made in the stomach travels up the esophagus. When that stomach acid gets to the throat, it is called laryngopharyngeal reflux.

Lower motor neuron: a nerve cell that goes from the spinal cord to a muscle. The cell body of a lower motor neuron is in the spinal cord, and its termination is in a skeletal muscle. The loss of lower motor neurons leads to weakness, twitching of muscle (fasciculation), and loss of muscle mass (muscle atrophy). A **lower motor neuron lesion** is a lesion in nerve fibers traveling from the anterior grey column of the spinal cord to a specific muscle or muscles—the lower motor neuron. One major characteristic used to identify a lower motor neuron lesion is flaccid paralysis —paralysis accompanied by loss of muscle tone.

Lung abscess: a pus-filled cavity in the lung surrounded by inflamed tissue and caused by an infection. Lung abscess is usually caused by bacteria that normally live in the mouth and are inhaled into the lungs. Symptoms include fatigue, loss of appetite, night sweats, fever, weight loss, and a cough that brings up sputum. Diagnosis is usually determined with a chest x-ray. People usually need to take antibiotics for several weeks before a lung abscess clears up.

Lyme disease: a bacterial illness caused by a bacterium called a "spirochete." Lyme disease is spread by ticks when they bite the skin. Lyme disease can cause abnormalities in the skin, joints, heart, and nervous system.

Macroglossia: the abnormal enlargement of the tongue. In rare cases, macroglossia occurs as an isolated finding that is present at birth (congenital). In many cases, macroglossia may occur secondary to a primary disorder that may be either congenital (e.g., Down syndrome or Beckwith-Wiedemann syndrome) or acquired (e.g., as a result of trauma or malignancy).

Magnetic resonance imaging (MRI): a special radiology technique designed to image internal structures of the body using magnetism, radio waves, and a computer to produce the images of body structures. In MRI, the scanner is a tube surrounded by a giant circular magnet. The patient is placed on a movable bed that is inserted into the magnet. The magnet creates a strong magnetic field that aligns the protons of hydrogen atoms, which are then exposed to a beam of radio waves. This spins the various protons of the body, and they produce a faint signal that is detected by the receiver portion of the MRI scanner. A computer processes the receiver information, and an image is produced. The image and resolution are quite detailed and can detect tiny changes of structures within the body, particularly in the soft tissue, brain and spinal cord, abdomen, and joints. See also fMRI.

Malnutrition: poor nourishment of the body often due to not eating healthy foods, improper digestion, poor absorption of nutrients, or a combination of these factors.

Manometry: measurement of pressure using a device called a manometer. Esophageal manometry is done to measure muscle pressure and movements in the esophagus in the evaluation of achalasia.

Mastication: the act of chewing.

Maxillectomy: a surgical procedure to remove all or part of the maxilla and is used to treat oral cavity cancer and cancers affecting the jaw and sinus cavity.

Medialization laryngoplasty: a procedure that provides support to a vocal fold that lacks the bulk, the mobility, or both, to achieve full adduction during vocalization and/or swallowing. A medialization laryngoplasty is done by inserting a silastic shim or surgical Gore-Tex into the lateral portion of the vocal fold. It is also frequently called a thyroplasty since the procedure is performed through the thyroid cartilage.

Modified barium swallow (MBS)/videofluoroscopic swallow study (VFSS): a fluoroscopic procedure designed to determine whether food or liquid is entering a person's lungs, also known as aspiration. It permits the medical team to observe the coordination of anatomical structures in the mouth and throat, as they are actively functioning when chewing, drinking, and swallowing. It also identifies the reason for aspiration.

Motor apraxia: inability to carry out, on command, a complex or skilled movement, though the purpose thereof is clear to the patient. Also known as kinesthetic apraxia; limb-kinetic apraxia.

Myositis: inflammation of muscle tissue. There are many causes of myositis, including injury, medications, and diseases.

Myotomy: the dissection or cutting of a muscle, performed to gain access to underlying tissues or to relieve constriction in a sphincter, such as in severe esophagitis or pyloric stenosis. With the patient under general anesthesia, a longitudinal cut is made through the sphincter muscle to create a relaxed state in the muscle.

Nasoduodenal tubes: feeding tubes that are inserted transnasally and end in the first section of the small intestines.

Nasojejunal tubes: feeding tubes that are inserted transnasally and end in the second section of the small intestines.

Nasopharyngoscope: a telescopic instrument, electrically lighted, for examination of the nasal passages and the nasopharynx.

Nd:YAG (neodymium-doped yttrium aluminum garnet; Nd:Y$_3$Al$_5$O$_1$): a crystal that is used as a lasing medium for solid-state lasers.

Neoplasia: new growth, usually refers to abnormal new growth and thus means the same as tumor, which may be benign or malignant. Unlike hyperplasia, neoplastic proliferation persists even in the absence of the original stimulus.

Neoplasm: an abnormal growth of tissue in animals or plants. Neoplasms can be benign or malignant. It is also called *tumor*.

Neural control: the process used by the nervous system to control everything from movement to physiological processes. The body is a series of complex interconnected systems that work together to sustain life on a variety of ways, and neural control is the underpinning of these systems.

Neuroplasticity: the brain's ability to reorganize itself by forming new neural connections throughout life. Neuroplasticity allows the neurons (nerve cells) in the brain to compensate for injury and disease and to adjust their activities in response to new situations or to changes in their environment.

Nonnutritive sucking: considered a natural reflex to satisfy a child's need for contact and may include unrestricted sucking on a breast, digit, pacifier, or other object like a blanket or toy. This nonnutritive sucking may make a child feel secure and relaxed, and allow the child to learn about the environment through mouthing objects.

Normal deglutition: consists of a succession of muscular contractions from above downward or from the front backward, which propel food from the oral cavity toward the stomach. The action is generally initiated at the lips; it proceeds back through the oral cavity, and the food is moved automatically along the dorsum of the tongue. When the food is ready for swallowing, it is passed back through the fauces. Once the food is beyond the fauces and in the pharynx, the soft palate closes off the nasopharynx, and the hyoid bone and larynx are elevated upward and forward. This action keeps food out of the larynx and dilates the esophageal opening so that the food may be passed quickly toward the stomach by peristaltic contractions. The separation between the voluntary and involuntary characteristics of this wave of contractions is not sharply defined. At birth the process is already well established as a highly coordinated activity, i.e., the swallowing reflex.

Nosocomial: originating or taking place in a hospital, acquired in a hospital, especially in reference to an infection or pneumonia.

Nosocomial pneumonia (NP; also known as hospital-acquired pneumonia [HAP] or health care—associated pneumonia [HCAP]): pneumonia that occurs more than 48 hours after admission but that was not incubating at the time of admission.

Nucleus ambiguus: on each side is a motor nucleus within the medulla of the brainstem. It lies dorsomedial to the spinal lemniscus and ventral to the nucleus of tractus solitarius. It supplies skeletal muscle fibers via 3 cranial nerves:

- Glossopharyngeal nerve: stylopharyngeus muscle
- Vagus and cranial root of accessory nerve
  - □ Pharyngeal branch to the muscles of the base of the tongue
  - □ Superior laryngeal nerve to cricothyroid muscle
- Recurrent laryngeal nerve to intrinsic muscles of the larynx

Nucleus of tractus solitarius: a brainstem nucleus on each side of the upper medulla. It lies lateral to the dorsal nucleus of the vagus, to which it has many connecting neurons, and medial to the spinal tract and the nucleus of the trigeminal nerve. The nucleus has afferent fibers that extend inferiorly within the upper medulla as the tract of solitarius.

The superior part of the nucleus receives fibers from the:

- Chorda tympani branch of the facial nerve; involved with taste sensation from the anterior two-thirds of the tongue
- Lingual branch of the glossopharyngeal nerve; involved with taste from the posterior third of the tongue
- Internal laryngeal branch of vagus nerve; involved with taste in the region of the valleculae

The inferior part of the nucleus receives fibers from the:

■ Vagus nerve
■ Glossopharyngeal nerve

Functionally, cells of the nucleus play a role in:

■ Blood pressure regulation
■ Cough reflex
■ Gag reflex
■ Sneeze reflex
■ Vomiting
■ Inspiration

Obturator: as related to dentistry, an obturator refers to a replacement prosthetic device that is used to replace upper teeth or associated structures (palate, gingiva, etc.) that may have been damaged in surgery, trauma, or altered development.

Odynophagia: a severe sensation of burning, squeezing pain while swallowing caused by irritation of the mucosa or a muscular disorder of the esophagus, such as gastroesophageal reflux, bacterial or fungal infection, tumor, achalasia, or chemical irritation.

Parenchyma: the tissue characteristic of an organ, as distinguished from associated connective or supporting tissues.

Parenteral nutrition: also known as intravenous feeding, is a method of getting nutrition into the body through the veins. While it is most commonly referred to as total parenteral nutrition (TPN), some patients need to get only certain types of nutrients intravenously. Also called parenteral alimentation. Parenteral nutrition is often used for patients with Crohn disease, cancer, short bowel syndrome, and ischemic bowel disease.

Parkinson's disease: a progressive disorder of the nervous system that affects movement. It develops gradually, sometimes starting with a barely noticeable tremor in just one hand. But while a tremor may be the most well-known sign of Parkinson's disease, the disorder also commonly causes stiffness or slowing of movement. In the early stages of Parkinson's disease, the face may show little or no expression, or the patient's arms may not swing when he or she walks. Speech may become soft or slurred. Parkinson's disease symptoms worsen as the condition progresses over time. Although Parkinson's disease cannot be cured, medications may markedly improve symptoms. In occasional cases, surgery to regulate certain regions of the brain and improve symptoms may be suggested.

Passavant ridge: a prominence seen during swallowing on the nasopharyngeal wall by contraction of the superior pharyngeal constrictor; also called Passavant pad. When the palate is not optimally functioning during swallowing, this deficiency may be compensated for by a greater convergence of Passavant ridge.

Pemphigus: One of a group of chronic, relapsing autoimmune skin diseases that causes blisters and erosions of the skin and mucous membranes. The immune system mistakenly regards the cells in the skin and mucous membranes as foreign and attacks them.

Penetration: inhalation of either oropharyngeal or gastric contents into the airway above the vocal folds; can indicate high risk for aspiration.

Pepsin: an enzyme produced in the mucosal lining of the stomach, acts to degrade protein. Pepsin is 1 of 3 principal protein-degrading, or proteolytic, enzymes in the digestive system, the other 2 being chymotrypsin and trypsin. The 3 enzymes were among the first to be isolated in crystalline form. During the process of digestion, these enzymes, each of which is particularly effective in severing links between particular types of amino acids, collaborate to break down dietary proteins to their components (i.e., peptides and amino acids), which can be readily absorbed by the intestinal lining.

Percutaneous endoscopic gastrostomy or **percutaneous endogastrostomy (PEG):** an endoscopic medical procedure in which a tube (PEG tube) is passed into a patient's stomach through the abdominal wall, most commonly to provide a means of feeding when oral intake is not adequate. The procedure does not require a general anesthetic; mild sedation is typically used. PEG tubes may also be extended into the small intestine by passing a jejunal extension tube (PEG-J tube) through the PEG tube and into the jejunum via the pylorus.

Peristalsis: a series of organized muscle contractions that occur throughout the digestive tract. Peristalsis is also seen in the tubular organs that connect the kidneys to the bladder. Peristalsis is an automatic and important process that moves food through the digestive system.

Primary peristalsis: the peristaltic wave triggered by the swallowing center. The peristaltic contraction wave travels at a speed of 2 cm/s and correlates with manometry-recorded contractions. The relationship of contraction and food bolus is more complex because of intrabolus pressures from above (contraction from above) and the resistance from below (outflow resistance).

Photodynamic therapy (PDT): a treatment that uses special drugs, called *photosensitizing agents,* along with light to kill cancer cells. The drugs only work after they have been activated or "turned on" by certain kinds of light.

Pierre Robin sequence or complex: Pierre Robin was a French physician who first reported the combination of small lower jaw, cleft palate, and tongue displacement in 1923. Pierre Robin sequence or complex is the name given to a birth condition that involves the lower jaw being either small in size (micrognathia) or set back from the upper jaw (retrognathia). As a result, the tongue tends to be displaced back toward the throat, where it can fall back and obstruct the airway (glossoptosis). Most infants, but not all, will also have a cleft palate, but none will have a cleft lip. Almost all will have swallowing problems due to the anatomy of the oral cavity. Pierre Robin sequence/complex, like most birth defects, varies in severity from child to child. Problems in breathing and feeding in early infancy are the most common. Parents need to know how to position the infant in order to minimize problems (i.e., not placing the infant on his or her back). For severely affected children, positioning alone may not be sufficient, and the pediatrician may recommend specially designed devices to protect the airway and facilitate feeding. Some children who have severe breathing problems may require a surgical procedure to make satisfactory breathing possible.

Pilocarpine: a cholinergic drug—that is, a drug that mimics the effects of the chemical acetylcholine, which is produced by nerve cells

Polymethylmethacrylate (PMMA): a suspension of microscopic synthetic polymer beads (microspheres) in a vehicle such as bovine collagen, hyaluronic acid, or some other colloidal suspending agent. Artecoll (PMMA suspended in bovine collagen) and MetaCrill (PMMA suspended in a chemical colloid) are two brands of PMMA injectable augmentation products. The resin has long been used by orthopedic surgeons in bone cement for joint replacement or to replace a skull bone defect.

Pompe disease: a rare (estimated at 1 in every 40,000 births), inherited and often fatal disorder that disables the heart and skeletal muscles. It is caused by mutations in a gene that makes an enzyme called acid alpha-glucosidase (GAA). Normally, the body uses GAA to break down glycogen, a stored form of sugar used for energy. Excessive amounts of lysosomal glycogen accumulate everywhere in the body, but the cells of the heart and skeletal muscles are the most seriously affected. Researchers have identified up to 300 different mutations in the GAA gene that cause the symptoms of Pompe disease, which can vary widely in terms of age of onset and severity. The severity of the disease and the age of onset are related to the degree of enzyme deficiency. The swallowing problems relate to muscle weakness and muscle fatigue.

Postprandial: after eating.

Prader-Willi syndrome (PWS): a genetic disorder that occurs in approximately 1 out of every 15,000 births. PWS affects males and females with equal frequency and affects all races and ethnicities. PWS is recognized as the most common genetic cause of life-threatening childhood obesity. PWS was first described by Swiss doctors Andrea Prader, Alexis Labhart, and Heinrich Willi in 1956 based on the clinical characteristics of 9 children they examined. The common characteristics defined in the initial report included small hands and feet, abnormal growth and body composition (small stature, very low lean body mass, and early onset childhood obesity), hypotonia (weak muscles) at birth, insatiable hunger, extreme obesity, and intellectual disability. PWS results from an abnormality of chromosome 15, and definitive diagnosis is now based on genetic testing.

Prandial aspiration: the entry of material from the oropharynx or gastrointestinal tract into the larynx and lower respiratory tract during food or liquid intake. A person may either inhale the material, or it may be delivered into the tracheobronchial tree during positive pressure ventilation. The aspirated material is often colloquially referred to as "going down the wrong pipe."

Progressive supranuclear palsy: a neurologic disorder of unknown origin that gradually destroys cells in many areas of the brain, leading to serious and permanent problems with the control of gait and balance. The most obvious sign of the disease is an inability to aim the eyes properly, which occurs because of damage in the area of the brain that coordinates eye movements. Some patients describe this effect as a blurring. Another common visual problem is an inability to maintain eye contact during a conversation. This can give the mistaken impression that the patient is hostile or uninterested. Patients also often show alterations of mood and behavior, including depression and apathy as well as progressive mild dementia, lack of appetite or dysphagia for solids. The disease is "progressive" because it worsens over time; "supranuclear" because the main problem is not in the nuclei (clusters of cells in the brainstem) that directly control eye movements, but in higher centers that control the nuclei; and "palsy," which means weakness, in this case of eye movement. Progressive supranuclear palsy (PSP) characteristically begins with loss of balance. Nearly all patients eventually develop the characteristic difficulty in moving the eyes up and down, the sign that often arouses a doctor's suspicion of the correct diagnosis. Although PSP gets progressively worse, no one dies from PSP itself. Difficulty swallowing can eventually permit aspiration of food into the trachea (windpipe). PSP may also be complicated by the effects of immobility, especially pneumonia, and by injuries from falls.

Prokinetic agents (or prokinetics): medications that help control acid reflux. Prokinetics help strengthen the lower esophageal sphincter (LES) and cause the contents of the stomach to empty faster. This allows less time for acid reflux to occur.

Prosthodontist: a prosthodontist is a dentist with advanced specialty training including the design and fitting of prosthetic appliances, dental implants, dentures, veneers, crowns, and teeth whitening.

Pseudobulbar palsy: bilateral corticobulbar tract damage in which speech and swallowing disorders are common.

Ptosis: also called *drooping eyelid*, is caused by weakness of the muscle responsible for raising the eyelid, damage to the nerves that control those muscles, or looseness of the skin of the upper eyelids.

Pulse oximetry: a technique to measure the oxygen saturation of arterial blood by means of a photoelectric technique.

Pulsed-dye laser (PDL): the pulsed-dye laser uses a beam of light at a specific wavelength; used for conditions or spots on the skin that are made up of blood and blood vessels.

Regurgitation: a backward flowing, for example, of food, or the sloshing of blood back into the heart (or between chambers of the heart) when a heart valve is incompetent and does not close effectively.

Reliability: a test's ability to measure the same thing consistently across multiple uses.

Rett syndrome: a uniform and striking, progressive neurologic developmental disorder and one of the most common causes of mental retardation in females. It is an X-linked dominant neurological disorder that affects girls only and is one of the most common causes of mental retardation in females. Girls with the syndrome show normal development during the first 6 to 18 months of life followed first by a period of stagnation and then by rapid regression in motor and language skills. The hallmark of Rett syndrome is the loss of purposeful hand use and its replacement with stereotyped hand-wringing. Screaming fits and inconsolable crying are common. Because of these autistic-like behaviors, feeding is highly irregular. Other key features include loss of speech, behavior reminiscent of autism, panic-like attacks, bruxism (grinding of teeth), rigid gait, tremors, intermittent hyperventilation, and microcephaly (small head).

Rheumatoid arthritis: a chronic inflammatory disorder that can affect more than just joints. In some people, the condition also can damage a wide variety of body systems, including the skin, eyes, lungs, heart and blood vessels. An autoimmune disorder, rheumatoid arthritis occurs when the immune system mistakenly attacks the body's tissues. Rheumatoid arthritis affects the lining of joints, causing a painful swelling that can eventually result in bone erosion and joint deformity.

Sarcoidosis: an autoimmune disease of unknown origin that causes small lumps (granulomas) due to chronic inflammation to develop in a great range of body tissues. Sarcoidosis can appear in almost any body organ, but most often starts in the lungs or lymph nodes. It also affects the eyes, liver, and skin; and less often the spleen, bones, joints, skeletal muscles, heart, and central nervous system (brain and spinal cord). In the majority of cases, the granulomas clear up with or without treatment. In cases where the granulomas do not heal and disappear, the tissues tend to remain inflamed and become scarred (fibrotic).

Schatzki ring: described by Richard Schatzki, M.D., in 1953; a narrowing of the lower part of the esophagus caused by changes in the esophageal mucosa. In the majority of cases, Schatzki ring is benign and asymptomatic; the condition is associated with hiatal hernias and can disrupt the normal esophageal functions. It has been suggested that long-term gastroesophageal reflux disease causes chronic inflammation and thus chronic damage to the lower esophagus. The damage will heal and form a scar that is the Schatzki ring.

Scleroderma: a disease of connective tissue with the formation of scar tissue (fibrosis) in the skin and sometimes also in other organs of the body. Scleroderma is classified into diffuse and limited forms. The CREST syndrome is a limited form of scleroderma. CREST stands for calcinosis (the formation of tiny deposits of calcium in the skin); Raynaud phenomenon (spasm of the tiny artery vessels supplying blood to the fingers, toes, nose, tongue, or ears); esophagus (esophageal involvement by the scleroderma); sclerodactyly (localized thickening and tightness of the skin of the fingers or toes); and telangiectasias (dilated capillaries that form tiny red areas, frequently on the face, hands, and in the mouth behind the lips).

Secondary peristalis: the peristaltic wave that is induced by esophageal distension from the retained bolus, refluxed material, or swallowed air. The primary role is to clear the esophagus of retained food or any gastroesophageal refluxate.

Sensitivity: a test's accuracy in identifying true cases of the target disorder.

Silent aspiration: aspiration without any obvious signs of swallowing difficulty, such as coughing or breathing difficulty. Silent aspiration is related to loss of sensation in the vagus nerve.

Sjögren's syndrome: an autoimmune disease of salivary and tear glands. Sjögren's syndrome involves inflammation of glands and other tissues of the body. Most patients with Sjögren's syndrome are female. Sjögren's syndrome can be complicated by infections of the eyes, breathing passages, and mouth. Sjögren's syndrome is typically associated with antibodies against a variety of body tissues (autoantibodies).

Slough: to separate from surrounding living tissue. Used of dead tissue.

Spasticity: stiff or rigid muscles with exaggerated, deep tendon reflexes (e.g., a knee-jerk reflex). The condition can interfere with walking, movement, or speech.

Specificity: a test's accuracy in rejecting cases that do not match the target disorder.

Squamous cell carcinoma: cancer that begins in squamous cells—thin, flat cells that look under the microscope like fish scales. Squamous cells are found in the tissue that forms the surface of the skin, the lining of hollow organs of the body, and the passages of the respiratory and digestive tracts. Squamous cell carcinomas may arise in any of these tissues.

Stenosis: an abnormal narrowing in a blood vessel or other tubular organ or structure. It is also sometimes called a stricture.

Stomatitis: inflammation of the mucous lining of any of the structures in the mouth, which may involve the cheeks, gums, tongue, lips, and roof or floor of the mouth. The word "stomatitis" literally means inflammation of the mouth.

Subluxation: partial dislocation of a joint. A complete dislocation is a luxation.

Suckling: motion than requires the tongue to move anterior to posterior. Usually the infant begins to swallow using this pattern. Compared to sucking which is an inferior to superior motion of the tongue that is acquired later in normal infancy.

Systemic lupus erythematosus (SLE): an autoimmune disease. In this disease, the body's immune system mistakenly attacks healthy tissue. It can affect the skin, joints, kidneys, brain, and other organs.

Tardive dyskinesia: a disorder that involves involuntary movements, especially of the lower face. Tardive means "delayed" and dyskinesia means "abnormal movement."

Tonic contraction: continuous contraction of a muscle.

Tractus solitarius: a tract composed of mostly sensory fibers that convey information from stretch receptors and chemoreceptors in the walls of the cardiovascular respiratory and intestinal tracts. Its fibers are distributed to the nucleus of the solitary tract.

Tracheostomy: a surgically created opening in the neck leading directly to the trachea (the breathing tube). It is maintained open with a hollow tube called a tracheostomy tube.

Tracheotomy: a surgical procedure that opens up the windpipe (trachea). It is performed in emergency situations, in the operating room, or at bedside of critically ill patients.

Transcutaneous: through the skin.

Transoral: by way of the mouth.

Treacher Collins syndrome: a condition that affects the development of bones and other tissues of the face. The signs and symptoms of this disorder vary greatly, ranging from almost unnoticeable to severe. Most affected individuals have underdeveloped facial bones, particularly the cheek bones, and a very small jaw and chin (micrognathia). Some people with this condition are also born with a cleft palate. In severe cases, underdevelopment of the facial bones may restrict an affected infant's airway, causing potentially life-threatening respiratory problems. People with Treacher Collins syndrome often have eyes that slant downward, sparse eyelashes, and a notch in the lower eyelids called an eyelid coloboma. Some affected individuals have additional eye abnormalities that can lead to vision loss. This condition is also characterized by absent, small, or unusually formed ears. Hearing loss occurs in about half of all affected individuals; hearing loss is caused by defects of the three small bones in the middle ear or by underdevelopment of the ear canal.

Trigeminal nerve (CN V): responsible for sensation in the face. Sensory information from the face and body is processed by parallel pathways in the central nervous system. CN V is primarily a sensory nerve, but it also has certain motor functions (biting, chewing, and swallowing).

Trismus: inability to open the mouth fully. This may be due to spasm of the jaw muscles and be a symptom of tetanus (lockjaw) or it may be due to abnormally short jaw muscles, as in the trismus-pseudocamptodactyly syndrome.

Trisomy 21 syndrome: a common chromosome disorder, often called Down syndrome, due to an extra chromosome number 21 (trisomy 21). The chromosome abnormality affects both the physical and intellectual development of the individual. Trisomy 21 syndrome is associated with a major risk for heart malformations, a lesser risk of duodenal atresia (part of the small intestines is not developed), and a minor but still significant risk of acute leukemia. Children born with Down syndrome are often slow to acquire strong sucking ability; thus, they may be slow to thrive if the swallowing problem is not detected early. In Down syndrome, there are certain characteristic features in the appearance that may individually be quite subtle but together permit a clinical diagnosis of Down syndrome to be made at birth. These signs of Down syndrome include slight flattening of the face, minimal squaring off of the top of the ear, a low bridge of the nose (lower than the usually flat nasal bridge of the normal newborn), an epicanthic fold (a fold of skin over top of the inner corner of the eye, which can also be seen less frequently in normal babies), a ring of tiny harmless white spots around the iris, and a little narrowing of the palate.

Upper motor neuron: a neuron that starts in the motor cortex of the brain and terminates within the medulla (another part of the brain) or within the spinal cord. Damage to upper motor neurons can result in spasticity and exaggerated reflexes.

Vagus nerve: (CN X) a remarkable nerve that supplies nerve fibers to the pharynx (throat), larynx (voice box), trachea (windpipe), lungs, heart, esophagus, and the intestinal tract as far as the transverse portion of the colon. The vagus nerve also brings sensory information back to the brain from the ear, tongue, pharynx, and larynx. It originates in the medulla oblongata, a part of the brainstem, and wanders all the way down from the brainstem to the colon.

Validity: a test's ability to measure what it is designed to measure.

Velopharyngeal insufficiency: incomplete closure of the velopharyngeal sphincter between the oropharynx and the nasopharynx. Closure, normally achieved by the sphincteric action of the soft palate and the superior constrictor muscle, is impaired in patients with cleft palate, repaired cleft palate, congenitally short palate, submucous cleft palate, palatal paralysis, and, sometimes, enlarged tonsils. The condition may also result when adenoidectomy or uvulopalatopharyngoplasty is done in a patient with a congenital underdevelopment (submucous cleft) or paralysis of the palate.

Velo-cardio facial syndrome (VCFS): a genetic condition characterized by abnormal pharyngeal arch development that results in defective development of the parathyroid glands, thymus, and conotruncal region of the heart. Shprintzen and colleagues first described the syndrome in 1978. More than 180 different clinical features are associated with velocardiofacial syndrome, with no single anomaly present in every patient. Some abnormalities are more common than others. Affected individuals may present with structural or functional palatal abnormalities, cardiac defects, unique facial characteristics, hypernasal speech, hypotonia, and defective thymic development. Palatal abnormalities predispose to speech and feeding difficulties.

Verbal apraxia: a motor speech disorder. It is caused by damage to the parts of the brain related to speaking. Other terms include apraxia of speech, acquired speech apraxia, verbal apraxia, and dyspraxia.

Vocal fold paresis: a condition of the vocal fold when it has lost partial neural innervation. Mobil-

ity of adduction and abduction is reduced and slower compared to normal function.

Wallenberg syndrome: also called lateral medullary syndrome, is a neurological condition caused by a stroke in the vertebral or posterior inferior cerebellar artery of the brainstem. Symptoms include difficulties with swallowing, hoarseness, dizziness, nausea and vomiting, rapid involuntary movements of the eyes (nystagmus), and problems with balance and gait coordination. Some individuals will experience a lack of pain and temperature sensation on only one side of the face, or a pattern of symptoms on opposite sides of the body, such as paralysis or numbness in the right side of the face, with weak or numb limbs on the left side. Uncontrollable hiccups may also occur, and some individuals will lose their sense of taste on one side of the tongue, while preserving taste sensations on the other side.

Wegener granulomatosis: characterized by a granulomatous arteritis involving the upper and lower respiratory tracts, a progressive glomerulonephritis, and extra respiratory symptoms attributable to systemic small-vessel arteritis. Wegener granulomatosis often affects the hard and soft palate and may lead to extensive ulceration, oronasal fistulas, and velopharyngeal insufficiency

Xanthum gum: a polysaccharide that is used as food additives and liquid thickeners; an addition or alternative to starch-based liquid thickeners.

Xerophonia: a dry-sounding voice caused by diabetes medication.

Xerostomia: more commonly known as dry mouth, is not a disease in itself. Rather, it is a symptom of many other diseases and conditions. These conditions cause saliva production to decrease or stop.

Zenker diverticulum: named in 1877 by German pathologist Friedrich Albert von Zenker; a diverticulum of the mucosa of the pharynx, just above the cricopharyngeal muscle. It is also called *pharyngoesophageal diverticulum* or *a pulsion diverticulum of the esophagus.*

Reflux Symptom Index (RSI)

A score of greater than 10 strongly suggests that the patient has laryngopharyngeal reflux.

Within the last MONTH, how did the following problems affect you?	0 = No problem; 5 = Severe problem					
1. Hoarseness or problem with voice	0	1	2	3	4	5
2. Clearing your throat	0	1	2	3	4	5
3. Excess throat mucus or postnasal drip	0	1	2	3	4	5
4. Difficulty swallowing foods, liquids, or pills	0	1	2	3	4	5
5. Coughing after you ate or after lying down	0	1	2	3	4	5
6. Breathing difficulties or choking episodes	0	1	2	3	4	5
7. Troublesome or annoying cough	0	1	2	3	4	5
8. Something sticking in throat or lump in throat	0	1	2	3	4	5
9. Heartburn, chest pain, indigestion	0	1	2	3	4	5
Total RSI:						

Reflux Finding Score (RFS)

A score of greater than 5 strongly suggests laryngopharyngeal reflux disease.

Findings	Scoring			
Subglottic edema (pseudosulcus vocalis)		2 If present		
Ventricular obliteration		2 If partial		4 If complete
Erythema/hyperemia		2 If arytenoid only		4 If diffuse
Vocal fold edema	1 Mild	2 Moderate	3 Severe	4 Polyp
Arytenoid/interarytenoid edema	1 Mild	2 Moderate	3 Severe	4 Obstruction
Posterior commissure hypertrophy	1 Mild	2 Moderate	3 Severe	4 Obstruction
Granuloma/granulation		2 If present		
Thick endolaryngeal mucus		2 If present		
Total RFS:				

Burke Dysphagia Screening Test

Patient Name:

ID Number:

Date of Evaluation:

1. Bilateral stroke   _____

2. Brainstem stroke   _____

3. History of pneumonia following acute stroke phase   _____

4. Coughing associated with feeding or during a 3-oz water swallow test   _____

5. Failure to consume one-half of meals   _____

6. Prolonged time required for feeding   _____

7. Nonoral feeding program in progress   _____

Presence of one or more of these features is scored as failing the Burke Dysphagia Screening Test.

Results: **Pass   Fail**   **Signature** _____

The MD Anderson Dysphagia Inventory

This questionnaire asks for your views about your swallowing ability. This information will help us understand how you feel about swallowing.

The following statements have been made by people who have problems with their swallowing. Some of the statements may apply to you.

Please read each statement and circle the response that best reflects your experience in the past week.

My swallowing ability limits my day-to-day activities.

| Strongly Agree | Agree | No Opinion | Disagree | Strongly Disagree |

E2. I am embarrassed by my eating habits.

| Strongly Agree | Agree | No Opinion | Disagree | Strongly Disagree |

F1. People have difficulty cooking for me.

| Strongly Agree | Agree | No Opinion | Disagree | Strongly Disagree |

P2. Swallowing is more difficult at the end of the day.

| Strongly Agree | Agree | No Opinion | Disagree | Strongly Disagree |

*E7. I do not feel self-conscious when I eat.

| Strongly Agree | Agree | No Opinion | Disagree | Strongly Disagree |

E4. I am upset by my swallowing problem.

| Strongly Agree | Agree | No Opinion | Disagree | Strongly Disagree |

P6. Swallowing takes great effort.

| Strongly Agree | Agree | No Opinion | Disagree | Strongly Disagree |

continues

E5. I do not go out because of my swallowing problem.

Strongly Agree   Agree   No Opinion   Disagree   Strongly Disagree

F5. My swallowing difficulty has caused me to lose income.

Strongly Agree   Agree   No Opinion   Disagree   Strongly Disagree

P7. It takes me longer to eat because of my swallowing problem.

Strongly Agree   Agree   No Opinion   Disagree   Strongly Disagree

P3. People ask me, "Why can't you eat that?"

Strongly Agree   Agree   No Opinion   Disagree   Strongly Disagree

E3. Other people are irritated by my eating problem.

Strongly Agree   Agree   No Opinion   Disagree   Strongly Disagree

P8. I cough when I try to drink liquids.

Strongly Agree   Agree   No Opinion   Disagree   Strongly Disagree

F3. My swallowing problems limit my social and personal life.

Strongly Agree   Agree   No Opinion   Disagree   Strongly Disagree

*F2. I feel free to go out to eat with my friends, neighbors, and relatives.

Strongly Agree   Agree   No Opinion   Disagree   Strongly Disagree

P5. I limit my food intake because of my swallowing difficulty.

Strongly Agree   Agree   No Opinion   Disagree   Strongly Disagree

P1. I cannot maintain my weight because of my swallowing problem.

Strongly Agree   Agree   No Opinion   Disagree   Strongly Disagree

E6. I have low self-esteem because of my swallowing problem.

Strongly Agree   Agree   No Opinion   Disagree   Strongly Disagree

P4. I feel that I am swallowing a huge amount of food.

Strongly Agree   Agree   No Opinion   Disagree   Strongly Disagree

F4. I feel excluded because of my eating habits.

Strongly Agree   Agree   No Opinion   Disagree   Strongly Disagree

Thank you for completing this questionnaire!

Scoring: All items, except for E7 and F2, are scored as 1 point for "strongly agree" and 5 points for "strongly disagree." Items E7 and F2 are scored as 5 points for "strongly agree" and 1 point for "strongly disagree."

Eating Assessment Tool (EAT-10)

Date: _____

Name: _____ MR#: _____

Height: _____ Weight: _____

Please briefly describe your swallowing problem.

_____

_____

Please list any swallowing tests you have had, including where, when, and the results.

_____

_____

To what extent are the following scenarios problematic for you?

Circle the appropriate response	0 = No problem; 4 = Severe problem				
1. My swallowing problem has caused me to lose weight.	0	1	2	3	4
2. My swallowing problem interferes with my ability to go out for meals.	0	1	2	3	4
3. Swallowing liquids takes extra effort.	0	1	2	3	4
4. Swallowing solids takes extra effort.	0	1	2	3	4
5. Swallowing pills takes extra effort.	0	1	2	3	4
6. Swallowing is painful.	0	1	2	3	4
7. The pleasure of eating is affected by my swallowing.	0	1	2	3	4
8. When I swallow, food sticks in my throat.	0	1	2	3	4
9. I cough when I eat.	0	1	2	3	4
10. Swallowing is stressful.	0	1	2	3	4
Total EAT-10:					

Dysphagia Handicap Index (DHI)

Please place a check in the box that describes your swallowing difficulty.

	Never	Sometimes	Always
1P. I cough when I drink liquids.			
2P. I cough when I eat solid food.			
3P. My mouth is dry.			
4P. I need to drink fluids to wash food down.			
5P. I've lost weight because of my swallowing problem.			
1F. I avoid some foods because of my swallowing problem.			
2F. I have changed the way I swallow to make it easier to eat.			
1E. I'm embarrassed to eat in public.			
3F. It takes me longer to eat a meal than it used to.			
4F. I eat smaller meals more often due to my swallowing problem.			
6P. I have to swallow again before food will go down.			
2E. I feel depressed because I can't eat what I want.			
3E. I don't enjoy eating as much as I used to.			
5F. I don't socialize as much due to my swallowing problem.			
6F. I avoid eating because of my swallowing problem.			
7F. I eat less because of my swallowing problem.			
4E. I am nervous because of my swallowing problem.			

continues

	Never	Sometimes	Always
5E. I feel handicapped because of my swallowing problem.			
6E. I get angry at myself because of my swallowing problem.			
7P. I choke when I take my medication.			
7E. I'm afraid that I'll choke and stop breathing because of my swallowing problem.			
8F. I must eat another way (eg, feeding tube) because of my swallowing problem.			
9F. I've changed my diet due to my swallowing problem.			
8P. I feel a strangling sensation when I swallow.			
9P. I cough up food after I swallow.			

1	2	3	4	5	6	7
Normal			Moderate Problem			Severe Problem

Please circle the number that matches the severity of your swallowing difficulty
(1 = no difficulty at all; 4 = somewhat of a problem; 7 = the worse problem you could have).

Voice Handicap Index-10 (VHI-10)

Instructions: These are statements that many people have used to describe their voices and the effects of their voices on their lives. Circle the response that indicates **within the past month** how frequently you have the same experience.

0 = Never; 1 = Almost Never; 2 = Sometimes; 3 = Almost Always; 4 = Always

1. My voice makes it difficult for people to hear me.	0	1	2	3	4
2. People have difficulty understanding me in a noisy room.	0	1	2	3	4
3. My voice difficulties restrict personal and social life.	0	1	2	3	4
4. I feel left out of conversations because of my voice.	0	1	2	3	4
5. My voice problem causes me to lose income.	0	1	2	3	4
6. I feel as though I have to strain to produce voice.	0	1	2	3	4
7. The clarity of my voice is unpredictable.	0	1	2	3	4
8. My voice problems upset me.	0	1	2	3	4
9. My voice makes me feel handicapped.	0	1	2	3	4
10. People ask, "What's wrong with your voice?"	0	1	2	3	4
Total:					

Answers to Study Questions

Chapter 1

1. **B**
2. **C**
3. **B**
4. **D**
5. **C**

Chapter 2

1. **C**
2. Age   **T**
   Type of bolus   **T**
   Quality of dentition   **F**
3. **C**
4. **C**

Chapter 3

1. **C**
2. **C**
3. **B**
4. **D**
5. **B**

Chapter 4

1. **D**
2. **E**
3. **D**
4. **C**
5. **A**

Chapter 5

1. **C**
2. **B**
3. **B**

Chapter 6

1. **B**
2. **C**
3. **C**

Chapter 7

1. **D**
2. **A**
3. **C**

Chapter 8

1. **C**
2. **B**
3. **D**

Chapter 9

1. **D**
2. **B**
3. **C**
4. **C**
5. **B**

Chapter 10

1. **B**
2. **B**
3. **D**
4. **D**
5. **D**

Chapter 11

1. **E**
2. **D**
3. **D**
4. **B**
5. **C**

Chapter 12

1. **C**
2. **A**
3. **D**
4. **D**
5. **B**

Index

Note: Page numbers in **bold** reference non-text material.